Women and Children First

Women and Children First

The Trailblazing Life
of Susan Dimock, M.D.

SUSAN WILSON

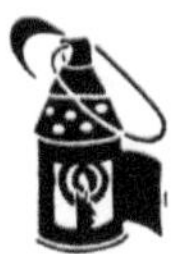

McFarland & Company, Inc., Publishers
Jefferson, North Carolina

ISBN (print) 978-1-4766-9248-7
ISBN (ebook) 978-1-4766-5046-3

Library of Congress and British Library
cataloguing data are available

Library of Congress Control Number 2023042885

Front cover image of the posthumously painted oil portrait
of Dr. Dimock by Swiss-born Boston painter Edward L. Custer
(used by permission of the Dimock Center, Roxbury, Massachusetts;
photograph © the author); a basket of babies delivered
at the New England Hospital for Women and Children
(used by permission of the Dimock Center, Roxbury, Massachusetts);
background The century dictionary and cyclopedia,
a work of universal reference in all departments of knowledge
with a new atlas of the world (1896) (14589808949) Wikimedia commons

Printed in the United States of America

McFarland & Company, Inc., Publishers
Box 611, Jefferson, North Carolina 28640
www.mcfarlandpub.com

To the women who persisted

Table of Contents

Acknowledgments

There's no question that it took a village to complete this biography. Both old and new friends and colleagues scattered around the world played a variety of essential roles in helping me collect stories and images, follow fascinating threads, and unravel countless mysteries in the process of researching and writing this first full-length biography of Susan Dimock.

Without my colleagues at the Women's Studies Research Center at Brandeis University in Waltham, Massachusetts, there would have been no home base or regular support system for my work. Thanks especially to the women in my two study groups, Writing Women's Lives and Issues in Historical Research, for reading and commenting on my manuscript over a period of six years. It was Kristen Mullin at the WSRC who paired me with two undergraduate students, Megan Catalano and Arianna Unger, both of whom provided invaluable research assistance as part of the center's Student Scholar Partner program.

Without my old friend Mary Smoyer, this book project might never have even begun. It was she who convinced me to dig out my old Susan Dimock lecture notes and slides from 1995 and rework them into a new PowerPoint lecture for the Jamaica Plain Historical Society twenty years later. Thanks also to that Society—especially Gretchen Grozier and Michael Reiskind—who gracefully hosted my first Dimock lecture in two decades and have continued to support the project ever since. Once I determined to make Susan Dimock's story into a full-length book, it was Mary Smoyer again who, along with the board of the Boston Women's Heritage Trail and the Forest Hills Educational Trust, provided early funding enabling me to begin research travels. Thank you all for believing in me and in this project.

My inaugural excursion was to Washington, North Carolina, where Susan Dimock spent her first seventeen years. I cannot over-emphasize how much I gained from the learned assistance of Claudia Dahlen of the Brown Library, Leesa Jones of the Washington Waterfront Underground

Railroad Museum, educator Ed Hodges, and editor Vail Stewart Rumley. Thanks for providing me with such a firm foundation and ongoing support. Thanks also to Ray Midgett of the Historic Port of Washington Project, Jennifer Spivey of St. Peter's Episcopal Church, Leonard and Johanna Huber, Carolyn Worsley, Billie-Jean Elliott Mallison, Betty Cochran, Debra Torrence, the Washington Visitors Bureau, and the Beaufort Country Register of Deeds. I am indebted to Reference Specialist/Genealogist Stephen Farrell of the Brown Library, who helped me clarify and correct information about the Dimock family's real estate and the formerly enslaved teens who traveled North with Susan's family.

While visiting the Isles of Scilly in Cornwall, England, and investigating Susan Dimock's death in the wreck of the S.S. *Schiller*, I asked Amanda Martin, then curator of the Isles of Scilly Museum, if I could interview her for perhaps a half an hour. Despite her packed schedule, she ended up spending more than four hours with me, as we moved from the books and maps in her home office to the compact yet exceptional museum, then on to Old Town Cemetery on St. Mary's Island. Through Amanda, I was introduced to insights, artifacts, and information that could not have been found elsewhere. Deep sea diver Todd Stevens and historic shipwreck expert/diver Richard Larn of St. Mary's, both of whom had personally explored the battered and scattered remains of *Schiller*, were exceptionally generous in sharing their time, tales, and artifacts. In Penzance, back on the Cornwall mainland, librarian Lisa Di Tommaso of the Morrab Library and Oliver Hawker of Oliver's Photography helped me gather vital images and info on *Schiller*, shipwrecks, and treacherous tides. My old friend Joan Orr, who owns The Art House in St. Ives, was generous with her time and knowledge as she toured us through much of central Cornwall.

With guidance from my old college suite-mate, Elizabeth Borner, I found convenient lodging in Zurich and learned how to navigate the local roads and trolleys, enabling me to access all the essential archival collections. While in Zurich I was able to sift through numerous primary sources with the aid of Martin Akeret at the University Archives, Nadine Schwaldat at the Stadtarchiv Zürich (City Archives), Esther Fuchs and Rudolf Vögele at the Baugeschichtliches Archiv (BAZ), Gudrun Kling at the Archiv für Medizingeschichte Universität Zürich, and Dr. Karin Huser at the Staatsarchiv des Kantons Zürich (State Archive).

Dr. Huser suggested that I connect with Swiss biographer Verena E. Müller, who soon after became my great friend, periodic editor and adviser, and a source of numerous stories about Susan Dimock's life in Zurich. Verena wrote a biography of Dimock's closest medical school colleague, Marie Vögtlin, filled with vivid written accounts of the duo's adventures together, both on and off campus. These stories complemented Susan's own writings and proved essential to understanding her Zurich sojourn. I cannot thank you enough, Verena, for your immeasurable assistance and perennial belief in me and this project. Kudos to Aina Lagor and Inez Hedges for assisting us in translating Verena's text from German to English.

Numerous individuals and institutions helped me piece together Susan Dimock's late teenage years in central Massachusetts. Heartfelt thanks to David Gibbs and the Sterling Historical Society for helping me uncover information about Susan's abolitionist aunt and to Kathy Bogosian for guiding me through the secret passages in her Sterling home. In the town of Hopkinton, my gratitude goes to Linda Connelly who assisted me in visualizing nineteenth-century Hopkinton through her work with both the Hopkinton Historical Society and the Hopkinton Public Library. Thanks also to Anne Mattina, who sleuthed the long-lost whereabouts of the Dimocks' Hopkinton hotel, and to Cobi Wallace, Shannon Soares, Anna Rogers, and John Palmer, who provided resources from Hopkinton Town Hall.

The Dimock Center in Roxbury is the modern incarnation of the New England Hospital for Women and Children. Though the institution's structures, services, and staff have changed and evolved over the decades, it is rather extraordinary to realize that the actual hospital building where Susan Dimock worked is still a centerpiece of the campus. Each time I walk the halls of that Zakrzewska Building, especially when no one is around, I can envision nineteenth-century women doctors and nurses conferring, consoling, treating, operating, and darting about as they assist their sisters in need. Since my initial discovery of the Dimock story in 1994, every administration at the Dimock Center has supported my work and buoyed my vision of sharing this adventure with a much wider audience. Without the Center's archival resources, and especially without the constant backing of Dimock perennials like Raquel Rosenblatt, I would have had far fewer resources and a far weaker foundation for my work.

Numerous archival collections outside the Dimock Center were indispensable to my research. My gratitude goes to the librarians at the Sophia Smith Collection at Smith College in Northampton, Massachusetts—the repository of most of the New England Hospital's nineteenth-century papers—and to Stephanie Krauss at the Countway Library of Medicine, who went above and beyond to help me and my student assistant locate and copy obscure medical and surgical records. Other indispensable primary resources were made available through the Massachusetts Historical Society, Forest Hills Cemetery, the Jamaica Plain Historical Society, the American Antiquarian Society in Worcester, Marta Crilly at the City of Boston Archives, Caitlin Jones of the Massachusetts Archives, Samantha Nelson of Boston by Foot, Kathy Kottaridis of Historic Boston

Incorporated, and Lucy Ross and Tegan Kehoe of Massachusetts General Hospital. In North Carolina, the numerous treasures stored at the Brown Library in Washington were supplemented by those found at the North Carolina Museum of History, Raleigh, and the Louis Round Wilson Special Collections Library at the University of North Carolina, Chapel Hill, where Jason Tomberlin helped me locate period engravings from the Civil War in North Carolina.

Back in the Northeast, I was able to untangle various family histories and ancestral connections with the expert assistance of Sally Zimmerman and Patrick McNamara of Historic New England, Wayne McCarthy of the Waltham Historical Society, librarians at the Waltham Public Library, Michael Bavaro of Waltham, and Kathleen Haley in Limington, Maine. Dana Echelberger at the Newburyport Public Library in Massachusetts, Stephanie Diorio at the Hoboken Public Library, Robert Forster at the Hoboken Historical Museum, and staff at both the New York Public Library and the Bowdoin College Library led me to collections where obscure yet vital details could be found. My deepest gratitude to all these institutions and individuals.

When I first began researching Susan Dimock's life and death back in 1994, I discovered that Kay Hicks of Lynchburg, Virginia, was a distant cousin through Susan's mother, Mary Malvina Owens Dimock. Kay generously provided copies of both letters and images held by her family since the nineteenth century, which were a boon to me and to the other archives where she later donated these same materials. It was through Kay that a previously unknown and unpublished photo of Susan—taken in Boston and depicting the doctor with her dog, Dotty—was given to me and eventually shared everywhere. Kay and her daughter Mary also graciously gave me copies of an 1898 photo of "Grandma Dimock," Susan's mother, that had never before been published. While mentioning relatives of the characters in my book, I must give a nod to Nick C. Greene in the U.K., who wholeheartedly supported my work in uncovering details about another member of his extended family, Bessie Greene.

More than a year before I began this book project in earnest, my great friends Dori Hale and Diana Rowan Rockefeller invited me to create a little literary salon with them. The original intent was for the three of us to write poetry, which we would periodically read and evaluate in soirees enhanced by Kim Crawford Sauvignon Blanc and scrumptious food. When I hatched the idea of tackling Susan Dimock's biography, they graciously allowed me to stop laboring over poems (a good idea) and to arrive at our salons instead with newly-written chapters which they gently dissected and generally improved. I cannot thank you enough, my self-styled Muse-keteers, for being there from beginning to end.

I am lucky to count as friends and colleagues a number of historians, independent scholars, archivists, educators, authors, poets, and artists who have supported me and my obsession with the Susan Dimock story for longer than some of them can remember. Among the valiant souls who read part or all of my manuscript, geared me towards valuable sources, or corrected my historic or literary errors were Jim Vrabel, Charlie Bahne, Susan Porter, Kate Larson, Ann Caldwell, Jen Manion, Ann Wadsworth, Arianna Unger, Megan Catalano, Bob Krim, Shane Snowden, David Gibbs, Kathy Bogosian, Bud Hanson, Amanda Martin, Leesa Jones, Stephen Farrell, Ray Midgett, Ed Hodges, Joyce Creswell, Kathy Goodman, Michael Strauss, Lucile Burt, Maura Condrick, and the aforementioned Verena Müller. Maura Condrick is a neighbor and a talented illustrator who also provided invaluable help in selecting appropriate images to run with the final text and happily improved the visual quality of a few.

While in college, I majored in history, minored in education and French, and barely scraped through a grueling year of Kiddie Chem. A scientist I was not. I was thus quite fortunate that retired surgeon, Jane Petro, became enchanted with my Dimock project after attending an early lecture and thereafter became my *de facto* medical editor and consultant. In 2020, it was Jane who convinced me and my student assistant, Megan Catalano, to enter an illustrated story about one of Dr. Dimock's more exceptional surgeries into a poster contest sponsored by the American College of Surgeons for their annual Clinical Congress. Though there were more than 180 entries, our little team—the three of us plus graphic designer Pat Nieshoff—was awarded first prize and asked to write an accompanying article for the March 2021 *Bulletin of the ACS*. Because of this excellent exposure, *Annals of Surgery Open* asked us to create an even longer article on Dr. Dimock for their highly acclaimed medical journal in 2022. Receiving such ongoing support from the medical community has been an honor as well as a boon to getting out a story that remained largely untold for far too long.

Finally, I have no way to adequately express my gratitude to my partner, Rebecca Strauss, who has nobly spent the last six years as editor, critical commentator, travel companion, videographer, still photographer, recording engineer, life coach, and cheerleader for what turned out to be the single largest project I have ever attempted.

I couldn't have done this without all of you.

Preface

My fascination with Susan Dimock began back in 1994, when I was writing local history columns for the *Boston Globe*. I had stumbled upon the story of Dr. Dimock's death while scrolling through nineteenth-century newspaper headlines in the microfilm room of the Boston Public Library. As I read the continued coverage of her death and funeral, then expanded my search into other journals, I was struck by the fact that Boston had fallen into deep mourning for a woman who was a most beloved and exceptionally talented Boston surgeon.

And I wondered why I had never heard her name.

Hooked on the mystery, I began to dig deeper. I discovered that there were no biographies of Dr. Dimock, but there was a community health center and a street bearing her name in the Roxbury neighborhood of Boston. There was also a gravesite at Forest Hills Cemetery in Jamaica Plain, though Dimock's stone was so worn by the elements that it was hard to decipher. After researching and writing the well-received *Globe* article, I spent the next year helping to establish the Dimock Heritage Fund and corralling my friends and colleagues into fundraising to replace Dimock's decaying headstone, spread her story, and celebrate her long-forgotten accomplishments and pioneering role as a woman surgeon. Then I moved on to other projects, including numerous articles and several books on other aspects of Boston history.

Two decades later, Susan Dimock came back to haunt me. A friend from the Boston Women's Heritage Trail asked me to pull out my old notes and slides and deliver a talk on Dr. Dimock's life for Women's History Month. Though I felt terribly rusty on the subject, I agreed, scanned my old slides, scoured my old notes, and delivered a PowerPoint to a packed and appreciative house. After the talk, numerous guests—who were as fascinated by Susan Dimock's adventurous life as I had originally been—asked if they could buy the book. I went home that night and began doing research. And I was frankly shocked to find that, despite the fact that there was an ever-growing number of books about pioneering nineteenth-century women doctors and their woman-run hospitals, there was *still* no biography about Dr. Dimock.

Writing Susan Dimock's life story now shot to the top of my personal bucket list. In 2016, I applied to the Women's Studies Research Center at Brandeis University in Waltham, Massachusetts, with Dr. Dimock's first full-length biography as my proposed project. For the next six years, I immersed myself in uncovering long lost details about Dimock's life, death, and legacy. There were no childhood diaries or letters left by Susan or her family members—if they ever existed, they may well have been lost when the Dimocks' home burned down as the Civil War literally played out in their front yard. Thankfully, letters from her young adult and professional years had been saved, many in a memorial volume that was published following her death. Filling in the substantial gaps were clues, leads, tangible objects, peripheral facts, and, most importantly, personal reminiscences from her friends and colleagues that could be pieced together bit by bit.

In the process of research, I waded through scores of books, annual reports, articles, censuses, online resources, and—most importantly—archives and other repositories spread around the world. Sometimes the research had dead ends. Other times, items miraculously and unexpectedly appeared, like an obscure 1858 church newsletter clipping about Dimock's childhood proclivity for healing that fell out of a family Bible donated to her hometown library in Washington, North Carolina, in 2017. In the research process I met, interviewed, and befriended archivists, librarians, historians, museum curators, doctors, deep sea divers, and people from all walks of life in her North Carolina hometown and in her adopted homes in Boston, Sterling, and Hopkinton, Massachusetts. I spent weeks scouring through archives and cemeteries in those towns as well as in Northampton and Worcester, Massachusetts, and Limington, Maine, and made fruitful excursions as I trailed her life journey through Hoboken, New Jersey, New York City, Zurich, Paris, London, and the Isles of Scilly, off the coast of mainland Cornwall, U.K.

It's been a long voyage from that 1994 article in the *Boston Globe* to the completion of this book. No one could have asked for a more thrilling ride with so many remarkable companions, both living and long-gone. Thank you, Susan Dimock, for inspiring us all.

Introduction

In nineteenth-century America, it was commonly assumed that the words "woman" and "doctor" did not belong in the same sentence.

It was acceptable, of course, for any woman to be treated by a doctor, especially by an upstanding white male doctor from a respectable white family. But the idea of a "woman doctor" was deemed by many to lie somewhere between unfathomable and repugnant. Women's place, it was argued, was in the home, where mothers and daughters could certainly bandage small wounds or administer hot compresses for family members. These were respectable middle- and upper-class women—a stark contrast to those improper ladies who pursued professional careers and were probably "unsexed," "manly," or perhaps even bearded.

Then along came Susan Dimock.

A young North Carolinian who dreamed of becoming a doctor, then grew up to practice medicine in late nineteenth-century Boston, Dimock was not the first American woman to battle the patriarchal medical establishment. But in the 1870s, she was arguably the best-educated, most-skilled woman surgeon in the nation as well as living proof that a woman could be competent, smart, womanly, lovely, and kind—all in the same package.

As resident physician and chief surgeon at the New England Hospital for Women and Children, the second hospital in the U.S. run by women and for women, Dr. Dimock impressed all who watched her work. A colleague observed that "anyone who saw Dr. Dimock at the operating table, where she was as calm and self-possessed as in the morning visit; who watched the extreme delicacy and skill with which she handled the tools, and the loving care with which she guarded the sensibilities of the patient,—must have recognized the eternal fitness of things, and seen that she was in her rightful place."

This ambitious biography, the first to chronicle the doctor's entire life journey, aspires to give Susan Dimock her equally rightful place in medical, women's, and world history. Throughout the book, Dimock's life reads like an adventure story—from recoiling at slave auctions and witnessing Civil War battles to escaping her fire-engulfed Southern hometown, then finding her place among Boston's most enterprising women. She studied medicine in Zurich and Vienna, hiked the Swiss Alps, executed complex surgeries, and trained America's first professional nurses, ultimately inspiring a new generation of female surgeons. It's no surprise that a prestigious Viennese medical professor, when asked for advice to aspiring young doctors, replied simply, "Make yourself to be like Miss Dimock."

In 1860, there were some 55,000 men and only 300 women practicing medicine in the United States. Today, more than 50 percent of the nation's medical students are women. Dr. Susan Dimock—with her patience, persistence, empathy, and excellence—was a fascinating and trailblazing figure in the all-too-long battle from there to here. As such, she is both a charismatic nineteenth-century role model and a thoroughly modern woman for a twenty-first century-reader.

This is her story.

CHAPTER 1

Early Years

It was the damn Yankees who started the fire, and everyone knew it.[1]

The Union soldiers were finally in retreat, ordered to evacuate the coastal town of Washington, North Carolina, as Confederate forces moved closer.

"The soldiers stole everything they could," cried local resident Martha Fowle. "And what could not be carried off—they destroyed. They got something to drink and behaved badly. Ladies were threatened, almost everything was done to alarm us."[2] The looting? That was probably to be expected from the frustrated and fleeing Federal troops, despite official orders specifically forbidding pillaging. But the fire? That was a disturbing surprise. Three days and nights of scuffling and shuffling of troops had passed—convincing some townsfolk that the worst was over—when the last Yankee attachment began embarking on ships in the harbor and the fire alarms first sounded.

On the front balcony of the Lafayette Hotel, seventeen-year-old Susan Dimock stood, transfixed and confused by the clanging alarms. A pretty girl of medium height, with dark hair and gray eyes, Susan was known to be ladylike, soft-spoken, and exceptionally smart. But today, the only child of hotel-keeper Mary Malvina Owens Dimock was about to call on her other strengths. When the alarm bells grew louder, just which strengths those were, and how best to use them, were still in question.

As clusters of friends and neighbors began bolting up and down the streets, Susan heard someone shout that the stables on William DeMille's wharf, just a few short blocks away, had been set aflame.[3] Her neighbor Martha Fowle suggested, "It was not done by orders but it was winked at, and no attempt made to stop it. The wind blew it away from us, it ran up this block, crossed the street at Mr. Hoyt's, and almost spread to the woods in an hour … the roaring could be heard for miles in the country. I can find no words to tell you how horrible it was."

Meanwhile, the bridge crossing the Pamlico River was also set ablaze, hurling fiery missiles into homes and warehouses along the riverway. Up

Bridge Street and east along Main, spreading up Van Norden and Gladden streets, the flames began consuming four church buildings—Methodist Episcopal, African Methodist Episcopal, Catholic, and Presbyterian. Human casualties were also part of the frightening scene. Mr. Havens was severely burned after blowing up some adjacent buildings—a common method for blocking the spread of fire—while trying to save his own house. And poor Mrs. Winnie Balance fainted right into the flames, burning to death before neighbors could catch her fall.

Some locals, including the inquisitive and curious Susan, clearly wondered if the Great Fire that roared through Washington on Saturday, April 30, 1864, was part of an actual Yankee attack. Even the exuberant Martha Fowle admitted that torching her once-vibrant town might not have been a deliberate act of war or vengeance. A friend of hers had stopped a Union officer and asked if it was done by order. "He said it was an accident," admitted Fowle. "The soldiers were ordered not to go near the fire and we could not do anything until they left...."

Susan was among those who knew that not all Federal troops were the villains that some Washingtonians chose to portray. Susan's late father, Henry Dimock, was a Northerner after all, born and bred in the state of Maine. Moreover, several Union officers had been lodging at the Dimock family's Lafayette Hotel for more than a year and were generally civil—and often polite. Many, in fact, had been openly friendly and even empathetic to the plight of the locals. On the day of the fire, one resident later recalled, "the soldiers crowding on the porch spoke to us several times, begging us to go away on their boats as the town was then on fire."

No matter. At this precise moment, there was a swiftly spreading inferno that needed to be tamed and contained. And contained it eventually was. The first break came with the southeasterly wind. Its welcome gusts blew back the flames and spared portions of upper Main Street, including the Dimocks' hotel and many private homes. The second break came with the "fireproof" Bank of Washington and the row of brick stores owned by the Bonner family. These sturdier stone and brick structures proved quite resilient, helping to arrest a blaze that otherwise swept through wooden houses and walkways, igniting the grand elms lining Main Street into a surreal stream of Biblical burning bushes.

Part of Washington's ultimate salvation was also due to local initiative. The few neighbors left in town responded swiftly when asked to grab buckets, run to the docks, and haul water from the Pamlico River to save their neighbors' stores and homes. Though able-bodied men were scarce during wartime, many women joined the Washington bucket brigade, including Susan Dimock, her mother Mary Malvina, and Mrs. Dimock's sister, Fannie Owens. Susan, her mother, and her aunt joined a bevy of friends who rolled up their sleeves, filled and lugged a slew of wooden buckets, then hurled river water onto the wooden facades. This spirited ad hoc team effort effectively saved some of the structures and minimized the damage to others.

"God blessed our feeble efforts," remembered Martha Fowle. By the end of the day, the soldiers were long gone and the conflagration had finally been halted or burned out. Martha, Susan, and their neighbors were relieved and finally able to "go up town to look for our friends there, that had suffered more than we."

Yet sadly, there was more to come.

Confederate troops, which had periodically hammered at the occupying Union forces for the past two years, soon marched into town in victory. But for Susan and the other remaining townspeople, that victory seemed a Pyrrhic one at best. On May 9, 1864, just nine days after that unimaginably Great Fire, a second blaze erupted. And this time it was clearly both an accident and a death knell for the town of Washington.

The second fire started in the trash area behind the Lafayette Hotel, a gracious lodging house perched on the northeast corner of Market and Main streets. The hotel's legal proprietor was Frances Owens—known affectionately as Fannie—aided by her sister, Mary Malvina Owens Dimock, the mother of teenaged Susan.

No one was sure exactly how it happened, but a servant may have accidentally ignited the flame while working in the garbage bins and stable area behind the hotel.[4] Since the town's firefighting equipment had been vandalized during the Union troop evacuation, no tools were available to stop the flames, which were increasingly fanned by high winds. The conflagration took up where the April 30 fire left off, roaring north up Market Street and further east on Main, taking the Lafayette Hotel itself as well as one more church as it swept onward and eastward. A handful of the faithful from St. Peter's Episcopal salvaged the baptismal font and crystal chandelier. As the church tower sizzled and burned, the heat caused the church bell to toll one last time before plummeting into the embers below. According to popular legend, an African American parishioner named Abram Allen pulled the metal bell from the ashes and saved it for future rebuilding.[5]

Ultimately, whether it was deliberate destruction or pure accident, the wartime retreat of the "damn Yankees" had initiated a chain of events that resulted in irreparable damage. In a period of less than two weeks, many of the finest architectural elements and historic structures of Washington, North Carolina, had gone up in flames, from churches, schools, and storage buildings to businesses, public facilities, and private homes. From the once-mighty warehouses on the riverfront to the wooded northern outskirts of town, almost half of the town had been reduced to soot and ashes, with little but gaunt, charred tree trunks and ghostly chimneys marking the paths of destruction.

One of North Carolina's most vibrant ports stood eerily still. And for some locals—including the now-homeless Dimock-Owens family—the choice seemed clear. It was time to leave town.

In the decades before the Civil War, Washington, was a peaceful little town with a bustling port. It was the *original* Washington in the colonies, having taken that name back in 1776, when hallowed George was still General of the Continental Army. But in 1791, when another Washington was named the site for the nation's new capital, its North Carolina namesake was downgraded to "Little Washington" by some.

Despite the slight, Washington, North Carolina, carried on without a backward glance. Life, in fact, appeared to be very, very good for its more than 3,000 inhabitants. As Susan Dimock walked through town each day on her way to classes at Washington Academy or on visits with her medical mentor, Dr. Solomon Satchwell, she enjoyed a truly bucolic view.

Washington's wide main streets, paralleling the busy waterfront, were surfaced with hard-packed earth, well shaded from the burning summer sun by rows of giant elms and the occasional sycamore or cedar that formed what one local described as "a perfect arch the whole length of the streets."[6] When rains rendered those streets muddy, wooden planks provided convenient sidewalks for pedestrian traffic.

Much of the traffic through mid–nineteenth-century Washington was indeed by foot, though horses, carriages, carts, and canvas-covered freight wagons clip-clopped, crunched, and rolled through on any given day. Susan knew well that a four-horse stagecoach, with regular routes to the nearby towns of New Bern and Plymouth, could take you all the way to New York if you had three days to spare. Railroads would later cut that time down, though no rails were laid in town until a dozen years after the war.

The streets that ran at right angles to the main thoroughfares were home to pleasant, often romantically old-fashioned Southern houses, some with lush gardens, ornamental shrubs, and arbored walkways. "An exterior view of the town presents nothing but a few steeples, peering out from a thick grove of trees," wrote David Hunter Strother, on assignment for *Harper*'s magazine in the 1850s, "and the street views only continuous archways of verdure. In fact, its modest white wooden houses are completely buried in trees; and when the weather is hot the effect is highly pleasing."[7]

The charming homes, churches, walkways, and trees—as well as the Dimock family's own Lafayette Hotel—were all indebted to the waterfront for their collective survival. Washington was set some sixty miles upriver from the Atlantic Coastline, on the northern banks of the Pamlico River. An important strategic and commercial center since the time of the American Revolution, the port of Washington buoyed not only the economy of the town itself, but also that of the broad region surrounding the entire Pamlico River basin.

As Susan strolled from Main and Second streets toward Washington's waterfront, the smells of freshly baked bread, smoking hams, summer flowers, grazing cows, sweating horses, and the musky hints of hay and woodchips gave way to more distinctly seaside odors. Predictable portside scents of fresh oysters and the daily catch—accompanied by cries of "Fresh Fish" from crusty fishmongers pushing their carts—joined with the warm, oily, and strong odors of tar mixed with the resinous and piney hints of turpentine and fresh timber.

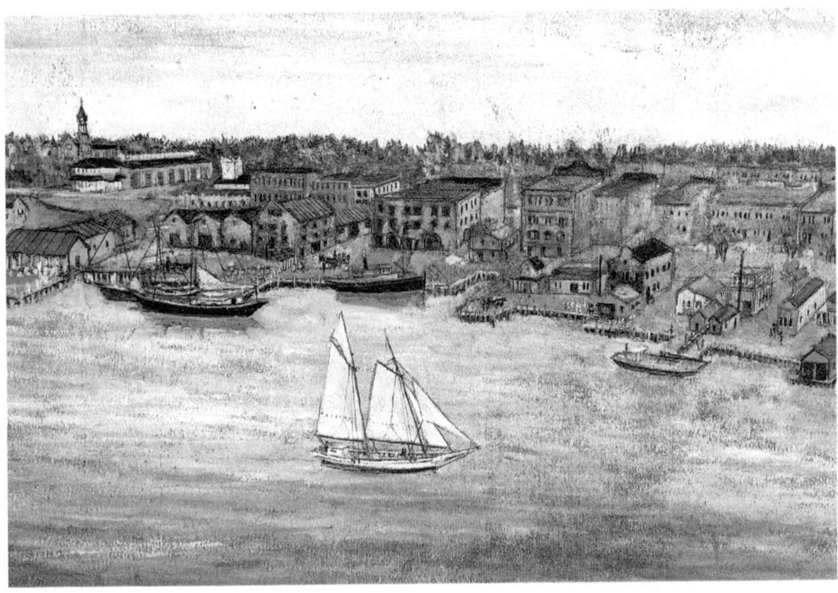

Washington, North Carolina, was set some sixty miles upriver from the Atlantic Coastline, on the northern banks of the Pamlico River. An important strategic and commercial center since the time of the American Revolution, the port of Washington buoyed not only the economy of the town itself, but also that of the broad region surrounding the entire Pamlico River basin (*Historic Washington Waterfront 1880–1920*, painted by Douglas A. Alvord; cropped from the original panorama; used by permission of the Historic Port of Washington, Inc.).

"Naval stores" like timber, tar, pitch, and turpentine—the stuff with which sailing ships were made and repaired—were a mainstay of the economy here before the Civil War. Agricultural products, primarily corn and cotton, were also shipped out of the busy port of Washington. Although some of these products were brought from inland sectors of the state in canvas-topped wagons, others were ferried downriver to the docks. Bales of cotton, barrels of tar, and stacks of shingles or bricks arrived on barges manned by half a dozen or more African Americans—sometimes enslaved, sometimes free—who propelled the flatboats by plunging their sturdy poles into the Pamlico as they chanted what Susan's neighbor Lucy Myers remembered as "a most peculiar mournful song."[8]

What shipped in to Washington was as impressive as that which shipped out. Each day, majestic sailing vessels voyaged up the Pamlico from the Atlantic Ocean, bringing anything from great blocks of natural ice cut from frozen Maine ponds and fashionable ladies' bonnets made in New York and Baltimore to exotic produce like sugar, molasses, oranges, limes, and tamarinds from the West Indies.[9] These ships and their cargo may have inspired Susan and her childhood friends to imagine someday visiting a world far bigger than the one they lived in day-to-day.

Among the earliest families to create and grow the shipping, ship-building, and warehousing businesses were the Fowles, Havens, Blounts, Marshes, and Myers. Brothers Josiah, Luke, and Samuel Fowle—proud sons of an old New England family—developed a primary trade with Boston and New York, and brisk secondary markets in Europe, the West Indies, and South America. John Myers and his sons specialized in exchanges with the northern states.

It was into this vibrant and ostensibly idyllic Southern environment that another proud son of an old New England family, Henry Robinson Dimock, had deliberately inserted himself more than two decades before the infamous fires. Dimock was born in Limington, Maine, on November 3, 1809, the second of Dr. Henry Dimock's and Nancy Whitmore Dimock's nine children. None of father Henry's offspring were drawn to his career path as a surgeon and physician. Young William, for example, became a successful Limington businessman and merchant, establishing a village store there that was later expanded by his own son, Charles.[10] Dr. Henry Dimock's namesake son, Henry, was similarly disinterested in medicine. That was something he would pass on to his own future daughter, Susan. Instead, Henry-the-Younger initially spent three years at Bowdoin College in Brunswick, Maine—a private school whose recent graduates included Henry Wadsworth Longfellow, Nathaniel Hawthorne, and future U.S. President Franklin Pierce. Seeking adventures that school failed to offer, Henry dropped out of college in 1831 and moved to Boston, Massachusetts, where for two years he served as headmaster of the Lower Jamaica, District No. 5, public school in Roxbury.[11]

During this antebellum era, a number of male students from prestigious northern schools like Harvard, Yale, Dartmouth, and Tufts began seeking business and marital opportunities in the South. Brimming with skill, ambition, and more than a modicum of self-confidence, these young entrepreneurs sought fame, fortune, opportunity, and willing Southern belles from old Southern families.[12] Henry Dimock joined that collegiate fray, removing himself from Roxbury to Beaufort County, North Carolina. His career choice was still in transition. He first taught at a school for young gentlemen, then briefly studied law.

While at Bowdoin, Henry had been a member of the Athenaean Society, a self-styled "literary and debating club"—the sort of organization that predated fraternities on college campuses. It was perhaps this penchant for debate and literature that interested him in buying an influential Washington newspaper called the *Whig*, founded in 1834 by Henry Machen. Eight years and several newspaper name-changes after its founding, Henry Dimock purchased the journal and renamed it *The North State Whig*. Dimock's penchant for debate and literature was also manifested in an infamous pistol duel he fell into when Congressional candidate Henry S. Clark felt maligned by a story in Henry's paper. Happily, both men emerged from the duel unscathed and repentant.[13] Dimock's paper was one of at least nine antebellum journals based in Washington. Since the region's dominant political party at the time was the Whigs, *The North State Whig* presumably wielded more clout than its competitors—and flourished as long as the Whig Party lasted.[14]

Flush with funds from the success of his newspaper, 37-year-old Henry Dimock married 24-year-old Mary Malvina Owens on July 30, 1846, with bondsman Samuel W. Wallace and witness J.G. Stanly in attendance.[15] Mary Malvina Owens was from local stock, the daughter of Elizabeth Young and Stephen Owens, who hailed from Cowhead Springs, three miles northeast of Washington, in Beaufort County, North Carolina. Father Stephen was well known in the area, having served as the county sheriff multiple times over the first three decades of the nineteenth century.[16] Daughter Mary Malvina made a name for herself as well. She was something of a powerhouse, remembered by neighbors as a hard mistress, a hard worker, and a woman of talent and brains with no tolerance for idleness.

"Tradition ... is rich in stories of Mrs. Dimock, whose name in Washington is a synonym for energy, character and determination," wrote Pauline Worthy in a 1937 article. "One, which is quite characteristic, says that she was so particular that she allowed her chickens only to pack [sic] in certain spots and then trained them so thoroughly that they kept to those spots."[17]

A decade after Henry and Mary were married, Mary Malvina Dimock's older sister, Fannie Owens, began leasing the Lafayette Hotel, on the northeast corner of Main and Market streets. Henceforth, the Lafayette would serve as both home and workplace for the extended Dimock-Owens family. Named for the popular French Marquis de Lafayette—who was feted at the hotel during his Stateside tour of 1825, the fiftieth anniversary of America's War for Independence—the Lafayette Hotel featured a grand 40-foot square dining room on its first floor, and, directly above it, a ballroom of the same size. Though its front door opened on Main Street, originally called First Street, and the hotel extended across two town lots, the backyard stretched to a third lot on Second Street, where both stables and servants quarters were located.

While no records exist of the Lafayette's bathroom facilities, it's probable that they were comparable to the elaborate Hanks family outhouse recalled by Edmund Harding. Generally set in the back of the yard's garden, these facilities were euphemistically referred to as "Garden Houses." "It was a [*sic*] eight-holer, four for grown folks, two for children and on the other side of the partition were two holes for the servants. A box of newspapers and a keg of lime were regular equipment. Several men or several women would visit the facility at the same time, but never in mixed company."[18]

Well before the Dimock-Owens family's lease of the Lafayette, the hotel was heralded as Washington's finest lodging. Built by entrepreneur Howard Wiswall to reflect the town's elevated status as the Beaufort County seat, the Lafayette had long been a popular site to entertain distinguished visitors, including President James Monroe and his Secretary of War John C. Calhoun in 1819 and the aforementioned Lafayette in 1825.

"Washington was always known as a hospitable town and there were always parties, dinations and big suppers when the Bishop, the Judge, or some famous soldier or person came to town," recalled local resident Edmund Harding. "A typical dination, as the big dinners were called, would include a six weeks old suckling pig, roasted with a red apple in its mouth, a roast turkey on one end of the table and a boiled turkey with a large bowl of egg dressing at the other. There was always a smoked or corned ham and a fresh ham. In season scalloped oysters were served. In the winter there was a big a dash of macaroni."

"It was poor taste to have macaroni in the summer."[19]

Some referred to little Susan Dimock as "a brilliant girl." Others insisted that the youngster—sometimes called Susie or Sue—was nothing short of "a precocious child."[20] Whatever her daughter's level of intelligence, Mary Malvina Dimock knew that developing and nurturing Susan's raw talent required someone with initiative and know-how—a role Mrs. Dimock readily assumed.

Before marrying Henry Dimock on July 30, 1846, Mary Malvina had been a teacher, working privately with select families who found value in "book-learning" for their youngsters. Henry and Mary Malvina's only child was born nine months after those nuptials, on April 24, 1847. And as the inquisitive, thoughtful, soft-spoken Susan began to grow, Mary Malvina feared that two major problems could impede her daughter's future. Since many Washingtonians were wary of free schooling, the town of Washington had no permanent, even minimally acceptable, public schools for younger children in the 1850s. Even worse, prevailing social opinion tended to frown on educating women.[21] Prevailing social opinion was also the reason why no schools were established for African Americans in Washington until after the Civil War.

Facing those realities, Mary Malvina proved herself to be an unusually independent, self-sufficient, and strong-willed Southern mother. She tutored Susan at home for a few years and, months before her daughter turned seven, provided her with supportive and competitive comrades and classmates by opening her own private "school for young ladies." Dimock's advertisement in the *North State Whig*, run during the summer of 1853, promised a school year divided into two twenty-week sessions and an impressive roster of subjects: reading, writing, and arithmetic ($8 per session); geography, grammar, and history ($10 per session); natural philosophy, chemistry, and botany ($12 per session); and music lessons on piano or guitar ($20 per session). Running the Lafayette Hotel also gave her the opportunity to promise that "a few young ladies can be accommodated in the family with board."[22]

Located across the street from the town jail, Mrs. Dimock's was not the only privately-run girls' school in town. For many years before the Civil War, a variety of men and women had helped fill the void of educational facilities in Washington, both for girls and for boys. Their ever-changing ranks included Mr. Joseph Blount, Miss Betty Patterson, Mrs. George Duran, Miss Louise Worthington, Mr. John Beckwith, one "Miss Nancy Richmond from Massachusetts," as well as an Englishman named Lewellyn and a Frenchman from the West Indies known as Monsieur Chapeau. Monsieur Chapeau, fondly remembered as "a very accomplished gentleman," taught French language and dance, with a specialty in the minuet, "for which the young ladies had a skirt especially made."[23]

Despite the legion of would-be instructors, the two local women noted as especially good teachers were Mrs. Dimock and Mrs. Sarah Nadal—the latter of whom held private classes for small children, first in the Masonic Lodge and later in a house on Respess Street, between Second and Main.

Though no records remain describing Mrs. Dimock's schoolroom, it's likely that it followed the typical model of both the era and area. Young Susan and her female classmates probably sat on shared benches and wrote their lessons on boards spaced along the sides of the room. They may well have enjoyed

---

Female School.

MRS. MARY M. DIMOCK respectfully informs the inhabitants of Washington and its vicinity, that she will open a Female School in this town, on the first Monday of October. The scholastic year will be divided into two Sessions of twenty two weeks each.

Terms of Tuition:

Reading, Writing & Arithmetic,	$8 per ses'n.
Geography, Grammar & History,	10 " "
Natural Philosophy, Chemistry and Botany,	12 " "
Music (Piano or Guitar)	20 " "

☞ A few young ladies can be accommodated in the family with board.

August 16. 1853 —33-tf.

SANS SOUCI

FEMALE BOARDING SCHOOL,
NEAR WASHINGTON, N. C.

Mary Malvina Owens Dimock tutored little Susan at home for a few years and, months before her daughter turned seven, provided her with supportive and competitive comrades and classmates by opening her own private "school for young ladies" (from the *North State Whig*, August 16, 1853; courtesy American Antiquarian Society, Worcester, Massachusetts; photograph © the author).

heat from a stove, but might have lacked a large blackboard. A desk at the front of the room was reserved for Mrs. Dimock, fortified with a long pointer and whatever books she could muster. If schoolbooks could be afforded, it's possible that she purchased them from local entrepreneurs like Demill & Brother, who advertised "a well selected assortment of such are used in schools of this vicinity; together with almost every article of Stationery."[24] The length of the school year was indeterminate—varying from teacher to teacher—though it often began in October and ran from just a few months up to nine months of any given calendar year. Mrs. Dimock's pair of twenty-week sessions was clearly lengthier and more ambitious than many of her peers.

Local lore suggests that the modest, unassuming Susan had a full, fair, and ruddy face that shone "like a gleam of sunshine."[25] Admired by others for her unusual intellect and drive, she enjoyed plenty of friends and playful childhood pastimes. "A happier group of children you will seldom see than that made up of Annie and Jennie Sparrow, Sue Dimock, Anne Blackwell and Anna Marsh Fowle," recalled a neighbor, reminiscing about a trip the girls took to a friend's seaside cottage in 1858, when Susan was eleven. Susan and her crew spent their mornings dressing dolls, reading story books, and writing to their absent mothers, while early evenings were filled "playing housekeeping in the yanpon [*sic*] bushes,"[26] making sand cakes, or frolicking in the surf in their "bathing costumes." Love of the seaside was something that would remain with Susan throughout her life. Later that night, the girls would spread their shawls on the parlor floor matting, and get down to playing Jack Straws or "a good game of checks."[27]

When back at school, Susan excelled at her studies with ease. Since she continually stood at the head of her class, she must have filled some of her classmates with a degree of envy. Still, friends noted that "her engaging manners made her always a pet among the older girls in the school"—a dynamic that was later repeated in her advanced schooling and professional work life.

After several years in her mother's school for young ladies, studious Susan moved on to the town's most notable antebellum educational facility for "older" children, who generally entered at ages 10 to 12. Built in 1808 on the corner of Bridge and Second streets, the large, private Washington Academy was a gem of an institution that prided itself in educating three or four generations of Washington's "most prominent citizens." The site was always a favorite for children, abounding in huckleberry bushes and chinquapins—tiny cousins of the American chestnut—that lined the small stream flowing behind the building.[28] By 1832, however, lack of funds and proper care had forced the Academy to close. Luckily for Susan, it was repaired and reopened a dozen years later, resuming its role as the educational center for white students until the start of the Civil War. Not surprisingly, schools were not racially integrated and free Black students in Washington had no educational facility of their own until a decade after war's end.

Susan's mentor at Washington Academy was a talented teacher and principal named Gilbert Bogart. Born in New York in 1804 and educated at Princeton College, Bogart had moved to North Carolina by 1840, where he married a Beaufort County native named Christiana Barden. Their son David was born in Washington in 1847, the same year Susan Dimock was born to a similar duo—a college man from the North and a strong-willed belle from the South.[29]

At age 56, the able and active Bogart ran 13-year-old Susan through her paces in arithmetic and grammar as well as "the classics," geography, and the formal English expected of "First Class" (first season) students. He may have found it curious that after a day of long and intense studies,

Susan chose to relax and amuse herself by reading. Seeing this exceptionally bright girl grow restless for more challenging studies, Bogart shepherded her toward Latin, which soon became her favorite subject. Her
father expressed the notion that her knowledge of Latin verse was even
better than his during his days at Bowdoin College.

Meanwhile, a future in medical studies was portended during Susan's
youth as well.

It's possible that Susan was inspired in part by tales of her grandfather, Henry Dimock, who made his living as a physician in Limington,
Maine. It's doubtful that she had personal reminiscences of Grandfather
Henry, however, since she was only five years old and living in North Carolina when Henry died in Maine. Still, reminiscences of an elder acquaintance named Luola suggest that Susan showed an interest in healing well
before her teen years. Back in 1858, while playing at the Marsh family's
beachside cottage with her friends Jennie, Annie, Anne, and Anna, Susan
found Jennie distraught with a painful toothache that none of the adults
could salve. She first tried to soothe Jennie by sitting with her and telling
stories. When that didn't work, Susan took action.

"Aunt Graham said the root of the pillentary was good for
tooth-ache," explained young Susan. "Annie Marsh and I went out on the
island to look for some. I think it did do her some good, for as soon as we
scraped some of the root and put it in her tooth, she fell asleep, and so we
left her." The next morning Jennie felt better but was fearful of going out
of doors. So Susan and her friends stayed nearby, "making and dressing
paper dolls for her amusement … and their attentions to Jennie did not
cease until she was well again."[30]

What may have been her natural inclination and warmth for compassionate healing was fanned into a full-blown flame by the time Susan
was thirteen. Susan's love for the ancient Latin texts given her by Gilbert
Bogart seems to have enticed her into reading *Materia Medica*—literally
"healing materials"—a term used for any of dozens of published works
produced from Roman to modern times on the therapeutic properties of
healing substances.[31] Having completed *Materia Medica*, she read every
medical book she could obtain and "never seems to have lost sight of her
purpose."[32] Her generally supportive parents held diametrically opposed
views on Susan's newfound dream of becoming a doctor. Mother Mary
Malvina saw it as a "childish fancy"—and strongly suggested Susan study
general literature, with the goal of becoming something reasonable, like a
teacher. Father Henry, however, observed his daughter's drive, and reck-
oned, "Sue says she wants to study medicine, and I tell her she may."[33]

Susan didn't have to walk far to find all those medical books. Across
Main Street from the Dimocks' Lafayette Hotel was the home of their

beloved family doctor, Dr. Solomon Sampson Satchwell—a handsome gentleman with thick dark hair, stylish mutton chop sideburns, sparkling eyes, and a welcoming grin. A solid rock of the community and favorite son of Beaufort County society, Dr. Satchwell was an unusually cosmopolitan, well-educated, and well-traveled gentleman, thanks in part to his strong survivor of a mother, Elizabeth Windley Satchwell.

Born in 1821 in Pea Ridge, not far from Pantego in Beaufort County, Solomon was still a youngster when his father James Satchwell died. Because of widow Elizabeth's perseverance and successful management, however, the family plantation thrived, providing the funds to send young Solomon to

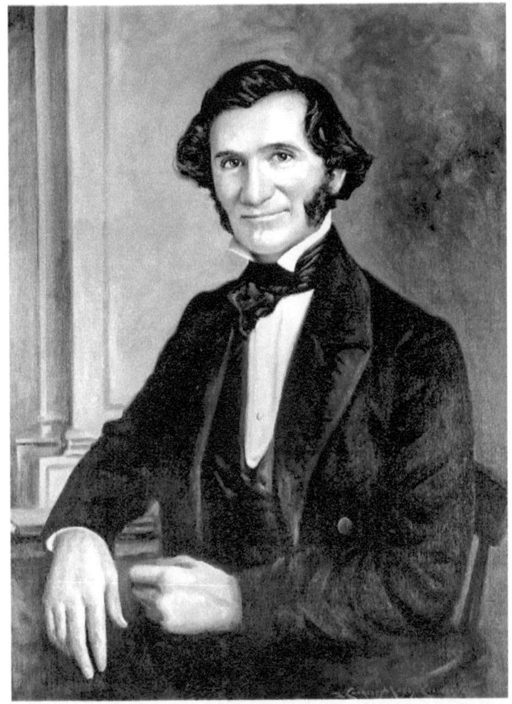

The Dimocks' beloved family doctor, Dr. Solomon Sampson Satchwell (1821–92), became Susan's mentor and friend, opening his medical library to the young girl and inviting her to make house calls with him in the rural countryside (oil portrait of S. Satchwell, photograph by the North Carolina Museum of History).

pursue his own passion for surgery and medicine at Wake Forest College and the University of New York, as well as post-graduate studies at the University of Paris.[34]

When young Susan Dimock raced across Main Street to Satchwell's office, the doctor was clearly taken by her interest in, and her obsession with, the world of medicine. He not only opened his medical library to the young girl, but invited her to make house calls with him in the rural countryside.

A popular tale relates how, at the age of thirteen, Susan was seen near a Washington watering-place, tucked cozily in the corner of a piazza for more than an hour while fully absorbed in a rather hefty book. "What interesting story has Susie got?" asked an inquisitive passerby. Standing

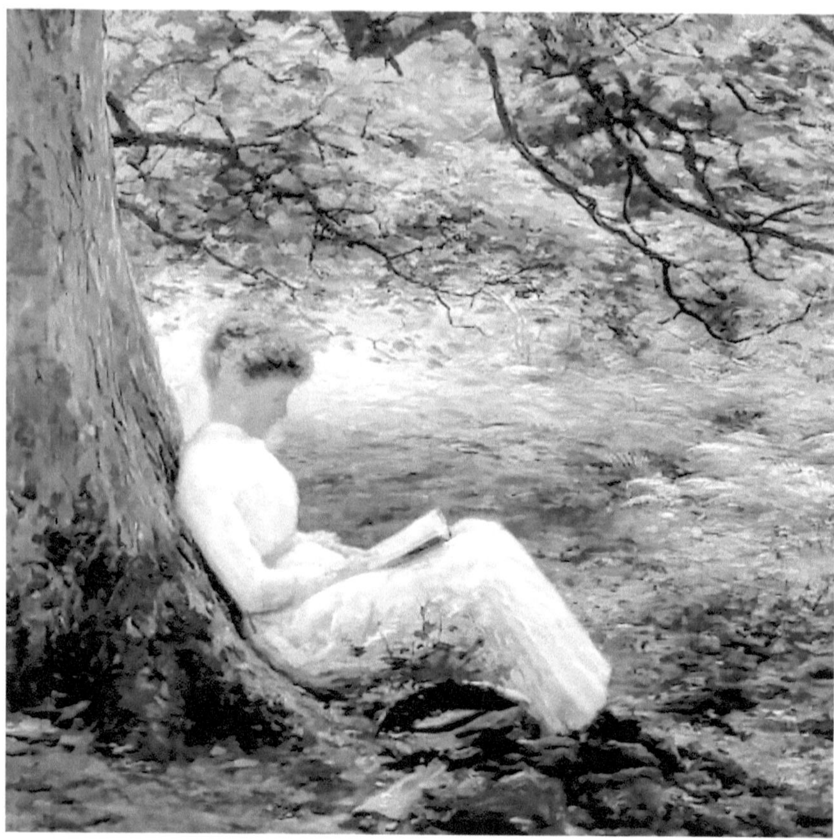

Though not an image of Susan Dimock, this painting perfectly depicts the way friends viewed her. After a day of long and intense studies at Washington Academy, young Susan was known to relax under a shade tree and amuse herself by reading medical books written in Latin (*Summertime* by Joseph Farquharson).

nearby, a doctor—presumably Satchwell—mused, "It is one of my medical books, which I have lent to her, and one of the driest, too."[35]

Whether Satchwell saw Susan as a daughter figure—or she saw him as a father figure—is not clear. His first wife, Elizabeth Norcum Van der Veer, had died in 1854, when Susan was only seven. The couple's daughter Elizabeth, known affectionately as Nannie, was born three months before her mother's death, then sent away to private school where, some years later, "she was disciplined for emptying a chamber pot out her window on some Union soldiers." "Father and daughter couldn't have known each other very well," surmised a descendant of Nannie more than a century later. "They couldn't have seen each other much."[36]

Satchwell remarried in 1859, in the second of what turned out to be three marriages. The following year he traveled to Paris, intent on enhancing his medical training with the superior facilities found in the French capital. By 1861, the Civil War had erupted and the good doctor returned home to become surgeon-in-charge at the Confederacy's General Military Hospital # 2 in Wilson, North Carolina, sixty miles west of Washington.[37] Whether or not Satchwell always was, or eventually became, Susan's father figure is probably moot, since he turned out to be a recurring blessing in Susan Dimock's life: first, as a mentor when Susan was an impressionable aspiring doctor; second, as a savior when fire leveled the Dimocks' hotel and home; and finally, as an advocate when Susan was seeking affirmation in her role as a professionally trained and eminently competent female surgeon.

It was just a matter of time.

Although the transatlantic slave trade had been abolished by both Britain and the U.S. by 1808, four decades before Susan's birth, the practice of selling African men, women, and children into forced labor persisted deep into the nineteenth century. The reason: though the transatlantic trade faded as the years wore on—or, in some cases, simply became more covert—a domestic slave trade grew in its place. During the end of the 1700s and the first half of the 1800s, an increased demand for slave labor in America's ever-expanding western territories coincided with an excess supply of enslaved people in the Upper South. Part of that "excess supply" was because children were continually being born into slavery, and part because the Upper South's economy simply didn't require as many laboring bodies as did the Deep South and the new western settlements.

The result was an extremely profitable interstate slave-trading system, especially in border states like Virginia, Maryland, Delaware, and Kentucky. The phrase "being sold down the river," which today means "betrayal," originated in this era, as enslaved workers from the Upper South were pulled from their homes and traded to large plantations in the Lower South. This domestic slave trade flourished in North Carolina as well, including in Susan Dimock's hometown of Washington.

The Dimock family's Lafayette Hotel was one block inland from the town's waterfront market. Both that riverside market and the county courthouse—the latter set two blocks up Market Street from the river— served as sites for private sales and public auctions of enslaved laborers. Since the Dimocks lived on the corner of Market and Main, halfway between these two locales, it's likely that Susan witnessed firsthand these dehumanizing exchanges of bonded labor. Like so many youngsters in

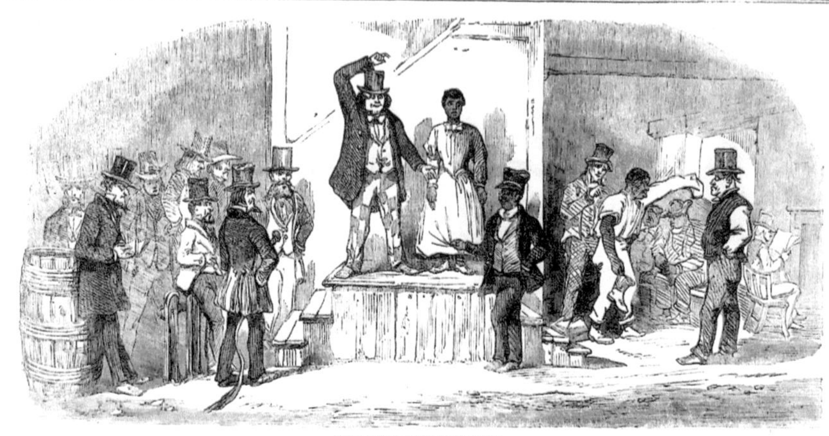

Although the transatlantic slave trade had been abolished by both Britain and the U.S. by 1808, the domestic slave trade flourished in North Carolina, including in Susan Dimock's hometown of Washington (Slave Auction at Richmond Virginia, *The Illustrated London News*, Sept. 27, 1856, 315).

the antebellum South, she may have internalized the horror of families degraded and torn apart as mothers, fathers, infants, and young adults were ogled, prodded, chained, bought, sold, and treated like cattle. Perhaps equally disturbing to Susan was learning that her own home, the Lafayette Hotel, had also been used for selling enslaved family members long before Aunt Fannie began leasing the hotel property from owner Howard Wiswall.

Typical of the ads posted on walls and run in local papers during this era—including in Henry Dimock's own *North State Whig*—were notices like the following:

> FOR SALE, TWO *likely male NEGROES—one about 33—the other between 12 and 14 years of age. For further particulars, inquire of Mr. Wiswell* [sic] *at the tavern....*
>
> NOTICE *... at the Court-house door in the town of Washington, on Tuesday the 30th day of April next.... I shall sell to the highest bidder One Likely Negro Girl named Mary, aged about nine years,—the property of Edmund Hoover and others.*[38]

Susan Dimock, of course, was exposed both to the cruelties of the slave trade and to the inhumanity of slavery itself. During her childhood, not only the town of Washington, but also the rest of North Carolina, depended on the enslavement of African Americans for its life and

TAKEN UP AS A RUNAWAY.

A negro girl has been taken up as a runaway, and committed to the jail of Beaufort County. She is about five feet high, 20 years old, of dark complexion, and says she belongs to George Westbrook. She appears not to have good sense.

HENRY CARROW, Jailor.

July 3. 1850—45-tf.

NOTICE.

PURSUANT to an order of Beaufort County Court, made at March Term, 1839—at the Court-house door in the town of Washington, on

Tuesday the 30th day of April next,

(being Superior Court week,) I shall sell to the highest bidder,

One Likely Negro Girl,

named Mary, aged about nine years,—the property of Edmund Hoover and others.—Terms: Six months credit will be given, the purchaser executing bond with approved security, or securities, for the purchase money.

WILL: C. EBORN, Cl'k. & Com.

P. S. Sale to commence at 12 o'clock of the day.

March 16, 1839—36 42

RANAWAY

FROM the subscriber on the 21st inst, a slave named OWEN. He is nineteen years old, about five feet eight or ten inches high, has dark and thick curling hair and dark eyes, but is of a very light complexion. He is probably lurking about the wharves in Newbern or Washington, or may be on Neuse. A suitable reward will be given for his arrest and confinement, so that I can get possession of him.

GAYER CHADWICK.

Beaufort, July 27th, 1849.

☞ As Owen may endeavor to get to sea on board the vessel of some Northern Abolitionist, the pilots and others at the Bar, are earnestly requested to aid in the effort to discover him.   G. C.

Negroes Wanted.

We are still in this place, for the purpose of buying Negroes, and will pay liberal prices for all such as will suit us. Any letters addressed to us on business will be promptly attend d to.

W. H. & J. M. HOLDERNESS.

Washington, February 1, 1850—24-tf.

Henry Dimock's *North State Whig* and other North Carolina newspapers regularly ran notices for slave auctions and ads offering monetary rewards for runaways (from the North Carolina Runaway Slave Advertisements Digital Collection, the University of North Carolina at Greensboro, and the *North State Whig*, courtesy American Antiquarian Society, Worcester, Massachusetts).

livelihood. "For 40 years before the War between the States," recalled U.S. Congressman Lindsay Warren of North Carolina, "Washington was a pleasure-loving but ambitious community…. Commerce teemed in the harbor and the docks were a busy scene. It was a day of large plantations, high living, fast horses, hard drinking, and political strife…. The people were hospitable … and entertained lavishly. *The slaves did the work.*"[39]

From the perspective of many of Susan Dimock's white Washingtonian neighbors, the fact that "the slaves did the work" did not pose a moral or ethical problem. For them, the local brand of slavery was not considered especially onerous nor their slave population particularly plentiful in the decades before the war. "There were not a large number of slaves owned in Washington," insisted Martha Wiswall, a contemporary of Susan's. "Those who dealt in naval stores [goods used in building and maintaining ships] kept a number of men. Some were coopers and made the barrels in which turpentine was shipped. Others loaded and unloaded the vessels as they came and went; others were carters. Of course, the domestic servants were generally owned by their employers. They were kindly treated, well clothed, and had the attendance of a good doctor whenever his services were needed."[40]

It was true that large plantations run by slave labor did not dominate Washington and the rest of Beaufort County as they did other sections of the deeper South or even other areas of eastern North Carolina. But Wiswall's claim that "there were not a large number of slaves owned in Washington" neglected to put numbers on the situation. According to the 1850 Federal Slave Census, the Grist family's large Elmwood Plantation on the western end of Washington had 116 enslaved persons, both male and female, ranging in age from one to ninety. In the 1860 census, 45 percent of Washington's residents were listed as white, 45 percent as slaves, and 10 percent as free men of color.[41]

Wiswall was correct, however, about the curious demographic of the downtown waterfront. Scores of Black men, both enslaved and free, had long worked as maritime laborers in and around the bustling port of Washington. Some were seasoned carpenters, constructing and repairing ships with locally sourced cedar and white oak. Others found toiling on the docks and wharves ranged from ropeworkers, riggers, and sailmakers to caulkers, painters, plasterers, and blacksmiths. Perhaps surprisingly, some of the African Americans who enjoyed personal freedom were known to have slaves of their own. Hull Anderson, for example, was a free Washingtonian who ran a successful shipyard from 1830 to 1841. Anderson owned four enslaved men, all of whom actively worked in his shipbuilding business.

According to historian David Cecelski, the African American presence in North Carolina waters actually stretched much farther inland than the port of Washington and other seaside towns like Wilmington, Beaufort, and New Bern. "Slave and free black boatmen were ubiquitous on these broad waters, dominating most maritime trades and playing major roles in all of them," Cecelski explained in his book, *The Waterman's Song*. In addition to the waterfront docks, noted Cecelski, "the intertidal marshes, blackwater creeks, and brackish rivers that flowed into the estuaries also teemed with black watermen."[42] Moreover, this network of waterways and web of Black watermen had long served as a source of communication and news-sharing for local African American populations.

Susan Dimock knew well that slavery was a topic of disagreement among Washingtonians, a disagreement that mirrored the diverse political opinions of North Carolina as a whole. Both before and during what locals called The War Between the States or The War of Northern Aggression—and that ardent abolitionists christened The War to Preserve Slavery—the townspeople of Washington had divided loyalties and differing opinions on both secession (initially referred to as "disunion") and the "peculiar institution," a popular euphemism for slavery.[43] To any close observer, it was predictable that the state of North Carolina itself was

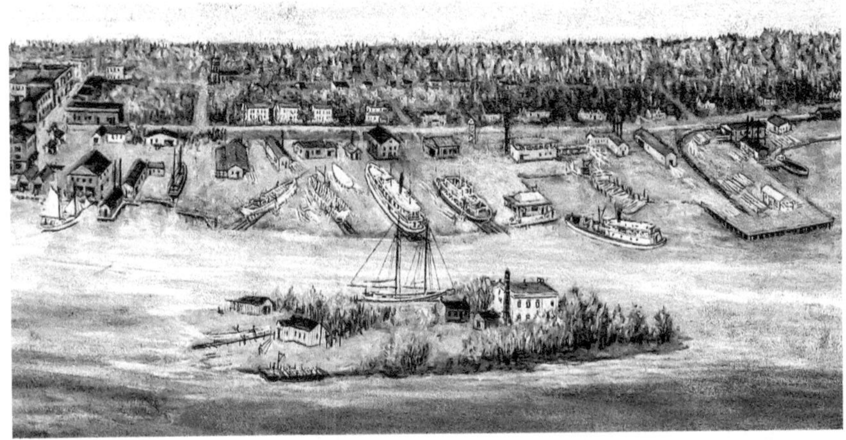

Shipbuilding and ship repairing were mainstays of the economy of Washington. Among those working as maritime laborers on the wharves of this bustling port town were scores of African American men, both enslaved and free (*Historic Washington Waterfront 1880–1920*, painted by Douglas A. Alvord; cropped from the original panorama; used by permission of the Historic Port of Washington, Inc.).

initially reluctant to secede from the Union—and became the tenth of eleven states to join the Confederacy, an act completed on May 20, 1861. Moreover, when Union troops entered Washington in 1862 and began a two-year wartime occupation, while many locals snubbed the intruders and shut their doors, others waved flags and cheered on the Yanks as they marched through town. Once the occupation had begun, many of the town's more commodious buildings, including the Dimocks' Lafayette Hotel, were used by ostensibly friendly Union troops as officers' quarters or military hospitals.

Recognizing her parents' dissimilar origins, Susan probably realized early on that slavery was an issue within the Dimock family as well. Her father Henry was a northerner, raised in a state where slave ownership had been outlawed for almost three decades before his birth—and where slavery was relatively rare even before then. When Henry Dimock agreed to lodge Union officers in the Lafayette Hotel during the occupation of Washington, he was jeered by staunch Confederate locals. In stark contrast was his wife Mary Malvina, who was born into a family and a society where slave labor was a fact of life. In the 1820 federal census, four years before Mary was born, her father Stephen Owens was listed as owning a dozen slaves—six males and six females, all but one under the age of 44. That there was discontent within his enslaved workforce is evidenced by reports of at least one effort at escape: in 1823, Mary Malvina's father ran an ad in local newspapers offering a fifteen dollar reward for the return of a 21-year-old runaway named Ruth. Whether Ruth fled because of long work hours, harsh conditions, whippings, or to find lost family members is not known. Yet by 1830, the Owenses were listed as owning nine enslaved persons, three fewer than a decade earlier.[44] Had those three successfully fled bondage, or did the Owens family simply require fewer hands by then? The record is not clear.

A journalist for the Raleigh *News & Observer* later shared local lore about Mr. and Mrs. Dimock's difference of opinion, noting that "Mary Malvina was accustomed to slaves and her husband, earning a comfortable income, bought house servants for her although he was bitterly opposed to slavery…." Years later, a northern apologist and friend of daughter Susan played down such marital disagreement, suggesting that "Although regretting the existence of slavery, they owned the few slaves necessary for the service of the household,—preferring to have control of them by purchase rather than to hire them of their masters."[45] The implication was that by owning their enslaved laborers the Dimocks knew exactly how well these Black women, men, and children were both trained and treated. At the time, "renting" Black laborers from other slaveowners was a popular alternative to owning them. Sometimes those who chose to rent simply lacked enough year-round work or money to purchase an enslaved laborer. Other renters may have wanted to avoid the stigma of slave ownership.

Whatever their individual opinions, the Dimocks did support the peculiar institution in their own way. The 1850 Federal Slave Census noted that Henry and Mary Malvina owned five enslaved persons at the time—four females, aged two, sixteen, thirty-one, and thirty-five years, plus one nine-year-old boy. The individuals' names are not known, since such information was not recorded in the federal census. The fact that the adults owned by the Dimocks were both female was symptomatic of one of slavery's more criminal aspects—the separation of mothers from fathers, of husbands from wives. When the parents of young slave children were sold, the offspring were generally purchased with their mother, while the father might well be traded elsewhere. If they were lucky, the enslaved-but-separated couple were owned by white families living in the same town or county, enabling them to periodically share visits. Many were not so fortunate. Curiously, recent scholarship indicates that by the time of the 1860 Federal Slave Census, the Dimock-Owens family did not actually own the enslaved laborers—or at least some of the enslaved laborers—who worked in their hotel. Instead, five of those African American workers were leased by Fannie Owens as part of the hotel property.[46]

That the number of domestic servants held by the Dimock-Owens was small does not erase the fact that Susan grew up in a privileged white family whose business clearly profited from the use of enslaved Black labor. Moreover, up until the *North State Whig* folded in 1854, Henry could hardly have been called an abolitionist editor. Although articles and ads in his newspaper reflected the Whig Party's disdain for "disunion," it also exposed the paper's weak stance on slavery. During the early 1850s, for example, multiple columns strongly denounced those Northerners (especially Bostonians) who defied the Fugitive Slave Law, and every issue featured ads offering rewards for the return of escapees.

Given this diversity of viewpoints within the Dimock family itself and among the townspeople in general, it's no surprise that while Washington was indeed a slave-owning town, it was also an important byway in the loose abolitionist web known as the Underground Railroad. Though the name suggests a service where steam locomotives pulled sturdy rail cars through subterranean tunnels, the Underground Railroad was actually a cooperative, clandestine, interlocking network of guides and safe-houses run by antislavery activists to help fugitives reach the Northern free states or Canada. The successes or failures of these escapes—and there were plenty of both—varied from station to station and from day to day.

As early as the turn of the nineteenth century, Washington, North Carolina, was known as a destination for those seeking freedom, a village where escapees from slavery could find support and sanctuary. The town's waterfront location and constant stops by northbound vessels were well-established means to possible escape. As noted earlier, an unusual number of enslaved and free laborers worked side-by-side in the waterfront shipyards, while numerous African Americans paddled or poled flatboats, barges, and smaller vessels in and out of connecting Carolina creeks, rivers, and marshes. While these rivers and their tributaries were important parts of the state's economy and transportation, they also served as "freedom roads" for Black fugitives. The fugitives' immediate reasons for flight were many, from trying to reunite with other family members or avoiding being sold, to running from harsh floggings or cruel sexual predation by their masters. At the core, of course, was a desire to be free from bondage and from exploitation—to be treated as equal human beings.[47]

If the runaway's goal was to stow away on a vessel heading to the North, he or she might shelter in woods or swamps near Washington, then sneak into town to clandestine alleys tucked between large waterfront warehouses like those found on Havens Wharf. Though the danger of detection was always present—and though punishment could range from a return to slavery to whippings or even death—many took their chances. Freedom seekers knew that oversight on the Washington waterfront tended to be looser than farther inland, where white planters held tight reins over their African American populations. Not only was the waterfront busier and more crowded than those rural areas, but interactions with free people of color, Black watermen, and abolitionists was more frequent there, leading to greater opportunities for escape.

North Carolina planters were well aware of the complex web that aided escapes on the Underground Railroad and the special appeal of port towns like Washington. This published plea to find a 19-year-old runaway named Owen was typical for the time:

> He is probably lurking about the wharves in Newbern or Washington. ... As Owen may endeavor to get to sea onboard the vessel of some Northern Abolitionist, the pilots and others at the Bar, are earnestly requested to aid in the effort to discover him.[48]

In the decades leading up to the Civil War, dozens of runaway slave advertisements echoed warnings that specifically cited the dangers and the appeal of the Washington waterfront. Comments like "he intends to go to a seaport town like Washington to board a vessel," "he was raised on the sea and wants to take shipping in Washington," or "he is a good sailor and broke jail once before in Washington" were typical in the published alerts. Frequently, slaveowners posting those ads described the fugitives as "lurking," "lurking around the wharves," or "lurking in Washington." The assumption that they were hiding among free Black citizens—or that those free Black citizens might be aiding and abetting their escapes—was also a common footnote in ads that speculated "they are among the free negroes in Fayetteville, Newbern, or Washington."[49]

Although countless fugitives drawn to the Washington waterfront fled enslavement on their own volition, some of their flights were choreographed with the aid of Black and white abolitionists in welcoming northern cities like Philadelphia, New York, and Boston. Some freedom seekers made arrangements with other Black fugitives, with compassionate white citizens in the South, or with the many free African Americans who worked the docks and riverside wharves. Even Black boatmen on the Washington waterfront who were themselves enslaved would sometimes help others to flee—then use their maritime skills and knowledge to orchestrate their own escapes. As a result, while some fugitives departing on northbound vessels stowed away in cargo holds, others were able to pass as free, either by presenting forged free papers or by using their maritime skills to work openly as hired shipmates.

If Susan Dimock's hometown was indeed a critical avenue to freedom—at the time, the second largest port in North Carolina—that position was only enhanced by the advent of hostilities in 1861. When both Alexandria, Virginia, and Charleston, South Carolina, were burned during the Civil War, Washington became an even more crucial wartime supply port and naval base where Union ships would stop to drop off or pick up supplies while moving them further north.[50]

Was Susan Dimock aware of the intrigues and intricacies of the Underground Railroad in her hometown? No record exists chronicling her knowledge on this subject. Still, Henry and Mary Malvina's daughter clearly developed a disdain for slavery, likely reinforced by her own experiences, readings, and astute observations. Her opinions may have emerged when she witnessed firsthand the scores of enslaved workers toiling in the scorchingly hot fields of large plantations like Elmwood. Her views may have come from the household slaves she observed working in her family's own Lafayette Hotel, as they toiled scrubbing laundry, preparing meals, cleaning rooms, washing floors, polishing furniture, and answering doors—while lacking the most basic of freedoms.

Whatever the cause and whatever psychic scars and doubts resulted from her observations and experiences, Susan later recalled regretfully, "I was always slow in taking in an idea; I did not feel the sin of slavery until I was eight years old." Considering how carefully this subject was excluded from general conversation in the South in the antebellum era, it was a remarkable comment coming from a youngster. Northern abolitionist Ednah Dow Cheney later noted that it showed "uncommon vigor and independence of thought, in a child of eight years, to perceive the evil of a social custom sanctioned by the example of those whom she most loved and respected."[51]

According to her friend, Lilian Freeman Clarke, by age fourteen the always reserved and often silent Susan had taken her political views on slavery a step further. "One day she sat by herself reading, while in the same room several persons were discussing the situation and bitterly denouncing the Abolitionists of the North. In a pause of the discussion, a soft, clear voice was heard saying, 'I am an Abolitionist.' Some of those present turned angrily upon her, saying, 'If that is the truth, you might at least be ashamed to own it!' She made no reply."[52]

As it turned out, this was only one of many ways in which Susan Dimock was not like the other girls.

CHAPTER 2

Transitions

On April 12, 1861, General P.G.T. Beauregard ordered his Confederate troops to open fire on the Union garrison at Fort Sumter in the harbor of Charleston, South Carolina. Though Fort Sumter was more than 250 miles south of Susan Dimock's home in Little Washington, Susan and her family were well aware that America's dreaded Civil War had begun. Five and a half weeks later, on May 20, 1861, North Carolina followed the states of the Deep South—and more significantly, of neighboring Virginia—and seceded from the Union. Once North Carolina formally joined the Confederacy, many of the Dimocks' prominent Washington neighbors began raising companies—small subdivisions of infantry battalions—and preparing them for military service. Men from Washington started departing *en masse* for Southern battlefields, leaving behind women, children, the elderly, the disabled, and the enslaved.

Eager to assist in the Confederate war effort during that first year of combat, local women joined together to make shirts for the soldiers. "Materials were purchased, I do not remember whether by a company fund or by citizens," recalled Susan's neighbor, Martha Fowle. "The ladies met and cut out all the garments, shirts, etc., and distributed them to be made. Many young ladies took their first lessons in shirt-making at this time, and those for their friends or especial favorite were sometimes ornamented by feather-stitching or embroidery."[1]

A wave of patriotic fervor also inspired the Washington seamstresses to buy flowing yards of silk from Mr. Parmalee's store, which they fashioned into flags designed by captain Daniel Reid for local companies like "The Washington Greys," "The Jeff Davis Rifles," "The Pamlico Guards," and "The Southern Guards." It's doubtful that Susan joined these Confederate women's flag-making efforts, due both to her father's pro-Northern sentiments and to her own firm but soft-spoken anti-slavery stance.

If she did assist in any way, it's more likely that it was along with other youngsters—and in the field of healing. "About the same time the flags were made Miss Mathilda Marsh gathered the young girls and children in the old Wiswall house, on the South East corner of Main and Respess streets," explained Martha Fowle. "[They] rolled bandages, scraped lint, and made cartridges." Though the rolling of bandages is familiar today, "scraping lint" was a popular project of Civil War–era relief groups that involved scratching a knife over a taut piece of flax or linen cloth. The resulting cotton "lint" was collected and used as a dressing for wounds and sores, held in place by those rolled cotton bandages. Later in 1861 and early '62, when the 31st Regiment of North Carolina Volunteers was stationed in Washington, Susan could easily have helped out when the old Presbyterian Parsonage was converted into an ad-hoc hospital and when many soldiers—either wounded in battle or stricken by an outbreak of measles—received nursing at that parsonage or in private homes.[2]

Almost a year after the attack on Fort Sumter, and just one month before Susan Dimock's fifteenth birthday, the war came home—and landed a stone's throw from the Dimocks' front door. On March 20, 1862, the 24th Massachusetts Regiment marched into Washington, North Carolina, beginning a Union occupation that lasted two years. As a fleet of Federal gunboats swept into the eerily calm harbor and flag-waving Union troops triumphantly flooded the tree-shaded earthen streets, Susan could hardly have imagined what would follow: two years of upheaval, uncertainty, and tragic loss for the Dimock family.

When Colonel Thomas G. Stevenson and the soldiers of the 24th Massachusetts entered town, Susan and her neighbors gazed in astonishment as a regimental band and several well-dressed companies landed on town docks and marched triumphantly and uninterrupted toward the Beaufort County Courthouse on North Market Street. The Dimock family's Lafayette Hotel was just down the street from that courthouse, enabling Susan to observe the invading Federal regiment raise a 34-star American flag while a widow with pro–Union sentiments spread out on the balustrade in front of her house a starry banner reading "Constitution and Union."[3]

Such a bloodless entry of Union troops into an ostensibly Confederate town might at first seem odd. But there was a logical explanation. "The Federal commander reported to the War Department that he had found Union sentiments among a few individuals," wrote U.S. Congressman Lindsay Warren.[4] The Boston *Journal* reported even more pro–Union feeling in town than had Congressman Warren, noting that two thirds of Washington's citizens had "seen fit to leave for the interior," while those remaining "met the troops with every expression of welcome."[5]

The actual proportion of pro–Union versus pro–Confederate sentiment in Washington that day may never be known. More significant is that those still living there put up no resistance to the 24th Massachusetts' occupation of their once-vibrant town. Part of the reason was the

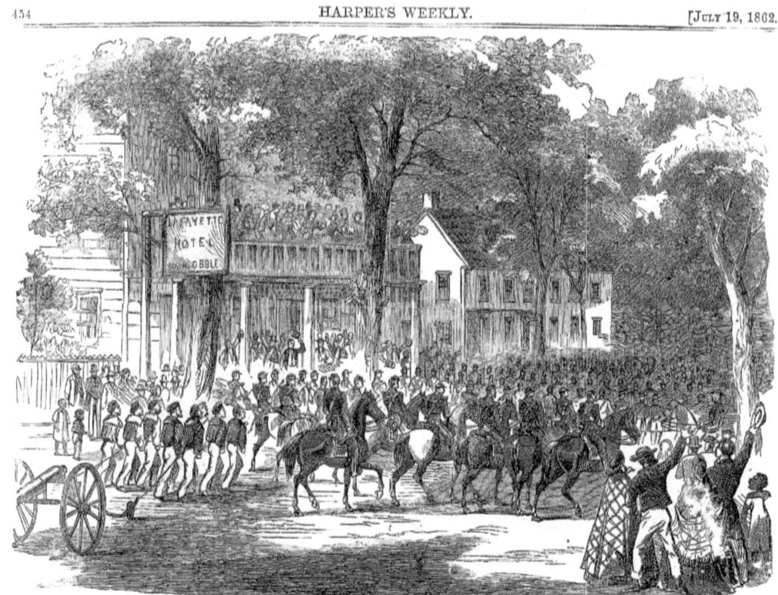

RECEPTION OF GOVERNOR STANLY AT WASHINGTON, NORTH CAROLINA.—SKETCHED BY MR. A. WISER.—[SEE PAGE 455.]

The Dimock-Owens family's Lafayette Hotel, on the northeast corner of Main and Market streets, was a central location for many events during the Union army occupation of Washington, North Carolina (reception of Governor Stanley at Washington, North Carolina, from *Harper's Weekly*, July 19, 1862, 454; image courtesy Wilson Special Collections Library, University of North Carolina at Chapel Hill).

diminished population noted in the Boston *Journal*: by the time the Federal occupation began, the town of more than 3,000 had already been reduced to some 700 individuals. As a result, a permanent Union garrison—with infantry, cavalry, artillery, and a fleet of gunboats—was easily established throughout Washington and its waterfront, and was able to endure for almost two years despite sporadic attempts at military siege by outlying Confederate troops.

As the weeks wore on, more and more of Washington's finest old residences were seized and converted for Federal wartime use. The Dimock's Lafayette Hotel, for example, and both the Myers and Marsh houses on Water Street were designated as officers' headquarters. The Hollyday House on West Second Street and the Fowle House on West Main were made into Union hospitals. Castle Island in the harbor—where the Fowle Brothers had created a shipbuilding yard back in 1818—became a Federal "battery," the term for a prepared artillery position.[6]

Though the housing of Union officers in the Dimocks' hotel/home was not threatening to Susan's family in any immediate way, to suggest that the Dimock family's life had any type of normality from that point on would be false. Because day after day, and piece by piece, Susan's world began disassembling.

Her formal schooling ended when the prestigious Washington Academy was terminated as a center of education and taken over by invading blue-uniformed Union troops as a military hospital and barracks. Her medical "internship" came to a halt as her family doctor, neighbor, and mentor, Dr. Solomon Satchwell, joined the war effort and moved sixty miles west to take charge of the Confederate Hospital in Wilson, North Carolina.[7] But the most devastating blow came seven months after the Union occupation began, on October 30, 1862, when Susan's beloved father Henry passed away at the age of 53.

Precisely how Henry Dimock died was not recorded by contemporaries or remembered by later generations. Neither the Beaufort County Register of Deeds nor the churchyard where he was buried, in the cemetery of Saint Peter's Episcopal Church near the Lafayette Hotel, has any written record of his death or interment.[8] Had he been killed in a military skirmish related to the war or the Union occupation, that fact would likely have passed down in local legend and lore. What is known is that the newspaper that consumed Henry's work life for a dozen years, the once powerful *North State Whig*, had folded eight years earlier, in 1854, as the Whig party began disbanding. Henry may well have been depressed since the paper's closure. Moreover, his personal finances could have fallen into disarray. Financial default would help explain why Henry was recorded as owning the family's enslaved laborers in the 1850 census, while his sister-in-law Fannie was shown as the family's official slaveowner in 1860. A ledger from the local general store run by Dave Fowle shows numerous "painkillers" listed under Henry Dimock's account, plus regular purchases of alcohol and camphor in the years after his newspaper shut down. Found in the wood of the camphor laurel, camphor was used medicinally to treat itching, knee pain, swelling, and diarrhea. Still, there is no proof that the painkillers were taken by Henry personally, and the alcohol and camphor could as easily been used for lighting lamps as for human consumption.[9]

The death of her beloved father—the man who wholeheartedly supported her dream of becoming a doctor—likely devastated teenaged Susan. Losing a parent is known to be one of the most shattering events a child can experience. A youngster's world, already in imbalance, could easily turn topsy-turvy. Since Susan was an only child, her immediate family was now reduced to her mother, Mary Malvina, her mother's sister, Fannie Owens, and Fannie's daughter, Virginia (Jenny). If young Susan ever wrote or talked about her sorrow, those records are long lost. Moreover, the fact

Henry Dimock

1858
Feby 17 Bt. Pain Killer 2/6 19th Colin...
Mar 1 Alcohol 5/— 4th Lotion for Sun...
" 6 Putty 1/— 10th Alcohol 5/— 16th Cal...
" 17 Alcohol 5/— 20th Quicksilver /6 c
" 27 K. Oil 3/6 April 7th Camos Si
April 7 Spts Turp /6 16th Assafœtida 1,

There is no record of why Susan's beloved father, Henry Dimock, died in 1862 at the age of fifty-three. A ledger from Dave Fowle's general store shows numerous "painkillers" listed under Henry's account, plus regular purchases of alcohol and camphor in the years after his newspaper shut down (Henry Dimock rolling account, 1856–59, ledger from Dave Fowle's General Store, Brown Library Archives, Washington, North Carolina; photograph © the author).

that the Civil War had finally come to the Dimocks' doorstep—and even come inside their home—probably gave scant time for the four women to fully mourn Henry's untimely death. Instead, they needed to survive the conflict, adapt to unforeseen dangers, and support themselves financially. It's possible, too, that Henry Dimock's death actually strengthened Susan's determination to become the successful professional woman her father believed she could someday be.[10]

At first, the wartime occupation by some 1,000 Union troops was probably just strange, strained, and inconvenient. Regular residents of the Dimock's Lafayette Hotel were forced to leave as army officers expropriated their rooms. Loyal Confederates in town derided the Dimocks for allowing traitorous Northern troops to lodge with them, though several other local homes and buildings were similarly seized by federal officers, medics, and prison wardens. Although no major aggressions or minor street battles occurred for weeks on end, Susan and her neighbors were continually aware that they lived in a state of war.

In the early days of the occupation, even families fiercely loyal to the Confederacy were more perturbed than seriously injured. Susan's childhood friend, Annie Blackwell Sparrow, recalled that "Consternation spread among our people when the dreaded enemy was at last in our midst, and we all expected little less than a general massacre. However, 'even the devil is not as black as he is painted,' and some of us still live to tell the tale of life in a town garrisoned by the enemy." In Sparrow's recollections, some of the worst initial offences were the rude stares and crude remarks made to local girls and ladies by occupying soldiers or the fact that men in the military headquarters opened and read as many incoming letters as they could seize. "Singing southern songs in private parlors was prohibited," she remembered with dismay, "and on one occasion, an officer called to tell my mother that if her daughters sang any more southern songs in their parlor, they would be arrested and put in jail."[11]

When news did arrive by mail—in letters sometimes hidden in egg baskets or tucked inside shoes or bonnets—it often described far-off military victories and losses, or chronicled the injuries and deaths of brothers, sons, and fathers. Equally disconcerting to many was the fact that unfamiliar faces were also flowing into Washington, from wounded soldiers and prisoners of war to ladies of the night, the latter ostensibly brought in to accommodate the troops.[12]

More threatening physical assaults on the town did sometimes occur—resulting in violence and chaos in the streets—most notably when Confederate forces attempted to recapture the quiet, riverside town from its Union occupiers.

The first major Confederate attack on Little Washington's Union outposts came early on Saturday morning, September 6, 1862, during Henry Dimock's last few weeks of life. As a heavy fog shrouded the landscape, Confederate Colonel S.D. Pool caught the Federal Garrison at Washington off guard by sweeping into town with segments of the 17th, 55th, and 8th North Carolina regiments and 10th artillery. Galloping in from several directions, the Confederates charged up and the down the streets, shouting like demons and brandishing their sabers. Soundly sleeping Union soldiers woke suddenly and tumbled out of their beds, as confused as Susan, her mother, and all the other terrified women and children who huddled by their windows and doors. "Imagine our fright and our hopes when we were awakened by the noise of the fight, not knowing at first what it was," remembered loyal Confederate Annie Blackwell Sparrow. "Peering through the closed shutters, early dawn as it was, we could at last distinguish dashing past, the grey uniform we loved so well. How madly our hearts beat and how earnestly we prayed."[13]

As the fog lifted, so did the confusion. This, everyone soon realized, was outright war. The Union gunboats *Picket* and *Louisiana* began firing on the Confederate attackers from the waterfront. A magazine (ammunition storage area) on the *Picket* accidentally exploded, sinking the ship and killing nineteen men and the captain. As the vessel exploded, Confederates began shouting "Little Washington is ours!"

But their claim to victory was short-lived.

The sound of gunfire had also reached the ears of Colonel Edward E. Potter, First Regiment North Carolina Union Volunteers, who was just outside of town, *en route* to Plymouth with cavalry and artillery in tow. Potter and company sped back to Washington, forged down Main Street, and broke into battle with the Confederates at the intersection of Market and Main—directly in front of the Dimocks' Lafayette Hotel.[14]

What Susan and her family witnessed during almost three brutal hours of cavalry and artillery battle must have been horrifying. Confederate and Federal troops advanced and retreated across town thoroughfares, charging in and out of the Dimocks' front yard. Shot and shells from gunboats in the harbor riddled homes and businesses, shattering and wrecking random structures in their wake. Tree limbs and branches were scattered everywhere, as heavy artillery scorched rows of mighty elms in full leaf. "The gunboats threw many shots into the town and afterwards into the woods beyond," explained Annie Blackwell Sparrow. "Our part of the town was badly injured. As the shells went whizzing over our roof, my mother assembled us all in a room downstairs. With her weeping children around her, she besought God to protect us. We were on our knees when a shell went crashing through the roof of our house and we clung together in speechless terror."[15]

By day's end, Union soldiers had defeated and driven away the Confederates. The occupation continued. And, surrounded by his loving family at the Lafayette Hotel, Henry Dimock was pushed that much closer to his death.

As the months rolled on in wartime Washington, the town's demographics changed even more dramatically than its landscape. Not only had the native population of 3,000 dwindled to 700, but the onslaught of what grew to be 1200 Union troops was augmented by hundreds of unexpected newcomers—most of them Black. The reason is a relatively unknown story in Civil War history.

While Union troops continued to march southward and occupy more North Carolina territory, many enslaved men and women took advantage of the confusion to flee their masters. Though their ultimate destination was Canada—or any safe haven north of the Mason-Dixon Line—the fleeing men, women, children, parents, and grandparents frequently had one immediate goal: to reach Union lines in North Carolina and settle into what came to be known as "contraband camps." Before President Lincoln's *Emancipation Proclamation* of January 1, 1863, enslaved people who escaped their masters were classified as "contrabands

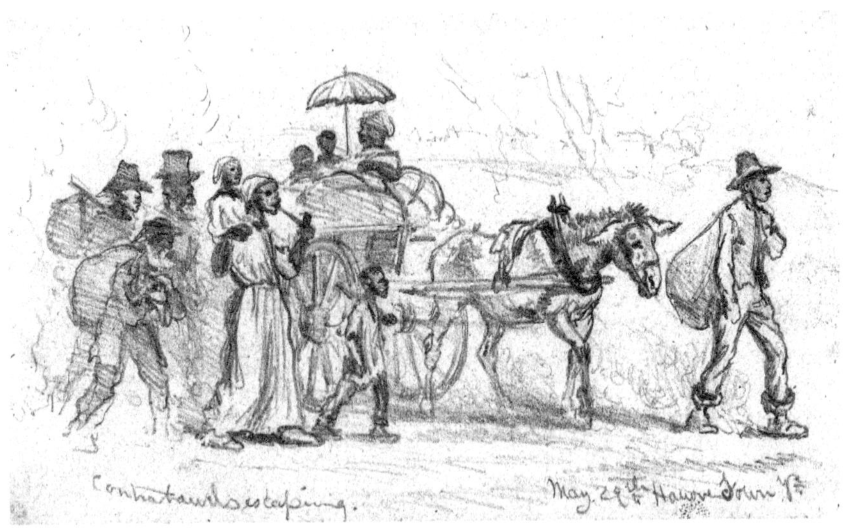

As Union troops occupied more North Carolina territory, many enslaved men and women took advantage of the confusion to flee their masters. Though their ultimate destination was Canada—or any safe haven north of the Mason-Dixon Line—those fleeing had one immediate goal: to reach Union lines in North Carolina and settle into what came to be known as "contraband camps" ("Contrabands escaping," by Edwin Forbes, 1864; public domain image courtesy Morgan collection of Civil War drawings, Library of Congress Prints and Photographs Division, Washington, D.C.).

of war." After the Proclamation declared "that all persons held as slaves" within the rebellious states "are, and henceforward shall be free," these same African Americans came to be called "freedmen." Located on the outskirts of Union military encampments, contraband camps were known to provide sanctuary, a rustic shelter, and either paid or unpaid work for those fleeing slavery. In Washington's case, that work included building Union fortifications and bearing arms to help fight off Confederate attacks. In some instances, camp directors even established schools and churches for the contrabands who managed to reach their retreats.

The largest contraband camp in eastern North Carolina was established in New Bern, some forty miles south of Little Washington. While New Bern shielded some 8,591 African American refugees, regional outposts also grew up in Beaufort, Plymouth, Roanoke Island, and Washington. The numbers grew so large that in April of 1863, Horace James, an evangelical Congregational minister and abolitionist from Worcester, Massachusetts, was appointed Superintendent of Negro Affairs to supervise these North Carolina outposts. By January of 1864, 17,419 contrabands/freedmen were living within Union lines, with 2,714 of them in Washington alone.[16]

Appalled that these towns were increasingly brimming with "Yankees, Negroes, and Traitors,"[17] Confederate General Robert E. Lee initially approved more attacks—including a second assault on Susan Dimock's hometown. Recently charged with leading the North Carolina troops, Confederate General D.H. (Daniel Harvey) Hill, the brother-in-law of Stonewall Jackson, planned a siege on Little Washington with two primary goals in mind: capturing the Union garrison embedded there—which would also effectively eliminate the contraband camp—and collecting supplies of meat and corn for Lee's armies in Virginia. When General Hill's earlier attack on New Bern proved a fiasco, he opted to move toward Washington with a less ambitious plan. The idea of a ferocious full-frontal assault on the Union garrison was replaced by simply harassing and distracting the Federal troops while gathering those sorely-needed food supplies.

As a result of this second siege, over the first two weeks of April 1863—only six months after Henry Dimock's death—constant dueling again disrupted the peace in Susan's battered town. In the recollections of Annie Blackwell Sparrow, "So dangerous was the firing from the gunboats, and from our own forts, that the people who had cellars and basements lived in them during the whole siege, inviting as many as they could accommodate to share their security."[18] Perhaps predictably, Confederate General Hill was effectively rebuffed by the well-prepared Union forces. Despite their valiant efforts, the gray-uniformed Confederates ultimately slogged out of town in an intense rainfall, with no success in dislodging or disrupting the Union encampment, but with a good deal of corn and bacon in hand.[19]

For Susan Dimock, her family, and her neighbors, this period of war must have seemed like a terrible dream. Every day, echoes of gunfire ricocheted past their Lafayette Hotel, coming to and from the Washington waterfront. The Forty-fourth Massachusetts regiment then camped in town had a band that periodically amused itself by playing "Dixie"—which, in turn, goaded Confederate troops into intensifying their fire. Meanwhile, one of the federal ships docked farther down the Pamlico River had a calliope on board, which soldiers played each night after dinner. The melodic climax to each concert was invariably the sound of bomb shells blasted at any Confederates nearby. Some nights, this odd wartime symphony was enhanced by an eruption of wildly clanging sounds. Well after nightfall, mischievous Confederates would tie cow bells around their horses' necks and dart into town, followed by Union gunfire once the occupying troops had figured out their game.[20]

Despite the endless occupation and the periodic chaos of active warfare, life for Susan Dimock went on. Over a period of less than two years, two Confederate attacks intent on recapturing Little Washington ultimately failed. As it turned out, their third and final attempt did in fact succeed—but at a price that was dear to Susan and her family.

The calendar read April 20, 1864, only four days before Susan's seventeenth birthday. On that memorable day, Confederate forces took the town of Plymouth, North Carolina. Sensing that their time was up and that the Grays' invasion was imminent, Union forces were ordered to evacuate Washington. Ten days later, as the last Federal detachment was preparing to embark from the Washington waterfront, a group of Union soldiers reportedly looted the town and torched Havens Wharf—either inadvertently or as a deliberate effort to prevent naval stores and other supplies from falling into Confederate hands.

From those waterfront warehouses, flames swiftly spread through town, ultimately charring as much as half of Washington's downtown area. Then, just nine days later, a second, purely accidental fire—reportedly started in the Dimocks' own backyard—engulfed even more of Washington, including the family's home and business, the Lafayette Hotel.

With nowhere to live, no way to support themselves, and no father to guide them, Susan, her mother, and their small entourage had no option but to flee the only home that Susan Dimock had ever known.

Precisely who comprised Susan Dimock's small entourage, and just how they escaped Washington after the great fires of late April and early May 1864, are still mysteries. Many secondary accounts read that Henry Dimock's "widow and child" fled their hometown to find relatives and relative safety.[21] Based on later census reports, however, it's likely that this group of native North Carolinians eventually included not only seventeen-year-old Susan and her mother Mary Malvina, but also her mother's older sister Fannie Owens and Fannie's twenty-one-year-old daughter, Jenny.

Particularly interesting is that by 1865, those four women were living in Massachusetts with fifteen-year-old "Ellen Dimmock" [*sic*] and twelve-year old "Lewis Dimmock," both of them Black. Recent research shows that, despite the alternate spelling (Susan and her mother were listed in the same census as Dimock with a single "m"), siblings Ellen and Lewis Dimmock had been enslaved houseworkers for Susan's family at the Lafayette Hotel—and were part of the "property" Aunt Fannie Owens leased from the hotel's legal owner, Howard Wiswall. It was common for enslaved individuals to bear their owners' surnames, both before and after emancipation. The fact that Ellen and Lewis were listed in the 1865 census as Dimmocks rather than Wiswalls brings up several questions. Had the Dimocks purchased these two Black youngsters from Howard Wiswall? Had Susan and her mother brought them along as de facto servants? Did they consider the youngsters free citizens in the wake of the Emancipation Proclamation? Or had they taken Ellen and Lewis on their northern journey to help them escape Wiswall and the bonds of southern slavery? No records have yet been found to answer those queries. Still, the result was that Ellen and Lewis Dimmock were now free Americans living in the Commonwealth of Massachusetts. And by bringing the siblings to a northern free state, Susan Dimock may have made tangible her claim that "I am an Abolitionist."[22]

What is known is that the fleeing Dimocks—however many there were—first traveled sixty miles inland, to the town of Wilson, North Carolina. If they had access to horses, carriages, or horse carts that had somehow survived the flames, or if they simply walked or hitched rides from compassionate locals to get there, is not clear. The stark reality was that the divided nation, as well as the Confederate State of North Carolina, was still engulfed by the bloodiest war in its history. Travel was treacherous at best. So for Susan and her band, it was vital to seek out friends, determine a final destination, then find a viable escape route to get there.

The farm market town of Wilson was a logical starting point. It's likely the Dimock clan went to Wilson to find shelter, aid, and advice from their old friend and family physician, Solomon Sampson Satchwell. Dr. Satchwell had relocated to Wilson earlier in the war to take command of the Confederate hospital there. More importantly, he always had been, and always would be, a dependable friend to Susan. Sometime during their stay—probably with Satchwell's input—Susan and her mother decided that their journey should end in the Union stronghold of Massachusetts. No military battles were taking place in the Commonwealth. More importantly, Maria Dimock Mann, the fifty-eight-year-old sister of Susan's late father, had a home in the rural town of Sterling, some forty miles west of Boston.

Accounts of Susan's life generally say the family "in some way"[23] traveled to Sterling but fail to mention the route or the means of transportation they chose for a perilous wartime trip of almost 700 miles. The fact that they went first to Wilson provides one clue. In addition to being Dr. Satchwell's home base, the town of Wilson was also a major railroad junction for the eastern part of the state. Trains did not come to the Dimocks' hometown of Washington, North Carolina, until a dozen years after the war.[24] At first, it sounds like a simple solution: If Susan and her mother were traveling by rail in the twenty-first century, they could easily catch an Amtrak sleeper from Wilson, North Carolina, to Boston, Massachusetts, with just one changeover in Washington, D.C., or New York. From Boston, they could take the Fitchburg Railroad Line to the outskirts of Sterling. In 1864, however, the route from Wilson to Sterling would have involved cobbling together a complex series of train rides from town to town and state to state, zigzagging northward through Confederate and Union lines on a variety of small, independent train lines and occasional ferryboats. There would be frequent transfers to distant depots, no way to coordinate arrivals and departures in advance, and the need to negotiate train schedules constantly muddled by the war.[25] If the family had somehow accessed a series of horse-drawn wagons, carts, or coaches, the routes would have been equally precarious.

The only other possible option would have been for the Dimocks to travel by sea, leaving a port like their hometown of Washington, then working their way up the coastline to New England. With both naval blockades and coastal battles in full swing—including the Battle of Albemarle Sound fought along the North Carolina coastline in May of 1864—that would have been an especially treacherous journey. In addition to heavily armed wooden vessels, Civil War naval battles included ominous "ironclad" warships, primitive submarines, underwater traps, and even torpedoes. Another fact that casts doubt on the "by sea" theory is that Susan and Mrs. Dimock had already travelled sixty miles westward to get to Wilson. To access sailing vessels on the eastern seaboard, they would have first had to backtrack that same sixty miles to Washington or another coastal town.

Though the trip north—whether by land or by sea—could not have been easy, Susan and her traveling companions finally reached Sterling, Massachusetts, by mid-1864. Sterling was a quintessential New England town, surrounded by rushing streams and dappled orchards. There was a town common—a flat, fenced, central area set aside for "common" use by the townsfolk—as well as three white clapboard churches with lofty spires. With a population of some 1,600, Sterling was roughly half the pre-war size of Susan's North Carolina hometown. Like Washington, Sterling's roads were packed with earth, though the town's tradesmen had decidedly more inland vocations. There were plentiful cottage industries producing wooden chairs, sewing machine needles, pottery, hats, leather goods, children's carriages, baskets, and harvested ice. Still, Sterling was primarily an agricultural community, best known for its apple orchards as well as its prize sheep and cattle. The Annual Cattle Show on the Town Common had been a popular local event since 1856.[26]

As different as Sterling, Massachusetts, was from Washington, North

Carolina, the two small American towns shared one curiosity in common. Both villages had enjoyed visits in 1824 by French icon and American Revolutionary War hero, the Marquis de Lafayette, during his "Farewell Tour" of all twenty-four United States. The Lafayette Hotel the Dimocks ran in North Carolina had been named in honor of the Marquis.

Local Sterling notables included Robert B. Thomas, who started the *Old Farmer's Almanac* in 1793, and Ebenezer Butterick, the founder of Butterick tissue-paper sewing patterns. Equally heralded was a 58-year-old woman named Mary Sawyer Tyler, who was the Mary of "Little Lamb" legend. As a nine-year-old schoolgirl in 1815, Mary Sawyer had indeed been followed to Sterling's Redstone Schoolhouse by an orphaned lamb she'd been caring for at her country homestead. Locals still proudly remembered that the endearing scene had inspired young John Roulstone to write a poem that was expanded and published by Sarah Josepha Hale in 1830, then set to music by Lowell Mason in 1831.[27] It's likely that as a child, Susan Dimock and her young friends had even sung "Mary Had a Little Lamb," since it was already a children's classic by the time of her birth in 1847.

Of far more immediate importance to Susan and her family than all this history, however, was finding the home of Daniel and Maria Mann. Susan's fifty-eight-year-old Aunt Maria had been married to sixty-three-year-old Daniel Mann for almost two decades. In 1845, seven years after the death of his first wife, Daniel had wedded the oldest of Henry Dimock's eight siblings, Maria Whitmore Dimock. A year later, happily settled into their cozy Sterling home, forty-year-old Maria bore the couple's only child, a son named Birney. Together, the family made a life on the picturesque farmland, which they shared with a bevy of oxen, cows, horses, swine, and whatever local farm hands were needed.[28]

Although the Manns lived on a farm, Daniel was not a farmer by trade. Instead, Uncle Daniel was a dentist and surgeon—a common combination at the time—with offices in downtown Boston.[29] He was also an ardent abolitionist whose dental clients included the nation's most prominent white anti-slavery advocate, William Lloyd Garrison. Mann reportedly pulled out five of Garrison's teeth in one sitting in 1865. Garrison bragged to his wife, "Of course, I went through it all without wincing, discarding ether and chloroform."[30] Members of the legendary Garrison family, who lived in the Roxbury Highlands on the outskirts of Boston, were frequent visitors to the Manns' Sterling farmhouse. A regular summer guest was William Lloyd's son, Frank Garrison, who was a close friend and former Boston Latin School classmate of Birney Mann. Despite the fact that they attended public schools, young Frank Garrison and his siblings mostly socialized with other abolitionists' children, for fear of attacks by violent anti-abolitionists.[31]

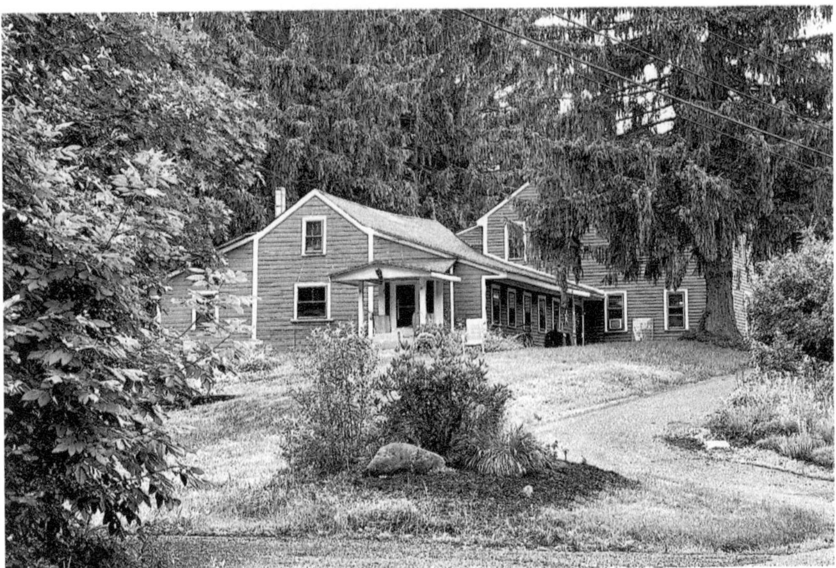

Susan's aunt, Maria Dimock Mann (1806–92), lived with her husband Daniel Mann on a picturesque farmland in the rural town of Sterling, forty miles west of Boston. This property was an abolitionist meeting place as well as a purported stop on the Underground Railroad (photograph © the author).

It was the late spring of 1864 when the weary travelers from North Carolina finally found the 190-acre Mann farmstead, three miles outside Sterling's town center. Undoubtedly, the Manns knew in advance that the Dimocks would be arriving. It's possible that they even "sponsored" the Southern family's arduous journey from a Confederate state to a Union stronghold. Set above the Stillwater River, the Mann farmstead perched on a country road in the southwest corner of town, near Oakdale village. When Susan's entourage arrived, the Mann house and its outbuildings were already considered antiquated. Built eight decades earlier, following America's War for Independence, the residence on the sprawling farm complex was a colonial-style New England salt-box house, with fieldstone foundation, weathered clapboard siding, a ridge roof, and a single, tall chimney in its center. The term "salt-box house" came from the structure's resemblance to the wooden salt containers popular in colonial times.

As Susan and family entered the Manns' farmhouse, they must have found the home cozy and comforting—a perfect ending to their arduous journey. The timber frame construction was plainly evident in the thick rustic beams that supported and stretched across the low-hung ceilings. A wide brick fireplace dominated the central room, and a broad wooden staircase led to chambers on the second floor.

Evidence of the Manns' abolitionist ventures was probably readily apparent to Susan and her mother, due both to the anti-slavery literature and broadsides lying about as well as to some unusual architectural elements in the home. Those architectural elements are still visible in the old Mann house, which remains in its original location to this day. "This property figured prominently in abolitionist activities, as well as being purported as a stop on the Underground Railroad," confirmed David W. Gibbs, curator of the Sterling Historical Society, during a 2016 visit to the site. "Most such claims are routinely dismissed," Gibbs agreed, "but this one I'm fairly certain was a stop."[32] The property's twenty-first-century owner, Kathy Bogosian, confirmed that theory. Graciously offering a tour of her colonial-era home, she escorted the author into the large main chamber, which seemed to be fundamentally unchanged over the generations. The ceilings were still low, the colonial fireplace still wide, and the chunky, hand-hewn, support beams still exposed. Though the main staircase leading to the second story was apparent upon entering the front door, a second, narrower stairwell was less obvious. A section of one side wall had been sliced open some three feet above the wooden floor to expose a once-boarded-over entrance to the attic. Climbing onto the hidden stairs by means of a chair placed beneath the wall opening, we ascended to find several small, unfinished chambers tucked under the sloping roof, including what Bogosian described as "a secret space behind the chimney."[33] No one knew when or why the steep staircase had been covered over and made essentially invisible. It looked like a perfect refuge for enslaved people fleeing their Southern masters.

Whether this was where the Manns and their abolitionist colleagues hid freedom seekers fleeing north may never be known for sure, but the questions it raises are many. Susan and her family had fled from Washington, North Carolina, a Union Army–occupied town that was a known stop on the Underground Railroad. Their entourage may have included two teenaged African Americans who shared the Dimock surname and were once enslaved. Their destination in Sterling, Massachusetts, was likely another station on that same Underground Railroad, and lodged in a community known for harboring runaways and hosting outspoken anti-slavery advocates.

If this all had a deliberate and conscious connection, it was not chronicled. The vast majority of information on that covert escape service—the stops, the stationmasters, the escapees, and the routes—was kept deliberately secret and unrecorded, both in the town of Sterling and throughout the divided nation.

Within a relatively short period of time—presumably aided by the Mann family—Susan and Mary Malvina Dimock re-established their lives in Sterling. Still only seventeen, Susan attended a local school for six months, while her mother worked on creating a modicum of financial and residential security. The most enduring benefit from this period of the Dimocks' journey, was however, not financial. "During her residence here," recalled one of Susan's colleagues year later, "she formed that acquaintance with Miss Bessie Greene which had so happy an influence on her ... life."[34] The relationship with Bessie Greene would be central for the rest of Susan's life.

Just seven months older than Susan Dimock, Elizabeth ("Bessie") Willard Greene undoubtedly made the acquaintance of the young North Carolinian through the town

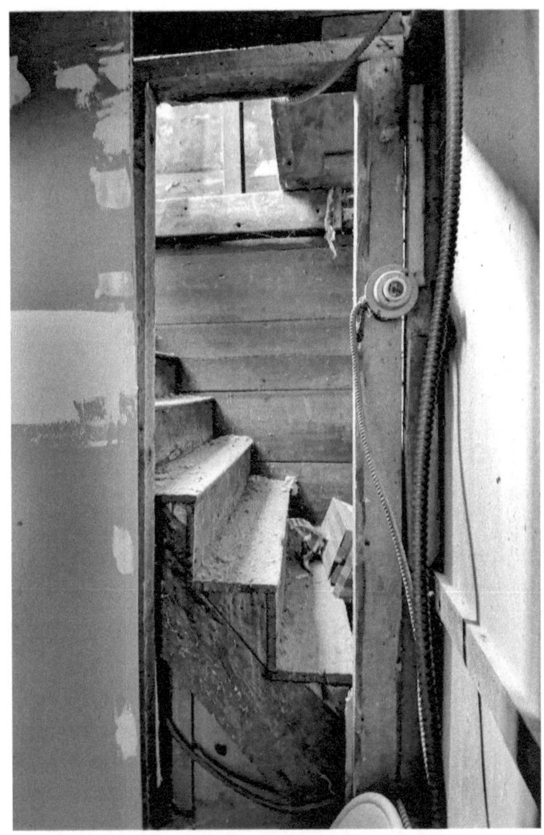

Inside the Mann farmhouse in Sterling is a once-boarded-over staircase leading to small attic chambers. The home's twenty-first century owner suspects it may have been a hidden refuge for enslaved people fleeing their Southern masters (photograph © the author).

of Sterling's extensive abolitionist circles. Bessie's parents were among the many liberal Bostonians who espoused abolitionism as well as women's suffrage, and who socialized with like-minded reformers. If they met thanks to progressive politics, Susan and Bessie bonded because of shared values and experiences. Both Susan and Bessie were beloved daughters, adored and supported by their respective families. Both had suffered familial losses in the past two years of wartime—Susan's father had died, while Bessie's first cousin, Colonel Robert Gould Shaw, had been killed while leading the all-black 54th Regiment into battle. Both Susan and Bessie were eloquent, studious, and well-read. Both were curious and talented.

And both were deemed attractive by their peers and admirers, who consistently described them with words like "feminine" and "womanly."

Lilian Freeman Clarke, a Bostonian who became close friends with the two young women, observed that it was not so much their similarities as their differences that made the companions most interesting. "Bessie Greene, this nearest and dearest friend, was as rare a character as Susan Dimock, but there was a strong contrast between them," noted Clarke. She saw Susan Dimock as "timid, silent, and full of reserved force—a deep well full of inexhaustible treasure." Bessie, however, was "all sunshine and brilliancy—a sparkling, flashing fountain, scattering the jewels of her rare mind with generous profusion."[35]

Bessie came by her beauty, brains, talent, and *joie de vivre* quite naturally. Her mother, Anna Blake Shaw, was related by birth and marriage to a multitude of Bostonians who considered themselves the "Brahmin elite," from the Shaws and Parkmans to the Willards, Howlands, and Greenes. Remembered as one of nineteenth-century Boston's most admired beauties, she was painted, drawn, and engraved by the city's most talented artists. Anna was also desired by many admiring men, most notably by her neighbor Theodore Parker—a powerhouse among Boston's abolitionist Unitarian preachers—who jeopardized his own marriage and created quite a scandal through his obsession with Anna.[36] Bessie's father, William Batchelder Greene, was as handsome as his wife was beautiful. His contemporaries described him as being an imposing figure, six feet tall, with black, penetrating eyes. One chronicler noted, "he was the center of attention in any group in which he took part, often accompanied by his wife, Anna, … a woman as fair as he was dark, nearly as tall as he and quite as distinguished in appearance."[37]

As with many in his progressive circle, William Batchelder Greene had been a Unitarian minister—in his case, in West Brookfield, Massachusetts, where daughter Bessie was born in 1846. Like his contemporaries, he enlisted in the Union army when the war erupted in 1861, serving as colonel of the 14th Massachusetts Infantry and the 1st Massachusetts Heavy Artillery. Not unlike other Unitarian ministers of his era, Colonel Greene espoused a number of classic liberal views. He lived briefly with the utopian community at Brook Farm, befriended Transcendentalists like Elizabeth Palmer Peabody and Ralph Waldo Emerson, championed socialism and labor unions, and advocated for both "woman suffrage" and the abolition of slavery. Greene was also an avowed anarchist and free-market libertarian who wrote and published profusely, including his treatises on Mutual Banking, an interest-free banking system.

It's well known that some of Boston's Brahmin families made their fortunes either directly or indirectly through the colonial-era slave trade or the fruits of nineteenth-century Southern slave labor. The mill owners of Lowell, Massachusetts, for example, were prominent among those who depended on Southern cotton to produce Northern textiles. Massachusetts Senator Charles Sumner, an ardent abolitionist and powerful orator, was among those who vehemently decried the "unholy union ... between the cotton planters and fleshmongers of Louisiana and Mississippi and the cotton spinners and traffickers of New England—between the lords of the lash and the lords of the loom."

Apart from a couple of distant in-laws, the Greene-Shaws seem to have avoided direct connections to the "peculiar institution."[38] More importantly, Bessie Greene's abolitionist parents were happy to share their extended families' vast holdings with liberal causes, institutions, and individuals. One of their friends, and the recipient of significant Shaw family funds, was Dr. Marie Zakrzewska. An abolitionist and suffragist herself, Dr. Zak was the founder of the New England Hospital for Women and Children in Boston, the first hospital in New England to be run by women and for women. Because of her unique mission and her espousal of such "radical" causes, Dr. Zak and her hospital had gained support from "a host of liberal social activists who called the Boston area home," ranging from William Lloyd Garrison and Theodore Parker to Lucy Stone and Julia Ward Howe.[39]

This last piece in a complex jigsaw puzzle of relationships turned out to be the capstone of Susan Dimock's northern excursion. Because Bessie Greene, once learning of her new companion's desire to become a physician, swiftly drew on her parents' close connection to Dr. Zakrzewska. "Miss Greene herself, a highly accomplished young girl, fond of deep and serious study, sympathized with the feelings of her new friend, and aided her to procure medical books to continue her favorite study," remembered one of the New England Hospital's benefactors, Ednah Dow Cheney. "Dr. Zakrzewska furnished to Miss Greene a list of medical books, which she procured and sent to her friend [Susan]."[40]

With that fortuitous link, and a stack of anatomy and physiology books in hand, Susan Dimock began the next phase of her life journey.

Three women shaped Susan Dimock's life over the next few years: Mary Malvina Dimock, Bessie Greene, and Dr. Marie Zakrzewska. The first of these women offered her a solid foundation, the second accompanied and supported her in her journey, and the third helped her launch a viable career.

Susan's mother, Mary Malvina Owens Dimock, was forty-two years old when the family fled from North Carolina to the Commonwealth of Massachusetts. In order to provide her extended family some stability, Mary Malvina found a more permanent home for them in Hopkinton, thirty miles southeast of Sterling. (Many also know Hopkinton as being 26.2 miles west of Boston, since it has been the starting point of the Boston Marathon since 1924.) Like Sterling, Hopkinton was another quintessential New England town with a town common, white-spired clapboard churches, and a scattering of old farmlands. Unlike Sterling, Hopkinton included the highest point in Middlesex County and a generally more "mountainous" terrain. "The land is hilly and rocky but well watered, the sources of branches of the Charles, Concord and Blackstone [rivers] being found there," recalled a local resident. In addition to rivers, three large ponds graced the area, as well as the famed Mineral Springs and Hotel. For many years, this fashionable resort, which advertised their springs' "magical healing powers," had attracted hordes of Bostonians and out-of-state dignitaries, who rumbled into town in handsome four-horse stagecoaches.[41]

By the time the Dimocks arrived in 1865, that popular resort was gone, lost to a devastating fire. More significantly, when the Dimocks came to town, Hopkinton was fully immersed in something Susan and her family had never experienced first-hand: the Industrial Revolution. Thanks to a new era of American innovation and mechanization, as well as a groundswell of Irish immigration, Hopkinton was a well-established and vibrant factory town. And though the 1865 census listed a wide variety of occupations among its 4,400 citizens—from harness- and carriage-makers, teamsters, and tailors to schoolteachers, saloon keepers, and plumbers—Hopkinton's biggest and richest employers were factory owners specializing in the fabrication of boots and shoes.[42]

Hearing that the town's population had nearly doubled in the previous decade and realizing that a veritable army of Irish bootmakers and traveling shoe salesmen would therefore be in constant need of lodging, Mary Malvina Dimock returned to a profession and source of income she knew well: that of hotel keeper. She located a lovely Greek Revival hotel at 112 Main Street that could accommodate her Washington family—including Ellen and Lewis Dimmock, the two African American teenagers in their party—as well as 35-year old, Irish-born bootmaker Michael Ragan, his wife Catherine, and their four small children.[43] Curiously, Mr. Ragan was the only individual in Dimock's boarding house registered to vote, since women, African Americans, and teenagers were all denied suffrage rights. Constructed around 1830 and surrounded by a flurry of small gable-end cottages, Mrs. Dimock's new hotel was visually striking: three-and-a-half stories tall, built of clapboard and brick, its façade

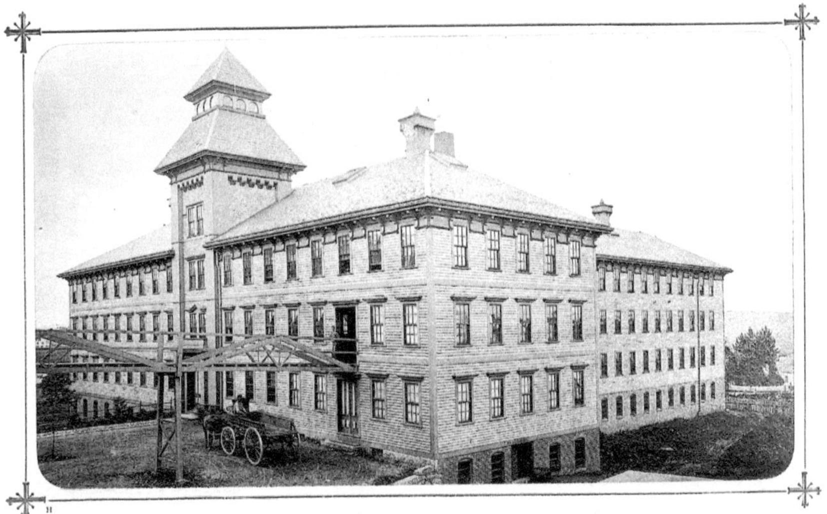

Hopkinton's biggest and richest employers were factory owners specializing in the fabrication of boots and shoes. Realizing that a veritable army of Irish bootmakers and traveling shoe salesmen would be in constant need of lodging, Mary Malvina Dimock returned to a profession and source of income she knew well: that of hotel keeper (D.T. Bridges Boot Factory circa 1880, used by permission of the Hopkinton Public Library, Hopkinton, Massachusetts).

featured an impressively broad central entry with a four-column Doric colonnade. Set on the central turnpike from Boston to Hartford, and just east of Wood Street, a popular route for those connected to the town's prosperous shoe and boot trade, the hotel was ideally located to attract transient as well as long-term lodgers.[44]

With her daughter now eighteen years old, Mrs. Dimock approved of Susan's decision to help with family finances by teaching at, rather than attending, one of Hopkinton's district schools. Susan Dimock never graduated from any high school. But in small-town, mid–nineteenth-century America, intelligence and the willingness to educate local children in morality, geography, and "The Three Rs"—reading, 'riting, and 'rithmetic—were deemed far more important, and more realistic, than requiring candidates to have a high school diploma, a Normal School (teachers' college) degree, or vast educational experience.[45] Moreover, public schools were always in need of unmarried young women to take up teaching, since women were forced to resign once they wed.

Each day on her way to district school, Susan undoubtedly passed some of Hopkinton's most distinctive buildings. Walking along downtown's

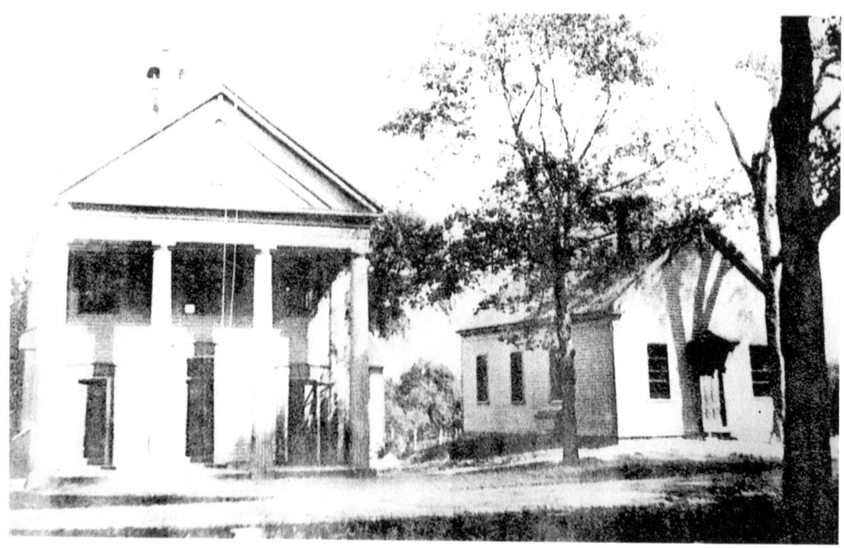

With her daughter now eighteen years old, Mrs. Dimock approved of Susan's decision to help with family finances by teaching at, rather than attending, one of Hopkinton's district schools (Hopkinton Primary School on Ash Street circa 1905, used by permission of the Hopkinton Public Library, Hopkinton, Massachusetts).

unpaved dirt roads, many lined with whitewashed picket fences and rows of shade trees, she may have marveled at the imposing four-story brick Central Coffee House, with its two-level front porch and ornate cupola, or the ancient-looking fortress called the Stone Tavern, owned by the Valentines, one of the town's richest families. Susan probably heard that the rustic Tavern, built in 1745, had been yet another stop on the seemingly ubiquitous Underground Railroad. There were several fine houses of worship, like the steepled, white clapboard Congregational Church or the Roman Catholic St. Malachi's, clearly built to accommodate the ever-growing Irish population. Both near the large central park and farther out from town center were the mammoth "boot manufactories" for which Hopkinton had become well known. The cacophony of sounds Susan experienced in these walks was surely a combination of barking dogs, resonant church bells, creaking carriage wheels, the rhythmic staccato of horses' hooves, and the taps, bangs, and whirs drifting from the windows of the bustling boot shops. Equally eclectic were the scents she encountered each day, mixing fresh-brewed coffee with the musky odor of leather, and the earthy smells of horse manure on dampened dirt roadways with the fragrant flowers and bushes lining the periphery of those very same streets.

Scattered about Hopkinton's boot factories were modest bungalows punctuated by premium lots where wealthy landowners and industrialists had built grand residences in the Federal or Greek Revival styles.[46] One of those homes—a splendid Greek Revival dwelling at 25 Main Street, with four imposing, fluted, Ionic columns gracing its portico—belonged to a wealthy landowner named Jefferson Pratt. Though the sixty-two-year-old Pratt was married to Harriet, eldest daughter of the well-to-do Joseph and Fanny Valentine, it was not Pratt's great wealth, impressive home, extensive landholdings, or celebrated relatives that most interested Susan Dimock. Pratt was also the local physician, and quickly became Susan's newest medical mentor. Born and educated in western Massachusetts, where he attended Berkshire Medical College, he had been practicing medicine in Hopkinton since 1827. Like Susan's mother, Dr. Pratt and his wife ran a household packed with members of their immediate and extended families as well as apparent lodgers. Unlike the Dimocks, the Pratts also had two Irish servants, Bridget Sullivan and Patrick Fitzgibbons.[47]

So while Susan's dear friend Bessie Greene was delivering books from Boston, culled from the list compiled by Dr. Marie Zakrzewska at the New England Hospital for Women and Children, Susan was studying those advanced medical texts under the supervision and guidance of her new friend, Dr. Jefferson Pratt.

Susan was thus willing—at least for a while—to balance teaching young Hopkinton students with being something of a student herself.

Bessie Greene, the second woman who helped Susan develop and grow in her new Massachusetts home, not only became Susan's closest companion, beloved confidante, and entrée to Dr. Zak and her woman-run hospital. She may also have been Susan's partner in what became known as a Boston Marriage.

It's long been argued that in the early nineteenth century, many middle- and upper-class American women were caught in a value system known as the Cult of True Womanhood, which delineated "the fairer sex's" Four Cardinal Virtues as piety, purity, submissiveness, and domesticity. The popular corollary was the notion that while females were rightfully confined to the "domestic sphere," the rough-and-tumble, money-making, political, and infinitely more exciting "public sphere" was a world reserved solely for men. Alfred Lord Tennyson, in his 1847 narrative poem, "The Princess," depicted this world view succinctly:

> *Man for the field and woman for the hearth:*
> *Man for the sword and for the needle she:*
> *Man with the head and woman with the heart:*
> *Man to command and woman to obey;*
> *All else confusion.*[48]

In the decades leading up to and through the Civil War, however, many women near vibrant urban centers like Boston "strayed" from their homes and their assigned spheres by joining abolitionist, temperance, and soldiers' aid groups in a quest for social improvement. These early ventures proved to be training fields for women's independence in the post-war years. Having pierced the public sphere—or, in some scholars' views, having begun to create their own "female public sphere"—and having found they were functioning there quite well, numerous middle- and upper-class women began actively pursuing careers and becoming increasingly self-supporting. As more and more women stepped outside the hearth and home, Boston in particular became a hotbed of independent female activity and enterprises led by women who defied social norms and sexual stereotypes. During this vibrant era, decades before American women had even won the right to vote in federal elections, Boston women created a world-class museum, a women's hospital, and a world religion. They also established schools, settlement houses, journals, clubs, associations, and businesses for women. Supportive men joined in the movement, creating opportunities for their "sisters" and encouraging them in new roles.[49]

The results did not go unnoticed. In the 1881 edition of Justin Winsor's classic four-volume *Memorial History of Boston*, a chapter dedicated to the status of contemporary women opened, "When an English gentleman was asked what seemed to him the most remarkable thing in Boston, he promptly answered, 'The Women!'"[50]

Granted, not everyone was impressed with these emboldened and seemingly "improper ladies." But despite the inevitable onslaught of disapproval, undermining tactics, and verbal attacks—including being called "manly" and "unsexed" by hostile men and women alike—they persisted. Some, like Louisa May Alcott (*Little Women*, 1868), became best-selling authors and remained adamantly unmarried. Others, like the widowed philanthropist and activist, Ednah Dow Cheney, used inherited family wealth to support progressive women's institutions and feminist causes. Some of these women married. Suffragist Lucy Stone, for example, wed the politically progressive and supportive Henry Blackwell. The duo used their Boston-based *Woman's Journal* to fight for "woman suffrage," women's enterprises, and equal rights. Stone *did* draw the line at taking her husband's last name, inspiring a bevy of like-minded women to follow suit and earn the moniker of "Lucy Stoners."

A certain subset of these ambitious women, however, decided that professional careers and conventional marriage were utterly incompatible. And a number of them chose to live, travel, and socialize with a member of the same sex in what came to be called the Boston Marriage, a term associated with Henry James' novel, *The Bostonians*.[51] Though some scholars have suggested that Boston Marriages were lesbian relationships—or nineteenth-century precursors to modern lesbian relationships—that's an unsubstantiated claim. Some undoubtedly were; some clearly were not. Between those two extremes lay a broad spectrum of experiences and reasons why two financially independent women would decide to share their lives.[52]

Susan and Bessie were acknowledged and loved by their contemporaries as constant companions and mutually adoring friends. "Women lived, worked, and traveled together at a time when emotional attachments between women did not evoke suspicion of a lesbian relationship," explained author Arleen Marcia Tuchman in *Science Has No Sex: The Life of Marie Zakrzewska, M.D.* "Quite the contrary,...," Tuchman continued, "nineteenth century women, whether single or married, young or old, frequently sustained loving, caring, and even romantic relationships with one another throughout their lives."[53] Moreover, "lesbianism" was neither in the lexicon of the English language, nor even a commonly held notion during their lifetime.

The question remains: Were Susan Dimock and Bessie Greene romantic friends or were they in a committed Boston Marriage, as suggested by many secondary sources today? It's well chronicled that from the time the two met in their late teens until the end of their lives, each was clearly the most significant individual in the other's life. When they traveled together, they happily shared a room and, most likely, a bed. And though both were considered exceptionally attractive and charismatic by their peers, neither is known to have had any romantic relationships with men or to have considered fitting conventional marriage into their adult lives and careers.[54]

Though no letters between them are known to exist today, there are clues to their relationship in the writings of several of their contemporaries. Some of their close friends—and, as a result, multiple twentieth-century scholars—compared Susan and Bessie to David and Jonathan, Biblical characters whose intimate bond was chronicled in Samuel 1 and 2 of the Hebrew Bible. In a memorial volume printed shortly after Susan's and Bessie's deaths, commentaries from the two women's peers repeatedly reference the David and Jonathan analogy. A 1937 article about Dimock, written by Pauline Worthy in the Raleigh *News & Observer,* observed that "Susan had never really had an intimate friend before.... She and Elizabeth [Bessie] were greatly attracted to each other and in time there developed between them a David and Jonathan friendship."[55]

The David in question was the heroic figure of both David and Goliath and King David fame. Jonathan was son of the King of Israel, and David's rival for the crown. Despite this confrontational situation, the Book of Samuel tells us, the two young soldiers were united by their common hatred of the Philistines and soon became drawn to one another. Then it got intense. The young men's unusual mutual affection included making a covenant together ("the soul of Jonathan was knit to the soul of David"), finding grace in one another's eyes, kissing one another, and even stripping off a robe to wrap around the other. Jonathan's father expressed anger that his son had "chosen" David, "which is a disgrace to yourself and the nakedness of your mother." Though both men married women and sired children, David went into deep mourning when Jonathan died, exclaiming, "Thy love to me was wonderful, passing the love of women."[56]

As might be expected, there have been dueling historic interpretations of this Biblical relationship. Were David and Jonathan—and by way of this comparison, Susan and Bessie—friends, lovers, or something in between? Traditional and Christian writers have insisted that the Biblical duo had a platonic relationship and were merely engaging in male bonding and homosociality. Contradictory modern accounts have argued that David and Jonathan shared romantic love and a homoerotic connection, whether physically consummated or not.[57] Even in the nineteenth century, the David and Jonathan story was sometimes used as a coded reference to homosexual relationships, given that same-sex connections between males were condemned or forbidden. In 1895, for example, British playwright and novelist Oscar Wilde referenced David and Jonathan and "the love that dare not speak its name" while under trial for the "gross indecency" of homosexuality.[58]

Predictably, the same vagaries apply to Susan Dimock and Bessie Greene. There is no written evidence that Susan and Bessie were lovers, and there is no written evidence that they were not. Over the years, the two friends socialized and worked with women in Boston Marriages, women in conventional heterosexual marriages, and women who chose to remain single. And though Susan and Bessie were clearly each other's most significant other, and did eventually work and travel together, they never actually lived in the same residence.[59] Ednah Dow Cheney observed of Susan that "very few claimed intimacy with her," adding, "Although genial and attractive on the surface, her nature was very reticent and reserved; and 'She still kept something to herself, She did not tell to any.'"[60]

It was Bessie Greene who introduced her companion to the third woman who had a profound influence on the development of teenage Susan Dimock's life, Dr. Marie Zakrzewska.

"In 1864, Miss Elizabeth Greene called upon me, requesting me to give her a list of books on anatomy and physiology for a friend of hers, who had come from the South to Oakdale, Mass.," recalled Dr. Zakrzewska, founder and attending physician of the New England Hospital for Women and Children in Boston. "She gave me the name of her young friend, Susan

Dimock, and said she was but sixteen years of age."[61] Realizing that reading medical books would not be enough to long satisfy Susan's intense curiosity and drive, Bessie eventually took her ideas for Susan's future—and her family connections—a step further. "By Miss Greene's advice and aid," explained Ednah Dow Cheney, "Miss Dimock applied to the New England Hospital for Women and Children, for admission as a student...."[62]

At the time of her application, Susan was teaching school in Hopkinton and studying those recommended medical texts under the direction of Dr. Jefferson Pratt. Susan's mother, Mary Malvina, had long thought that teaching might be a realistic and practical profession for her daughter—one that a nineteenth-century woman could pursue without societal disapproval. She had never agreed with Susan's late father, who famously declared, "Sue says she wants to study medicine, and I tell her she may." For many years, Mary Malvina had clearly accepted the prevailing notion that only men could pursue careers as physicians and surgeons. After Susan had taught school for a single term, however, her mother, "becoming convinced of her entire devotion to her medical pursuits," approved her daughter's application to study medicine at Dr. Zak's hospital, "and ever after gave her all the assistance in her power."[63]

Early in January 1866, following the end of her school semester in Hopkinton, Susan Dimock's application to study at the New England Hospital was accepted. And an exciting new chapter of her life began.

When Dr. Marie Elizabeth Zakrzewska (zak-SHEF'-ska) welcomed Susan Dimock into her New England Hospital for Women and Children, the hospital was not yet four years old. Dr. Zak, as her colleagues called her, was thirty-six at the time. Years later, Dr. Zak remembered the event well. "In the year 1866, Miss Susan Dimock called upon me to make application to enter the New England Hospital as a student. She was then nearly nineteen years old, and had been studying, entirely by herself, anatomy and physiology, to such an extent as to be thoroughly well informed on these subjects." Dr. Zak decided to admit her immediately despite the fact that young Susan had not so much as attended college—let alone graduated from such an institution. She was impressed, as she recalled, by Susan's "quiet determination to carry out her aims, and her decided taste for study...."[64]

"Quiet determination" was something that Marie Zakrzewska knew well. It had, in fact, been the guiding principle of her own life. Descended from Polish nobility, her grandparents had fled the Russian Tsar and settled in the nearby, and much safer, German States. Marie was born in

Berlin in 1829, with four sisters and one brother eventually to follow. Her father, Martin Ludwig Zakrzewski (the male spelling of the name), was a Prussian army officer, a civil servant, and a freethinker who stirred his daughter's independent nature and willful spirit. Marie's early interest in medicine, however, came from the maternal side of the family. Her grandmother was a veterinary surgeon and her mother, Caroline Fredericke Wilhelmina Urban, worked as a midwife. Even as a child, Marie was fascinated by her mother's mission and by the concept of healing in general.

Both in Europe and the United States, midwifery was considered outside—and inferior to—the overwhelmingly male field of professional medicine. Realizing that midwifery was the only somewhat comparable career open to women, Marie applied to the Royal Charité Hospital in Ber-

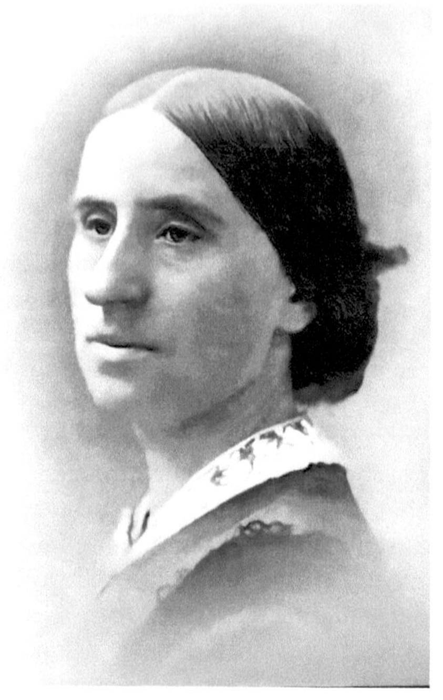

Dr. Marie Zakrzewska (1829–1902), of Polish ancestry and German birth, assisted the Blackwell sisters in setting up their infirmary for women in New York City before establishing her own hospital for women and children in Boston in 1862 (used by permission of the Dimock Center, Roxbury, Massachusetts).

lin to pursue formal studies. Turned away three years in a row because of her youth, she was finally admitted at age twenty. Bright, determined, and driven, she graduated with honors and was made chief midwife at the hospital in 1852 at the age of twenty-two. Her success, however, was short-lived. When her mentor and advocate, Dr. Joseph Hermann Schmidt, died on the day of Marie's confirmation as chief, Marie knew that her career had come to an abrupt end. It was clear that others at the Charité deemed her age too young and her gender inappropriate. These, she soon learned, were deeply engrained biases that scores of other young women, including Susan Dimock, would experience for generations thereafter.

Frustrated by Old World restrictions, Marie turned her sights on the United States. She recalled that the revered Dr. Schmidt had once told her, "In America, women will now become physicians, like the men; this shows that only in a republic can it be proved that science has no sex."[65] Inspired by that idea, Marie and her younger sister Anna emigrated to the United States in 1853, settled in New York City, and began a small embroidery business to make ends meet. It was not long before her deep interest in medicine drew Marie to sisters Elizabeth and Emily Blackwell. The Blackwells were pioneering female doctors whom she eventually assisted in setting up and operating the New York Infirmary for Women and Children, the first hospital in the nation both run and staffed by women. Impressed with Marie's intellect and drive, the Blackwells offered the young German immigrant two opportunities that would eventually change her life—and, more than a decade later, the life of Susan Dimock as well.

Although established American medical schools generally refused to admit women students, a few very determined females had gotten special dispensation to attend classes in select colleges. Inspired by that back-door approach, Elizabeth Blackwell arranged for Marie Zakrzewska to matriculate at Cleveland Medical College (now Western Reserve). Though the clever, hard-working Marie was still struggling with the English language, she graduated with honors in 1856. The male students were so upset by her presence that the college immediately slammed the door shut on any other females for the foreseeable future. Marie's father was equally unsupportive, lamenting in a letter from Berlin, "If you were a young man, I could not find words ... to express my satisfaction and pride in respect to your [medical career] ... but you are a woman, a weak woman; and all that I can do for you is to grieve and to weep. O my daughter! return from this unhappy path."[66]

The second opportunity the Blackwells gave Marie was a trip to Boston, ostensibly to fundraise for their New York Infirmary. Once in eastern Massachusetts, Marie encountered and impressed some of greater Boston's wealthiest and most progressive figures, many of whom shared her passion for liberal causes. They soon discovered that Marie was not only a fellow abolitionist, but also an ardent advocate for women's rights who had simply chosen the field of professional medicine as her primary battlefield. Among those who became Marie Zakrzewska's lifelong friends and supporters were social reformers like Ralph Waldo Emerson, William Lloyd Garrison, Theodore Parker, and Samuel E. Sewall.[67] As an added bonus, Marie's fundraising visit to the Sewall homestead inspired the family's 19-year-old daughter Lucy to pursue a career in medicine. Over the following decade, Lucy Sewall would study under Dr. Zak, earn a medical degree, work alongside Dr. Zak in an innovative Boston hospital, and take that hospital's newest student, Susan Dimock, under her wing.[68] Lucy's father, Samuel E. Sewall, was himself impressed by Dr. Zak. He was an abolitionist lawyer active with the Underground Railroad who became a lifelong friend and source of both financial and legal aid for her medical projects.

Word of Dr. Zak's presence in Boston spread rapidly around the city. One especially fortuitous connection ensued when Boston native Dr. Harriot K. Hunt—credited as the first American woman to practice medicine professionally—sent Dr. Zak to visit the recently widowed Ednah Dow Cheney. Like the Sewall clan, Cheney soon became a convert to the Zakrzewska cause. "The first thing that awoke me to the claims of duty outside of my own house was a visit from Dr. Zakrzewska, who was then in Boston on a mission to raise funds for the New York Infirmary," explained Cheney. "It seemed impossible to enter into her earnest, enthusiastic views at the time," observed Cheney of Dr. Zak, "but she would not let me rest in the indolence and selfishness of grief, but impressed me with her own noble and unselfish character. ... I must give my testimony to her large genius, and still larger heart."[69]

Ednah Dow Cheney was clearly captivated—and, like the Sewalls, spent the rest of her life supporting Marie Zakrzewska's medical ventures in tandem with her other feminist missions.

Numerous liberal Bostonians developed such an admiration for Marie Zakrzewska that in 1859 they encouraged her to move from New York to Boston, where she was offered a job as Professor of Obstetrics and Diseases of Women and Children at the New England Female Medical College. Founded by Samuel Gregory in 1848 as the Boston Female Medical School, the New England Female Medical College was originally formed to teach women to become midwives and instruct mothers on how to care for their children. A program was later added to train women for careers as physicians. Though she took the job, Dr. Zak soon became frustrated with the mediocrity of the school's medical education. She was dissatisfied with the college's inability to give its students adequate clinical experience—a failing quite common in all-male American medical schools as well—and objected to Samuel Gregory's insistence on calling his graduates "Doctress" rather than "Doctor." Dr. Zak was especially incensed at Gregory's resolve to graduate *all* his women students, rather than just those who excelled at their studies and passed their exams.[70]

Arguments between doctors Zak and Gregory led to a fallout, partly caused by Marie Zakrewska's sometimes aggressive and combative demeanor. Ednah Dow Cheney acknowledged that her friend Dr. Zak was "of quick, impatient temper, and brusque manners, somewhat characteristic of her country [Prussia/Germany]." The result, in Cheney's view, was that Dr. Zak "sometimes gave offence."[71] But part was simply due to the good doctor's desire for excellence. Mediocrity was something that Marie Zakrzewska despised. Like her future student Susan Dimock, she realized that women doctors would not be taken seriously in what was considered a "manly" profession unless they were as qualified as, if not *more* qualified than, their male peers.

In an effort to practice and teach the best medicine possible, Marie Zakrzewska decided to leave Samuel Gregory's school and to open her own women's hospital in Boston. Unlike Dr. Gregory, Dr. Zak did not attempt to create a medical college. Instead, she envisioned a working hospital that offered a hands-on post-graduate program for physicians as well as a nurses' training school. There, she would be able to teach practical as well as theoretical skills to her female students and even introduce scientific instruments like microscopes and thermometers into the curriculum— something that Dr. Gregory had resisted. There she could prove her professionalism in mainstream ("allopathic") medicine, while distancing herself from those increasingly disparaged purveyors of "irregular" alternative practices like homeopathy and phrenology, as well as from midwives, mesmerists, spiritual mediums, and clairvoyants. There she could also be living proof that the words "female physician" did not mean an untrained back-alley "abortionist."

It's not that Dr. Zak believed that mainstream medicine was significantly more successful in curing patients than alternative practices. It wasn't. Just a decade before Dr. Zak opened her hospital, medicine was still more a trade than a profession. In the mid–nineteenth century, America's allopathic doctors were only beginning to move away from eighteenth-century beliefs and ineffective practices, while inching toward the world of scientific medicine. Most still thought that putrid air, or "miasma," could cause disease. Many still engaged in what was known as "heroic" medicine, where the natural balance in a patient was allegedly restored by administering debilitating drugs or purging. Among the most popular purging practices were "bleeding" out evil toxins by slicing open veins, pressing warmed glass cups over open cuts until the cup filled with blood, or using hot plasters to create blisters, then methodically draining them. Doctors were frequently assisted by leeches and maggots, which they placed on patients' body parts to suck bad blood or feast on damaged flesh. Meanwhile, too much surgery remained in the bloody hands of barbers (the classic red-and-white striped barber pole symbolized red blood and white bandages). As might be expected, mainstream medical treatment of "women's diseases" was particularly primitive. Classic examples were those surgeons who inserted leeches into the vaginas of female patients to stimulate menstrual flow or to "cure" other feminine disorders (this was in stark contrast to the women/midwives who practiced "menstrual restoration" using herbs and other natural remedies).[72]

Dr. Marie Zakrzewska was personally more interested in the future of science than the medical traditions of the past. But she also realized that being accepted by, and someday even admitted to, the conservative and adamantly all-male Massachusetts Medical Society, founded in 1781, or the American Medical Association (1847) would require a firm, orthodox stance. What she thought might be her biggest hurdle—corralling enough local support for her hospital plan—turned out to be easier than she had imagined. When Dr. Zak walked out of the New England Female Medical College in 1861, she was accompanied and cheered on by many of the school's former advocates, medical allies, and financial backers, along with her coterie of liberal activists.

The result of Marie Zakrzewska's ambitious dream, the New England Hospital for Women and Children, opened its doors in a rented wooden house at 60 Pleasant Street (today's Stuart/Kneeland streets) in downtown Boston on July 1, 1862. The small but "sunny, airy" building cost $600 a year to lease and was sparsely furnished with $150 worth of items obtained second-hand from the clinic at the New England Female Medical College. Years later, board secretary Alice B. Crosby recalled fondly that "Our possessions ... were a few chairs, a few iron bedsteads and other necessary furniture, our earnest purpose, and our admirable Dr. Zakrzewska."[73]

Like many other hospitals of the era, Dr. Zak's facility was run essentially as a charity, catering primarily to the poor. As such, the New England Hospital was initially considered only a few steps above the almshouse, combining what would later be called "social work" with medical treatment. Hospitals of the mid–nineteenth century—when invasive and

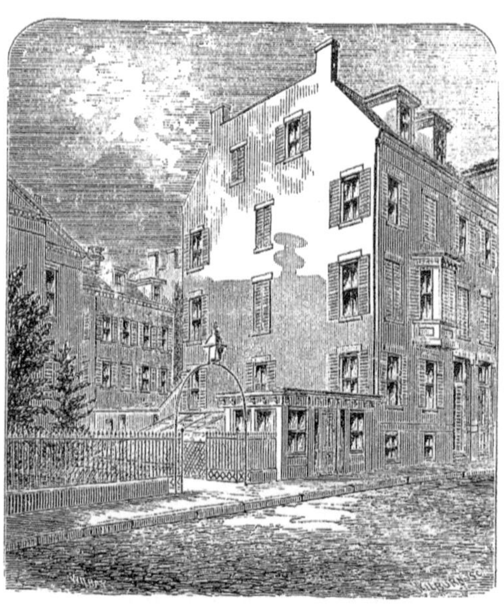

HOSPITAL BUILDING ON WARRENTON STREET

The New England Hospital for Women and Children opened its doors in a rented wooden house at 60 Pleasant Street in downtown Boston on July 1, 1862, later expanding into a nearby estate on 14 Warren Street (today's Warrenton Street) near the modern-day Charles Playhouse (used by permission of the Dimock Center, Roxbury, Massachusetts).

abdominal surgeries were quite rare—were often filled with patients suffering chronic illnesses that necessitated prolonged periods of both treatment and rehabilitation.

The New England Hospital for Women and Children was not the first or even the second medical training school for women in the United States. Samuel Gregory's Boston Female Medical College (1848) and the Female Medical College of Pennsylvania (1850) had earned those honors more than a decade earlier. Nor was Dr. Zak's New England Hospital the first medical facility in the nation run by women doctors who treated women patients. The Blackwell sisters had already done that with their New York Infirmary—ably assisted by young Marie Zakrzewska. What Dr. Zak created in Boston was the first female-run hospital and training school where women could get regular practical clinical experience instead of education gleaned primarily from lectures and books. As a result, many students from the Boston and Pennsylvania Female Medical Colleges applied to Dr. Zak's hospital following graduation, in an effort to complete and enhance their education with hands-on medical training. Dr. Zak's facility was innovative in other ways as well. It was, for example, the first hospital in Boston to offer obstetrics, gynecology, and pediatrics under one roof and the first to show no regard to race or socio-economic status of its patients.[74]

When the New England Hospital officially incorporated in March of 1863, Dr. Zak and her colleagues delineated three primary goals:

1st To provide for women medical aid of competent physicians of their own sex.
2nd To assist educated women in the practical study of medicine.
3rd To train nurses for the care of the sick.[75]

The third goal was yet another aspect of the hospital that set it apart from others of the era. Realizing that well-educated nurses were essential to the success of a hospital and the welfare of its patients, Dr. Zak inaugurated a nurses' training program in her facility. At the time, there was no way to know that one of her students—Susan Dimock from North Carolina—would eventually expand the modest program into the first professional training school for nurses in the United States.

On January 10, 1866, when Susan Dimock walked into the New England Hospital for Women and Children to begin life as a student, she was greeted by the hospital's already-iconic Marie Zakrzewska. At the time, Dimock was eighteen and Zakrzewska twice her age. Though both women sported the classic, conservative, Victorian coiffure of the day—long hair, neatly parted down the middle, then pulled back into a chignon at the nape of the neck—that's where any physical similarity ended. Dr. Zak tended to be quick, intense, and somewhat curt, with her German accent still quite pronounced. With a protuberant nose and a broad mouth, she was seen by her contemporaries as a plain, practical, no-nonsense professional. Dimock, in contrast, spoke with a gentle Southern drawl. Remembered for her quietly pretty face and gentle mannerisms, she was described by friends as "fresh and girlish" with "a certain flower-like beauty, a softness and elegance of appearance."[76] Yet the traits shared by these two determined women—intelligence, zeal, and an unflagging devotion to the science and practice of medicine—were far more important than these superficial physical differences.

Within her first few days of student work, Susan Dimock was shown how much had changed since the hospital's founding, only three-and-a-half years earlier. Most obvious was the building itself. Because the original structure at 60 Pleasant Street had proven too small and the hospital had proven of such value to the public, the facility had recently expanded into a nearby estate on 14 Warren Street, today's Warrenton Street, near the modern-day Charles Playhouse in Boston. With a larger house in front and three smaller ones opening onto Pleasant Street in the rear, there was much to celebrate—so much so that friends had just thrown the hospital a festive housewarming party that included a poetry reading by Julia Ward Howe of "Battle Hymn of the Republic" fame. Celebration was due in part because the original ten beds had now grown to forty. Moreover, the doctors and nurses acknowledged that the new, larger, intersecting buildings gave "much better opportunity for isolating the Maternity patients and more room for the Dispensary."

Isolation of female patients was vital to minimizing the scourge of nineteenth-century maternity wards, the dreaded and contagious puerperal (childbirth) fever. The enlarged Dispensary, in turn, was packed each morning with crowds of women from Boston, as well as many from outlying towns, all seeking free medical help. The hospital's secretary noted that the larger housing capacity offered yet another advantage that would help develop Susan's future medical career as a surgeon, since "here for the first time the Surgical Department became of importance."[77]

Susan found that the hospital, though still a struggling charity, was also on somewhat firmer financial footing than it had been just a few years back. When the New England Hospital opened in 1862, America's bloodiest war was raging—a reality that Susan had experienced firsthand in her hometown of Washington, North Carolina. While no Civil War battles took place on Massachusetts soil, almost 14,000 Massachusetts men eventually died in the war. Hence, an early hospital fundraising letter had to acknowledge, "True, it is in the midst of a terrible civil war, which drains our resources, that we make this appeal, but never has it been more necessary. While the soldier has been fighting our battles on distant fields, how often has his wife come pleading at our doors for that help in her hour of need...."[78] Though money was initially scarce, Dr. Zak's philanthropist friend, Ednah Dow Cheney, joined with three other women to bankroll the hospital's first year of rent. The Trustees of the Boston Lying-In Hospital Corporation, forced to close their own doors because of rampant epidemics in their maternity wards, contributed another $1,000 per year, specifically for maternity patients.

By the time Susan arrived on Warren Street in January 1866, the four-year Civil War had finally ended. It was nine months since Lee's surrender to Grant at Appomattox—and nine months since John Wilkes Booth, the brother of beloved Boston-based actor Edwin Booth, had assassinated President Abraham Lincoln. Like the nation as a whole, Boston was still reeling, balancing shock and mourning with the hope of eventual recovery. Despite this instability, Susan learned that the New England Hospital had actually gained some financial ground as hostilities waned. The Massachusetts State Legislature, for example, realized the importance of a hospital for women in such troubled times and awarded Dr. Zak's institution an impressive $5,000 grant, equal to more than $80,000 in purchasing power today. That grant was matched by a number of individual donors, spearheaded by many of Dr. Zakrzewska's loyal liberal followers like the Sewall, Garrison, Shaw, Agassiz, and Weld families, as well as other advocates for abolition, "woman suffrage," and women's rights.

Susan soon became aware that fundraising fairs—an idea borrowed from old abolitionist circles—were already surprisingly successful sources of revenue for the hospital. Equally unexpected was her delightful discovery that non-monetary gifts of all shapes and sizes were constantly flowing into the hospital's offices—from scissors, bandages, underclothes, old linens, flannel shirts, and flowers to cornstarch, tea, cooking pears, baskets of apples, and worn copies of the *Atlantic Monthly*. According to the hospital's Annual Report for 1866, the women patients of the New England Hospital appreciated those odds-and-ends gifts as much as the official Matron, who duly processed the curious daily intake. "The scent of early violets bears their thoughts away to the woods, and autumn's brilliant colors flame in their quiet chambers. The strawberry, the currant, the pear, the grape, the ruddy apple, the flowing cans of milk, are doubly welcome to the patient as the expression of loving remembrance outside their walls.... The Matron has many useful contributions to her linen press and clothes store, but she is a perpetual Oliver, always 'asking for more.'"[79]

The struggles and successes, the strengths and weaknesses, and the unfamiliar terrain of the New England Hospital proved a lot for eighteen-year-old Susan Dimock to absorb in her first few days on Warren

Street. But the best was yet to come. Because Marie Zakrzewska and Susan Dimock, the no-nonsense German and the soft-spoken Southerner, were about to get down to work.

Medical Training

For a young, impressionable pre-medical student like Susan Dimock, the days at the New England Hospital were long and the work eye-opening. Each morning, she and her fellow female students took their cues and instruction both from Dr. Zakrzewska and from Lucy Sewall, the hospital's twenty-four-year-old resident physician. The eldest daughter of liberal lawyer and New England Hospital benefactor Samuel Sewall—and the second cousin of an ambitious young local writer named Louisa May Alcott—Lucy Sewall had been inspired to pursue a career in medicine after meeting Dr. Zakrzewska at a fundraising event back in 1856. In the following years, she studied under Dr. Zak at Samuel Gregory's New England Female Medical College, then perfected her craft by interning in London and Paris hospitals. She returned to Boston during the Civil War and joined the estimated 300 American women who had successfully managed to pursue medical careers. Meanwhile, Sewall and her female colleagues were well aware that some 55,000 male physicians were practicing in the U.S. on the eve of the Civil War—and that many of these gentlemen had never actually graduated from a medical college.[1]

With smoothly pulled-back tresses and large blue eyes, the talented Dr. Sewall was yet another example of a woman who perplexed those detractors who imagined professional female doctors were invariably "manly," "unsexed," and possibly even bearded.[2] In stark contrast, Lucy Sewall was described by a student as humble, kind, and "singularly girlish in appearance ... so gentle and womanly that, until one knew her well, her reserves of strength were a source of repeated surprise."[3]

When Susan Dimock arrived in Boston, Dr. Lucy Sewall was firmly entrenched at the New England Hospital, balancing student instruction with managing the hospital and caring for patients at the Dispensary. Captivated by Sewall's demeanor and talent, Susan and the other students eagerly followed her everywhere. Susan and her handful of peers actually lived and slept at the hospital. On a typical day, they rose at 6:30 a.m., shared breakfast at 7:00, then began doing rounds through the forty-bed

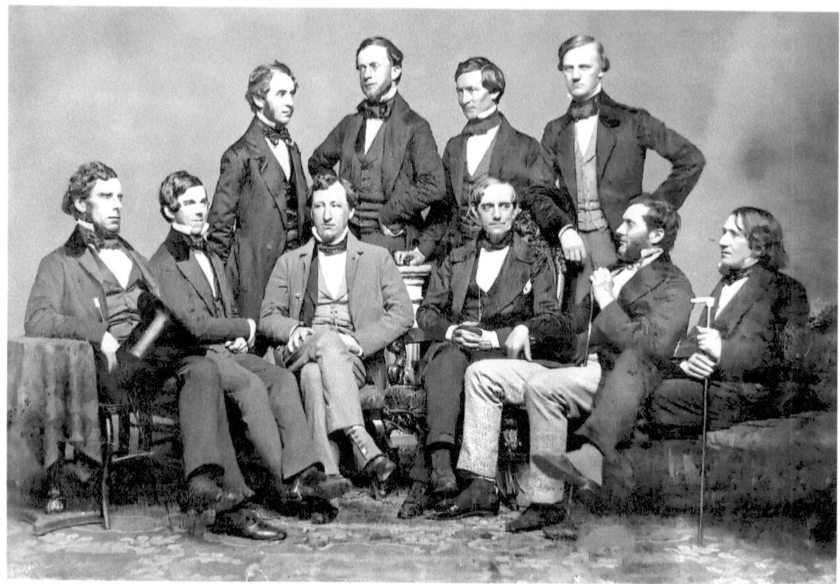

The Boston medical establishment was adamantly all-male, as shown in this 1853 photograph of the Boston Society for Medical Improvement. Countless patients attending the New England Hospital for Women and Children, however, expressed the importance of being treated by doctors of their own sex, exclaiming, "Oh, I *could not* go to a man." (Oliver Wendell Holmes and members of the Boston Society for Medical Improvement, ca 1853; image courtesy the Francis A. Countway Library of Medicine, Harvard University, Boston, Massachusetts).

hospital wards. Under the resident physician's gentle yet firm guidance, the students were then tasked with making up medicines in preparation for the opening of the Pleasant Street Dispensary at 9:00 a.m.

Over the next four hours, aided by her students and an assistant physician or nurse, Dr. Sewall met sixty or seventy patients at the hospital's free Dispensary. When not checking in patients, Susan and her comrades pulled medicines and lotions from the shelves, filling the prescriptions as fast as the doctor could write them. While some patients sought simple consultations or pickups, others required applications or surgical treatments. And if severe illness prevented some from coming to the Dispensary for medical help, Susan or other students were sent out to visit them in their homes.[4] Although nearby home visits could be done on foot, more distant locales required hopping onto one of the several horsecar and train lines that converged near modern-day Park Square. When Susan had the opportunity to accompany Dr. Zakrzewska on home visits, travel was a lot classier. Dr. Zak had recently purchased a horse and second-hand

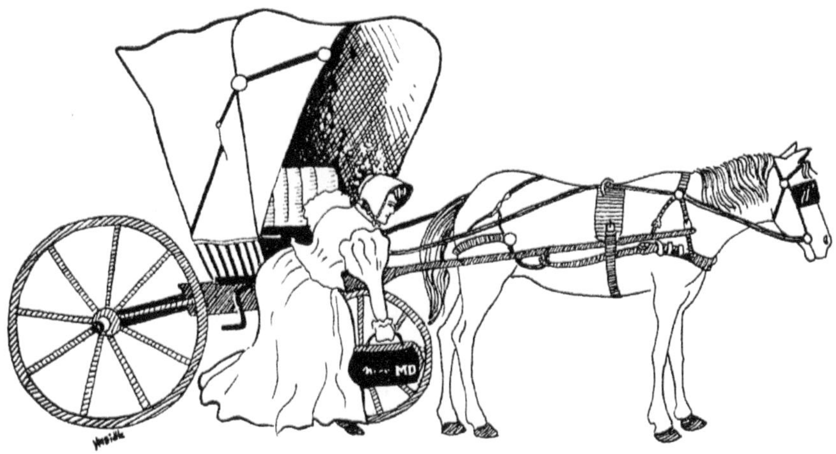

The New England Hospital's founder, Dr. Marie Zakrzewska (1829–1902) purchased a horse and second-hand buggy, partly as an efficient way to make distant medical calls and partly to appear as professional as her male peers (used by permission of the Dimock Center, Roxbury, Massachusetts).

buggy, partly as an efficient way to make distant medical calls and partly to appear as professional as her male peers.

At 1:00 p.m., following four intense hours in service of the Dispensary, Dr. Sewall and her medical apprentices broke for dinner. (In the nineteenth century, mid-day dinner was the main meal of the day, while evening "supper" was lighter fare.) As might be expected, all members of the team were generally exhausted. Still, they conversed with interest, discussing how patient after patient expressed the importance of being treated by a doctor of her own sex. "[I]n many cases of long standing and great suffering," explained Sewall, "my colleagues and I have inquired how the patient could have so long remained without treatment, and have been answered 'Oh, I *could not* go to a man,' in a tone so earnest as left no doubt that whether the feeling were wise or not, it was most undoubtedly sincere."[5]

In her 1867 Resident Physician's Report, Dr. Sewall touted the success of the hospital Dispensary. "That the benefits … are very fully appreciated by the poor is evident from the number of old patients who re-appear after absence, bringing with them friends who desire similar treatments." The official numbers confirmed her claim. During the 1867 fiscal year alone, the hospital's Dispensary had served, free of charge, an astonishing 4,576 patients and given out 16,024 prescriptions.[6]

When not at the Dispensary or visiting patients' homes, Susan was able to observe and assist with cases in the New England Hospital's medical, surgical, and lying-in (maternity) wards. As she walked from ward to ward, she invariably inhaled what was popularly known as "that good old hospital stink." Even though Dr. Zak's excellent German training had made staff aware of the medical advantages of clean surroundings, most mid–nineteenth-century hospitals had unavoidable and predictable odors. Patient rooms and hospital hallways often smelled of urine, vomit, feces, and dried blood, while surgical wards sometimes reeked of necrotic tissue, burning flesh, and a scent reminiscent of butcher shops. Coupled with everyday human body odor, the plentiful bouquets of flowers and baskets of fruit gifted by friends of the hospital were no match for the resulting olfactory assault.[7]

Though patients at the free Dispensary were from lower socioeconomic classes, those Susan met in the hospital wards were decidedly more diverse. Sometimes the maternity patients were women of wealth—a group that was heartily welcomed, since their cash payments helped offset pro-bono services for the less fortunate. During Susan's first year, one such affluent woman was sent to the hospital by a male physician who considered the case hopeless, since the woman had delivered three successive still-born children. Under Lucy Sewall's careful attendance, however, the patient gave birth to a healthy baby boy and left the hospital in joy, agreeing with her husband "that the $100 paid by her to its funds, represented but a portion of her gratitude."[8] Another young socialite arrived with sores covering her entire head. Her scalp had been shaved, causing her many days of "great pain and irritation as well as unsightliness." When she appeared in despair at the New England Hospital, she was treated by Dr. Sewall and the nursing staff with salves and ointments and, perhaps more importantly, constant attention. The socialite improved immediately, and was discharged in a month's time, "completely well" and utterly grateful.[9]

Sometimes the patients Susan encountered, especially in the lying-in wards, were women of limited means. These included a number of formerly enslaved African Americans who had recently moved from the South—and who often rejoiced as their infants were born into freedom. Having grown up in the slaveholding South—where she witnessed the "peculiar institution" firsthand and proclaimed herself an abolitionist— young Susan was undoubtedly heartened by the hospital's inclusive policies. She surely also appreciated the solidarity she found among her New England Hospital colleagues. "It is very funny to see the little black head and the fair white baby peeping out of their cribs side by side," mused Ednah Dow Cheney, the hospital's longtime volunteer secretary, adding, "Our Indian [Native American] patient was brought to us by a policeman from the Providence Railroad Station,—so that the three great races which divide the continent were represented in our wards."[10]

To suggest that Susan Dimock experienced only success during her student years at the New England Hospital would, of course, be false. On June 2, 1867, it might have been exciting to see the delivery of triplets at the hospital and read the coverage that local newspapers gave that joyous event. Joy turned to sorrow, however, when the three infants, born prematurely and exceptionally frail, "all died successively before the mother left the hospital."[11] While maternity patients like this typically spent upwards of three weeks at the New England Hospital's lying-in wards—a full week longer than at their local competitor, Boston Lying-In Hospital—patients in the medical and surgical wards were often chronic cases who sometimes stayed for months at a time.

Susan observed other disturbing cases as well. Many of the hospital's meticulously handwritten reports from the mid– to late–1860s (typewriters were not marketed until 1874) tell of women seeking help with irritated bowels, constipation, diarrhea, or intense pain in the lower back. Records indicate that rather than the "heroic surgeries" and toxic medicines often used at male-operated hospitals, the women doctors' treatments frequently consisted of administering botanical or mineral blends such as chamomile tea, castor oil, Rochelle Salt, zinc oxide, and bismuth nitrate, supplemented by beef tea, nourishing foods, hot baths, warm moistened bandages, and outdoor walks or carriage rides.[12] In the summer of 1868, one such woman was transferred from the Dispensary to the hospital ward, "having such an inflammation of the bowels that fears were entertained that she might not reach her home again alive." She was cared for immediately, and even seen by Dr. Samuel Cabot, one of a handful of well-respected, Harvard-educated, male physicians who happily consulted for the hospital free of charge. Despite that wealth of care and expertise, the medical team's efforts were in vain. "Whenever conscious," wrote Dr. Zakrzewska, "the poor woman was thanking every one around her for their kindness, and thus died, just a week after her admission."[13]

It was inevitable that Susan would bear witness to untimely deaths. Though best known for treating "diseases peculiar to women," Dr. Zak's hospital was also appreciated as one of the rare places where the terminally ill could spend their final days. During Susan's last year as a student, a dying patient arrived on the Pleasant Street doorstep. A local male physician had been treating the woman for debility "caused by blows from an insane husband," and was preparing to send her to a state institution. While that transfer was in process, the woman went into premature labor, was brought to the New England Hospital, "delivered of a sickly child," and died within a week of admission.[14] But she had done so in the comfort of compassionate private care, a fact that consoled Dr. Zak and her female colleagues.

It's likely that the medical cases Susan found most troubling as a student were those involving puerperal fever, the much feared and widely misunderstood "scourge" of nineteenth-century maternity wards. Since her early teenage years in North Carolina, where she taught herself Latin to study medical books, Susan had known that *puer* meant "boy" and *parere*, "to bring forth." Together they became *puerperium*, the period after the delivery of a baby. She also learned that lying-in hospitals and maternity wards around the world dreaded puerperal fever—also known as childbirth, childbed, and postpartum fever—which generally began a few days after delivery, then progressed rapidly, causing agonizing abdominal pain, high fever, enfeeblement, and even death. "Epidemics of puerperal fever are to women as war is to men," wrote French pediatrician and obstetrician, Jacques-François-Édouard Hervieux. "Like war, they cut down the healthiest, bravest, and most essential part of the population; like war, they strike their victims in the prime of their lives...."[15]

In the 1860s, Susan and her medical mentors could not have known that puerperal fever was caused by infection of the placental site within the uterus and that, once in the bloodstream, it became puerperal sepsis. That knowledge would come more than a decade later, with the development of germ theory. Still, there were already hints as to the nature of its deadly spread. Some physicians noted that childbed fever certainly existed during the centuries when female midwives delivered babies in women's homes. But they also observed that it had grown to epidemic proportions in the nineteenth century, as professional doctors and their hospitals expropriated the birthing process, while simultaneously denigrating midwifery.

The beloved Boston poet, Oliver Wendell Holmes, is best remembered as a columnist for the *Atlantic Monthly*, the author of "The Autocrat of the Breakfast-Table," and a member of the literary Saturday Club, whose roster included names like Longfellow, Emerson, and Hawthorne. But medical Boston knew Holmes equally well as professor of anatomy and physiology at Harvard and the author of the 1843 treatise, "On the Contagiousness of Puerperal Fever." In this seminal work, Dr. Holmes argued that his fellow physicians might be playing a part in spreading the disease as they moved, with unwashed hands and unsterilized instruments, from patient to patient—or, even worse, from diseased cadaver to the defenseless infirm. In Vienna, Dr. Ignace Semmelweis made similar arguments a few years later, insisting that those performing autopsies needed to scrub their hands in chlorinated lime before tending to maternity patients. This not only enraged obstetricians—whom Semmelweis ultimately likened to murderers—but it also ran counter to the popular disease theory that noxious fumes called "miasmas" were the cause of infections and their spread.[16]

Both Holmes and Semmelweis were ignored or ridiculed by the bulk of their medical contemporaries. As a result, puerperal fever continued to ravage maternity wards worldwide through the 1860s and even '70s. Both in 1866 and 1867, during Susan Dimock's first two student years, it spread rapidly in lying-in wards all over Boston. Susan's classmate, the English-born Sophia Jex-Blake, recalled seeing gangrenous vulvas and peritonitis in some of the afflicted patients, who were already in a "wretched state" of mental anxiety and physical suffering.[17]

Dr. Zakrzewska was among the physicians who believed hospital cleanliness and good health went hand-in-hand. Despite that commitment, the New England Hospital lost five patients during the 1867 outbreak alone. "The terribly contagious and fatal nature of this epidemic ren-

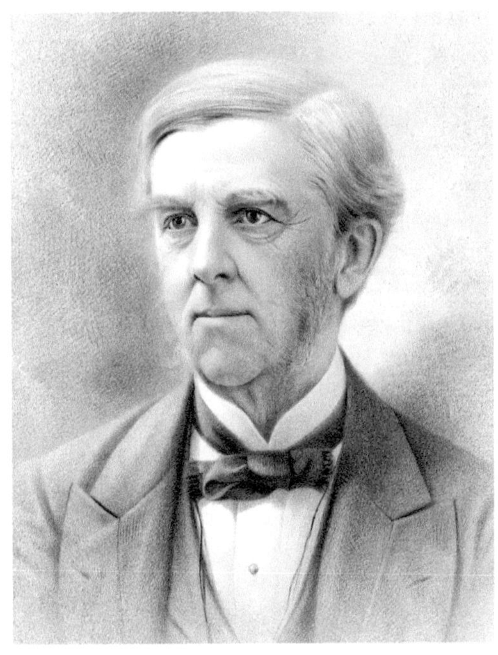

The beloved Boston poet, Oliver Wendell Holmes, Sr. (1809–1894), was also a professor of anatomy and physiology at Harvard and author of the 1843 treatise, "On the Contagiousness of Puerperal Fever," where he argued that his fellow physicians might be spreading the dread disease as they moved with unwashed hands from diseased cadaver to the defenseless infirm (Oliver Wendell Holmes, Sr, ca. 1879, by Armstrong & Company, Boston, Massachusetts; image via Wikimedia Commons).

dered it necessary to close [our] Wards for ... thorough cleansing and white-washing...," wrote Dr. Sewall in her year-end report.[18] Emma Call, yet another New England Hospital student, remembered Dr. Zak telling the directors that "it is thought that carelessness and want of thorough cleanliness is at the bottom of epidemics of puerperal fever." Still, Dr. Zak and her colleagues focused on disinfecting the rooms, without consciously disinfecting the doctors, their instruments, and the patients themselves. While these medical experts understood sanitation, they had no notion of antisepsis—using antiseptics to eliminate the microorganisms that caused disease. As a result, Dr. Zakrzewska's suggestion for a long-term solution was to decrease hospital size, increase the number of hospitals in Boston, then locate them in different parts of the city, "so that at times whole wards can be left empty for purification and thorough cleansing." As for poor women patients, she recommended that they simply remain at home during childbearing.[19]

Susan Dimock and Sophia Jex-Blake were clearly intrigued and perplexed by this ongoing conundrum—so much so that, years later, they both focused their medical school dissertations on the understanding and treatment of puerperal fever.[20]

During her two-and-a-half years studying at the New England Hospital, Susan's mission was to learn as much as possible, with the ultimate goal of applying to a first-rate medical school and earning a medical degree. As might be expected, her intense interest and exceptional drive did not go unnoticed. "Miss Dimock entered with great zeal and thoroughness into the work of the hospital," recalled Ednah Dow Cheney, "and was soon distinguished by her teachers as possessing remarkable abilities."[21] When not seeking out wisdom from female mentors like doctors Zak and Sewall, Susan looked to the handful of Harvard-educated male physicians who crossed the gender boundary and regularly consulted for the hospital—most notably, surgeon Samuel Cabot and Harvard's professor of clinical medicine, Henry Ingersoll Bowditch. "So eager for improvement was Miss Dimock," noted Cheney, "that she gladly seized every opportunity of taking the other students' work, when they wished to relinquish it from any cause; and she has often offered to take charge of a confinement case at night,—allowing the students who had charge of it to go to bed,—that she might gain experience from it."[22] In their spare time, both of the New England Hospital's notoriously over-achieving students—Susan Dimock and Sophia Jex-Blake—supplemented their hospital training by attending a "partial course" of lectures at the New England Female Medical College, located in Boston's South End.[23]

What was it that compelled Susan Dimock to join the world of professional medicine—a fellowship where women were clearly not welcomed? What propelled the young North Carolinian forward during an era when ambition and drive were deemed admirable traits for males, but unacceptable for their female counterparts? If she ever spoke about any of this to others, her thoughts were not recorded. "She still kept something to herself, She did not tell to any," observed Ednah Dow Cheney.[24] It's likely that Susan's drive was partly inspired by her mother, Mary Malvina, a hotel-keeper and teacher who was an unusually independent, self-sufficient, and strong-willed woman for the era. Susan may have been motivated to continue the medical legacy in the Dimock family itself: her grandfather, Dr. Henry Dimock, was a Maine physician who had died when Susan was only five; her cousin Helen later married John Lord, a graduate of the Bowdoin, Maine, medical school who became a practicing physician and surgeon.[25] It's possible that Susan's constant motion helped mask the pain of losing her father and her childhood home while enduring the horrors of the Civil War. It's probable that she kept replaying her late father's words, "Sue says she wants to study medicine, and I tell her she may."

Whatever the origins, Susan's relentless determination was clearly fueled by the growing legion of allies who supported, encouraged, and believed in her, from childhood through imminent adulthood. Marie Zakrzewska's first biographer, Agnes Vietor, could explain no more than this: "Susan Dimock differed from ... other students in that she had more initiative, or more self-dependence, or less fear of circumstances and convention, or some other temperamental quality."[26]

On the eve of her twentieth birthday, Susan's next major move was additional proof that she was not like the other girls. Or, at least, like precious few of them.

In the world of American medicine, Harvard Medical College was the gold standard. Founded in 1782 in the wake of America's War for Independence, it was the third medical school in the nation—but the first choice of elite New Englanders and others who were dazzled by the well-polished glow of Harvard. That glow, of course, appeared to be largely merited. Harvard's medical school was the first to introduce smallpox vaccinations in 1799, and the first to publicly demonstrate diethyl ether as a general anesthetic, in 1846. Its faculty, student body, and graduates included some of the finest minds and wealthiest families in eighteenth- and nineteenth-century medicine, including a long line of Warrens, all related to Revolutionary War hero, Joseph Warren, himself a physician.

When viewed through the lens of modern medicine, however, that glow appears far dimmer. In 1869, any man who paid the required fees could be admitted to Harvard Medical College. Only one fifth of the school's students held college degrees, and more than half could not write. Two four-month series of lectures constituted the curriculum, and there were no written exams. Classes depended almost exclusively on lectures, textbooks, and demonstrations, and students had only to pass five out of nine five-minute oral exams in order to graduate. Students in clinical subjects engaged in no patient care whatsoever, and whatever hands-on experience students were able to muster was thanks to the school's proximity to Massachusetts General Hospital.

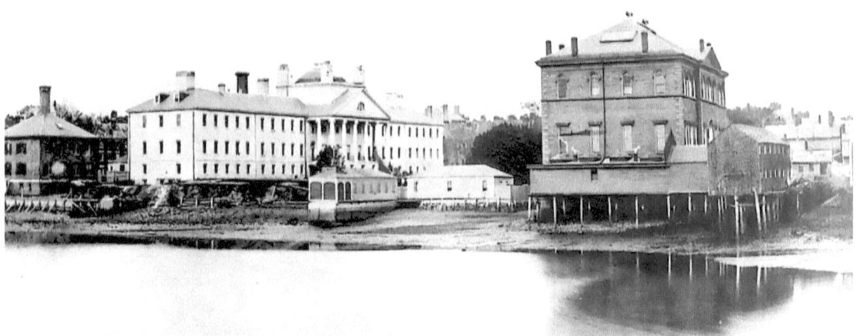

In 1866, the year Susan arrived in Boston, Harvard Medical College (right) was comfortably lodged in its fourth and newest home, on North Grove Street in Boston's West End. Directly next door, on the shores of the Charles River, was the Bulfinch Building of the Massachusetts General Hospital (left) (view of Massachusetts General Hospital and Harvard Medical School from the Charles River, ca. 1850; courtesy the Massachusetts General Hospital Archives).

Curiously, despite these flaws, Harvard Medical College was deemed superior to most American medical schools of the era. Henry Jacob Bigelow, a Harvard professor of surgery, admitted in 1871 that no successful medical school in the nation seemed willing to trade high student enrollment and high cash receipts for the dubious task of giving those students a more thorough education.[27]

Still, Harvard had that glow. And young Susan Dimock was drawn to the light.

The building that housed Harvard Medical College looked as well-groomed and prestigious as the men who worked within. In 1866, the year Susan arrived in Boston, the school was comfortably lodged in its fourth and newest home, on North Grove Street in Boston's West End. Constructed in the symmetrical Federal style, it featured classic brick walls, a hip roof topped by numerous tall chimneys, plus large double-hung palladian windows and decorative stone quoins. At the center of its perfectly balanced façade was a tall arched entrance and small front porch, accessed by matching railed staircases on the left and right. Since the school was set on the banks of the Charles River—and subject to tidal ebb and flow until the Charles was dammed in 1908—it perched on dozens of thick wooden pilings that vanished from view during high tide. The school's location, as Susan and her peers well knew, was quite deliberate, since directly next door was the Bulfinch Building of Massachusetts General Hospital. This side-by-side placement on the shores of the Charles provided an intimate physical connection that benefited both institutions. Moreover, it gave Harvard's medical students easy access to a clinical setting that the University did not have to purchase or own.

In sum, Harvard Medical College was in a perfect situation.

The problem with Harvard—at least for ambitious nineteenth-century women like Susan who wanted to earn an M.D. degree—was that it was a club built exclusively for men. It was no different from most of the nation's six-dozen-or-so existing medical schools, which were also adamantly men-only. Despite that bias, individual women had been able to able to sneak in through the back door of a handful of those single-sex medical schools by the time of the Civil War. Elizabeth Blackwell, for example, became the first American woman to earn a medical degree in 1849 when she graduated from Geneva Medical College in New York. It was Blackwell who arranged for Marie Zakrzewska to attend and graduate from Cleveland Medical College (Western Reserve) in 1856—though that school famously shut its doors to women after Dr. Zak's departure.

In 1850, women's rights advocate Harriot Kezia Hunt even briefly broke down hallowed Harvard's gender barrier. The forty-five-year-old Hunt had been practicing medicine in Boston for more than a decade, with no formal training. Finding that Hunt was both well-qualified and mature, the Harvard Medical faculty voted five-to-two to allow her to attend lectures—as long as she didn't pursue a degree. Three Black men were admitted at the same time, with the agreement that they would emigrate to Liberia once trained.[28] Harriot Hunt's much-publicized stay at Harvard Medical College was short, however, since "the faculty feared the students would leave Harvard and go to Yale upon the advent of a woman student." The students' unequivocal demand read, "*Resolved,* that we object to having the company of any female forced upon us, who is disposed to unsex herself, and to sacrifice her modesty, by appearing with men in the medical lecture room."[29]

A seemingly endless battle to matriculate and graduate from Harvard Medical College was waged by a variety of other women in subsequent years, including Doctors Lucy Sewall and Anita Tyng in 1866. Both Sewall and Tyng worked at the New England Hospital for Women and Children, Sewall as resident physician and Tyng as chief surgeon. Unlike many practicing male doctors of the era, both women had already earned medical degrees—Sewall from the New England Female Medical College in Boston and Tyng from the Female Medical College of Pennsylvania, located in Philadelphia.[30] The problem was the colleges themselves, which were the only medical schools in the nation created specifically to accommodate female students. The Boston school was the institution that Marie Zakrzewska had left in consternation because of its low standards.

The Philadelphia college lacked the excellence, the prestige, and the clout of Harvard, and—as with most male medical schools of the era—offered its students plenty of books and lectures, but no practical clinical experience. Nevertheless, Doctors Sewall and Tyng persisted in their efforts to obtain an additional, and a superior, education at Harvard. To no one's surprise, they were politely denied by the school's Dean, George Cheyne Shattuck.[31]

Undaunted, and perhaps even challenged, by these precedents, New England Hospital trainees Susan Dimock and Sophia Jex-Blake agreed in February of 1867 to follow in Sewall and Tyng's footsteps and to apply for admission into Harvard Medical College. The two envisioned themselves walking through downtown Boston along Tremont and Cambridge streets to North Grove Street, then buying tickets for their first classes. In that era, rather than pay for a semester's tuition, students purchased tickets to individual classes.

After being initially rebuffed by the Dean, the two penned a letter of intent directly to the President and Fellows of Harvard University on March 11, 1867.

> *GENTLEMEN,*
>
> *Finding it impossible to obtain elsewhere in New England a thoroughly competent medical education, we hereby request permission to enter the Harvard Medical School on the same terms and under the same conditions as other students, there being, as we understand, no university statute to the contrary.*
>
> *On applying for tickets for the course, we were informed by the Dean of the Medical Faculty that he and his coadjutors were unable to grant them to us in consequence of some previous action taken by the corporation, to whom now therefore we make request to remove any such existing disability. In full faith in the words recently spoken with reference to the University of Harvard,—"American colleges are not cloisters for the education of a few persons, but seats of learning whose hospitable doors should be always open to every seeker after knowledge"—we place our petition in your hands and subscribe ourselves,*
>
> *Your obedient servants,*
>
> *SOPHIA JEX-BLAKE.*
> *SUSAN DIMOCK.*[32]

A month later, on April 8, 1867, Sophia received Harvard's arguably predictable reply.

> *My Dear Madam,*
>
> *After consultation with the faculty of the Medical College, the corporation direct me to inform you and Miss Dimock that there is no provision for the education of women in any department of the university.*
>
> *Neither the corporation nor the faculty wish to express any opinion as to the right*

or expediency of the medical education of women, but simply to state the fact that in our school no provision for that purpose has been made, or is at present contemplated.

Very respectfully yours,

THOMAS HILL[33]

The Committee of the Faculty had voted down their request by a vote of seven to one.

The New England Hospital's two rising stars were not about to let the matter go. First, they approached the press, convincing the *Boston Daily Advertiser* to publish their correspondence, which was widely copied by a variety of newspapers and journals in the U.S. and abroad. Even Harvard's bi-weekly publication, *The Advocate,* took a jab at the university's unflinching sexism, noting, "We understand that the friends of female education have no notion of resting satisfied with their first rebuff; and that prominent Alumni of Boston are already taking measures for the prolonged agitation of the question."[34]

Emboldened by this support, Sophia Jex-Blake initiated a letter-writing campaign that systematically canvased individual Harvard

The Standing Committee of Harvard Medical College rejected the applications of Susan Dimock and Sophia Jex-Blake on the grounds that "no provision has been made, or now exists, for the education of women in any department of the University" (report, March 23, 1867, Harvard University, Corporation. Committee on Admitting Women to the Medical School, Harvard University Archives, Women Working, 1800–1930, Curiosity Collection, Harvard Library, Harvard University Archives, Creative Commons Attribution 4.0 International License).

faculty members. Among the handful of male doctors who responded in support of the women's right to attend classes was Dr. Oliver Wendell Holmes, the Parkman Professor of Anatomy and Physiology and former dean of the medical school. "I should not only be willing, but I should be much pleased, to lecture to any numbers of ladies for whom we can find accommodation in the anatomical lecture room," wrote Holmes, with the caveat, "always provided that any special subject which seemed not adapted for an audience of both sexes should be delivered to the male students alone." (Although Holmes was a towering presence in nineteenth-century Boston, he was a surprisingly small fellow: slender, with narrow shoulders, sparkling blue eyes, and a boyish face, he described himself as "five feet three inches when standing in a pair of substantial boots....")[35]

Despite their failure to gain admission to Harvard Medical College, Sophia and Susan briefly benefited from their well-publicized rejection and subsequent letter-writing campaign. In the spring of 1867, they were offered a limited amount of clinical experience at Massachusetts General Hospital and the Massachusetts Charitable Eye and Ear Infirmary. The two women were able to attend Mass Eye and Ear's popular 11:00 a.m. lectures for several weeks before being asked to leave. Pressured by the powerful Massachusetts Medical Society, then "the principal watchdog of purity of medicine in Massachusetts," Dr. Hasket Derby informed Jex-Blake in a letter dated June 1, 1867, that he and the other surgeons "cannot continue to allow female students to attend our cliniques. Ungracious as is the task, we therefore feel compelled to ask you to suspend your visits." His final sentence apologetically noted that "our intercourse with yourself and companions [has] been throughout most pleasant to us personally." In contrast, the Trustees of Mass General chose to ignore the Mass Medical Society and let individual physicians and surgeons welcome female students at their own discretion. Women had to be separated from the male students, however, and could only attend clinical practices in female wards. According to Jex-Blake's biographer, although Sophia and Susan were able to receive instruction at MGH for eight months, they "walked with a constant sense of insecurity, as one member of the staff was keenly opposed to the presence of women, and was on the look-out for causes of offence."[36]

Over the following year, the strong-willed and tenacious Sophia Jex-Blake continued to spearhead the two women's fight for admission to Harvard with what she characterized as "a sort of dull persistency."[37] The glass ceiling would not be broken in their lifetime. It would take, in fact, almost eight more decades to shatter; Harvard Medical School admitted its first female students in 1945. Meanwhile, Jex-Blake made plans to attend a new women's medical college founded by the Blackwell sisters in New York. As it turned out, that dream dissolved when her father fell ill and died, and she was compelled to return home to England. In 1869, she resumed her battles—this time in the British Isles—waging war to study medicine at the all-male University of Edinburgh. A prominent spokesperson for women's right to medical education, Jex-Blake eventually became the first practicing female doctor in Scotland and helped found medical schools for women in both London and Edinburgh.

In the aftermath of the Harvard rejections, Susan Dimock set her sights across the Atlantic as well. It was common knowledge that medical schools in nineteenth-century Europe were superior to those in the United States. As a result, many of America's most ambitious male physicians had chosen to take post-graduate courses in cities like Paris, Berlin, Zurich, and Vienna in order to learn the best in modern medicine. Knowing that Susan "showed so much real genius for the medical profession," Marie Zakrzewska and her colleagues urged their star student "to make efforts to obtain a European education, especially as her general education and knowledge of languages would facilitate her entrance into a European university."[38] In Susan's case, her goal was to attend one of the finest and most progressive medical schools on mainland Europe, at the University of Zurich. On March 17, 1868, she wrote a letter to the Dean of the Medical College there.

> *Dear Sir,*
>
> *I have heard that female students are admitted at the Medical School of Zurich, and being desirous to obtain certain particulars about such admission, apply to you.*
> *I should like to know in the first place if women, when received into the Medical School, have in all respects equal advantages with other students. How long is the course of instruction, what are the incident expenses, and what are the conditions, if any, of admission?*[39]

Susan went on to explain her lack of any college training, her two years of internship at the New England Hospital, and her desire for medical education. Seven weeks later, on May 6, 1868, Dean Anton Biermer replied from Zurich.

> *DEAR MADAM,—I reply to your letter of March 17th, which has just come to hand. I have the honor to inform you there exists in this University no lawful impediment to the matriculation of female students, and that female students enjoy equal advantages with male students.*
>
> *There is here full liberty, and every one can attend the lectures as long as he may desire. The majority of the students need from five to five and a half years' course, before taking their degree. In answer to other questions of yours, I send you some printed regulations of the University.*
>
> *I am, with great esteem, yours,*
>
> BIERMER
> Prof. and Dean of Med. Fac.[40]

After her rejection by Harvard, Susan Dimock wrote to the Medical College at the University of Zurich, wondering, "I have heard that female students are admitted at the Medical School of Zurich…. I should like to know in the first place if women, when received into the Medical School, have in all respects equal advantages with other students" (New England Hospital for Women and Children Records, Sophia Smith Collection, Smith College, Northampton, Massachusetts; used by permission of the Dimock Center, Roxbury, Massachusetts).

Susan's Boston supporters swiftly rallied behind the good news. Dr. Zakrzewska and another friend collected enough money for her to sail to Europe and begin her studies, while the Rev. James Freeman Clarke—the beloved Boston abolitionist, women's rights advocate, and New England Hospital supporter—wrote a glowing character reference. Clarke was the founder and pastor of the Church of the Disciples, whose congregation included liberal and literary luminaries like Bronson and Louisa May Alcott, Ralph Waldo Emerson, Nathaniel Hawthorne, Margaret Fuller, Julia Ward Howe, Horace Mann, and the Peabody sisters. His wife Anna Huidekoper Clarke served on the Board of the New England Hospital for several decades.

Knowing that the next step in her career was firmly established, Susan Dimock spent the four months between acceptance and setting sail for Europe determined to study German, to continue to work at the hospital, and to engage in leisure activities with her Boston friends and colleagues.

Both Susan and her classmate Sophia Jex-Blake had learned early on that Doctors Zak, Sewall, and their colleagues balanced their hard work with ample doses of hard play. "[C]an't you understand how refreshing it is to slip into the bright life of all these working people," wrote Sophia, "working hard all day, and then so ready for fun when work's over."[41]

Sometimes Susan and her friends went off on seaside excursions—refreshing jaunts that she had cherished since childhood. Sometimes that fun was had at the hospital itself, singing songs, playing "a most ridiculous game of cards called 'Muggins,'" and roaring in laughter.[42] Often it involved taking in the cultural diversions of downtown Boston, from enjoying fine ice cream or watching patrons flock into Boston's two newest restaurants—Jacob Wirth's and Marliave—to attending world-class theatrical presentations. Boston was slowly recovering from the sorrows of the Civil War and celebrating with an ever-growing roster of cultural events. Among the theatrical highlights was the triumphant return of Shakespearean actor Edwin Booth, who had gone into hiding as a precaution in the wake of his brother's assassination of President Lincoln. If not watching Booth play a brilliant "Othello" at the Boston Theatre, Susan likely attended one of novelist Charles Dickens' sold-out readings at Tremont Temple. During the winter of 1867–1868, the British superstar made his home base at Boston's Parker House while doing his second—and, as it turns out, final—reading tour of the United States. Meanwhile, Susan's love of music may have been satisfied by concerts at the Boston Conservatory of Music and the New England Conservatory of Music, both of which made their debut in 1867.

She couldn't help but have noticed the progress that women were making in Boston, both in the New England Hospital and beyond. During Susan's student years at the hospital, the Young Women's Christian Association of Boston and the New England Women's Club were established, the first woman was admitted to the M.I.T. School of Architecture, and the famed William Morris Hunt began offering art classes for women—which some felt a scandalous leap for proper ladies. Whatever the field of endeavor, all these events offered a broader concept of women's work and the women's sphere than she or her friends could ever have imagined.

During her final months in Boston, Susan and her medical peers were amused by the rumpus over the first monument erected in Boston's Public Garden. The object of controversy was a forty-foot tall, marble and granite "Ether Monument," commemorating the first public demonstration of ether anesthesia conducted at Massachusetts General Hospital in 1846. Since no one could agree on who actually deserved credit for the discovery of anesthesia—Boston dentist William Thomas Green Morton and Dr. John Collins Warren were but two of several claimants to the honor—it was finally decided to depict a generic biblical Good Samaritan rather than a specific doctor in the sculpture. Oliver Wendell Holmes, speaking as both poet and physician, mused that it should be called the "ether or either" monument, letting the viewer decide which man was actually being honored. Holmes actually had a stake in the conversation, since it was he who coined the term "anaesthesia."[43]

Many festive nights were also spent at Dr. Zakrzewska's home in Roxbury, an adjacent town annexed to the city of Boston in 1868. Dr. Zak's house had a large garden, a series of grape-vined terraces, a variety of fruit trees, and a scattering of outdoor seats and tables to accommodate her frequent guests. In the winter, she invited friends inside, and offered plentiful wine, dance, or games of chess and whist to her coterie of doctors, interns, and leading Boston radicals. Though notorious for her intense devotion to work and study, young Susan Dimock was also well-known as "among the happiest of guests, dropping all cares for the time being, in true German fashion." "When at a merry … party, she would frolic and dance with perfectly childlike enjoyment," recalled Ednah Dow Cheney. "On one such occasion she said, after dancing with great glee, 'Oh! one must be among Germans fully to enjoy one's self. Come, Doctor, one more waltz.'"[44]

The Germans in question were not only Dr. Zak, but Zak's younger sister Minna, as well as Karl Heinzen, publisher of the radical German journal *Pionier*, who lived at Dr. Zak's house along with his own wife and child. Marie Zakrzewska's eclectic "family" also included occasional invalids from the hospital, as well as the semi-invalid Julia Sprague, a leading woman reformer, a founding member of the New England Women's Club, and Dr. Zak's partner in a Boston Marriage that endured some forty years. At that time, two other frequent guests to the Zak galas—Dr. Lucy Sewall and student Sophia Jex-Blake—were also in a Boston Marriage, albeit a far shorter one. If Susan Dimock attended with her favorite companion, Bessie Greene, they must have felt right at home in this group of strong women and supportive men.[45]

By the late summer of 1868, however, what mattered most was what was about to happen next. The dismissiveness of Harvard was behind her. The welcoming embrace of the University of Zurich lay ahead. And the board of the New England Hospital capped off the joy by promising Susan the position of resident physician upon her return.

On September 7, 1868, twenty-one-year-old Susan Dimock set sail on one of the greatest voyages of her life. With months of German language study under her belt, loans from generous Boston patrons in her trunk, and the promise of full-time work in Boston following graduation, she boarded ship for medical studies in Europe.

Despite brief stops in London and Paris *en route* to Zurich, Susan was frugal with both her time and money. She paused in London to meet with Elizabeth Garrett Anderson, England's first woman doctor. Then Mary Putnam, a former student from the New England Hospital pursuing medical training in Paris, met her in the City of Light. "We urged her to spend a few days [in Paris] for the sake of the recreation to which American students usually consider themselves entitled before they settle down to their studies," Putnam recalled. But Dimock gently turned down the offer, explaining that having borrowed money to pursue her studies, she "should not feel justified in spending a cent of it for amusement or sight-seeing."[46]

As with many others who encountered Susan on her European journey, Putnam was struck by Susan's unique mixture of Yankee grit and Southern charm.[47] She found her friend "as fresh and girlish as if such qualities had never been pronounced by competent authorities to be incompatible with medical attainments." Marie Vögtlin, a fellow Zurich medical student, had a similar impression of Susan's persona when they first met: "The American is a remarkably accomplished person for her age; she seems so soft and childlike, and yet her whole manner is one of decisiveness in her thinking and acting."[48]

Zurich itself was as charming as Susan. And even though the beautiful Swiss city was more provincial than the Boston she had just departed— and had a population of only 25,000, one-tenth the size of Boston—there was a compatible sensibility in both cities. Both Boston and Zurich boasted an appealing architectural mixture of old and new. Both had a quaint combination of winding little roads and broader boulevards, many lit by oil or gas streetlamps. Both were important terminals for an ever-growing network of national railroads and shipping. In both towns, a large river was central to the town's allure, useful for transportation and recreation. Both were home to impressive new "polytechnic" schools, focusing on applied science and engineering.[49] And like Boston, the once-quiet Swiss town had become a center for banking, commercial activity, and liberal thought.

But substantially more than Boston, Zurich was also a haven for political dissidents and refugees, especially following the revolutionary uprisings of 1848 in France, Italy, Germany, and the Austrian Empire. And that, as it turned out, worked in Susan's favor.

A veritable onslaught of talented, liberal thinkers running from neighboring states benefited the University of Zurich in two significant ways. An exodus of German professors from the German States, not yet united into a single country, filled the ranks in the University, most notably in the medical faculty. "The reputation of the university grew as it provided shelter to those awaiting major appointments in Germany," observed historian Thomas Neville Bonner. As "a first-class waiting-station," Zurich's medical school in particular attracted "young scientists destined to play a commanding role in the changes overtaking medical science."[50] Many of those expatriate medical talents were soon to become Susan's professors, advisors, and mentors, including Adolf Gusserow, a noted gynecologist who served as both Susan's thesis director and president of the University of Zurich School of Medicine.

The liberalism for which the University of Zurich had become known was a reason why women like Susan—who had no paths to high quality professional medical training in their own countries—were invited to matriculate at the medical school.[51] A pivotal test case was a Russian native named Nadezhda Suslova, who was among the many women expelled from Russian universities as student radicals. Suslova was admitted as an auditor in Zurich's medical department in 1865, and by the 1866/67 winter semester was officially enrolled, eventually becoming the first woman to earn a doctorate in the German-speaking world and the first woman physician in Russia.

On the heels of Suslova came a handful of young women whose lives and aspirations intersected and overlapped during the next few years: Susan Dimock from the United States, Mariia Bokova from Russia, Frances Elizabeth Morgan and Louisa Atkins from England, Eliza Walker from Scotland, plus one local girl, Marie Vögtlin, from Switzerland. Together, this experimental female crew became known—and

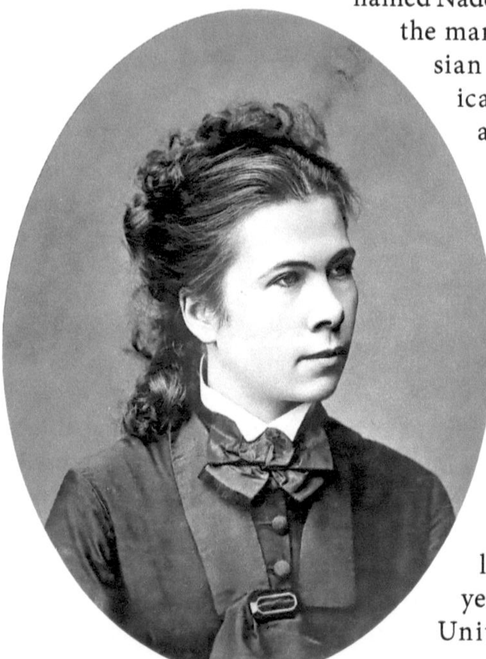

In 1867, Russian student Nadezhda Suslova (1843–1918), the first of The Zurich Seven to matriculate, was also the first to graduate. Credited as Russia's first female physician, she became a feminist legend in her homeland through her medical work, writings, and philanthropy (image via Wikimedia Commons).

internationally renowned—as "The Zurich Seven." By 1868, they were the only women out of forty-one students enrolled in the medical school.

It would be false to claim that The Zurich Seven were admitted to the University's medical school solely because of liberal thought and radical runaway professors. Part of the decision to pioneer this experiment with female students was simply financial: in the mid–nineteenth century, university education was not the highest priority for many Swiss themselves. Swiss universities discovered they could get high foreign-student fees from international students, so made the application process simple and the admission standards lower—in some cases, so low that the incoming students were too young or too poorly prepared for the task.[52] Of all The Zurich Seven, Marie Vögtlin of Switzerland had the highest bar to jump for admissions, precisely because she was Swiss.

When Susan Dimock first arrived in Zurich, she emerged from the 1847 train station—a terminus for a transit system growing so rapidly that it would be replaced by another in only a few years. As she left the station, she may not have realized that Zurich's main downtown street, the broad Bahnhofstrasse ("Train Station Street"), was only four years old and built over the old "Ditch of the Frogs."[53] Walking toward the scenic River Limmat, she was struck by the broad neoclassical Polytechnikum, sitting majestically on the hillside overlooking the river. Susan would soon learn that the uphill climb to the College of Medicine, situated in the Semper Building of the Polytechnikum, was a hefty trek that students and faculty alike simply took in stride. Boston had long ago been dubbed The City on the Hill. But Zurich was more like a city on a mountain—a mountain that would offer panoramic views of the Alps and pristine waterways as well as hours of athletic hiking for Susan and her peers when breaking from their intense medical studies.

By October 18, 1868, Susan had completed her first week of orientation—and seemed surprisingly well adjusted to all this newness. "Sunday finds me safely through with last week's herculean labors," she marveled in a letter to her mother. "You know I had a hundred formalities to go through with, and no German to speak of. Looking back upon it, I do not see how I managed it; however, it is all plain sailing now, and I have nothing to do except to listen to lectures, study hard, and learn German. &c. [sic]"[54]

Susan soon discovered that if she went through the necessary formalities and paid the fees, she had the same opportunities as her male counterparts. "And then I find also the warmth and protection and feeling of interest which a young man finds in a university," she concluded. "[I]t is delightful; the professors are all very kind to me." Most importantly, the young medical student was thrilled to finally have "what I have been

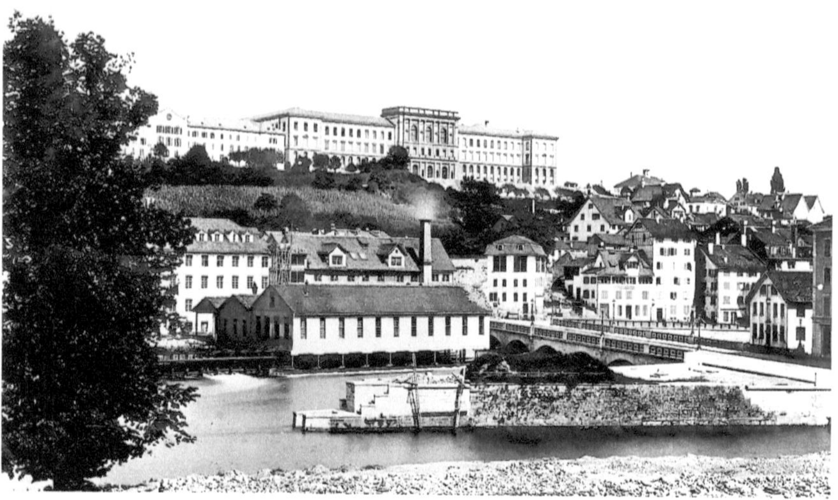

Susan soon learned that the uphill climb from the River Limmat and the Zurich railway bridge to the College of Medicine, situated in the Semper Building of the broad neoclassical Polytechnikum, was a hefty trek that students and faculty alike simply took in stride (image of the railway bridge and Polytechnikum in 1864, courtesy ETH-Bibliothek Zürich, Bildarchiv).

begging for in Boston for three years! I have every medical advantage that I can desire. I told the professor of anatomy, for instance, that I wanted a great deal of dissecting; and he immediately bowed, and said so kindly, 'You shall have it; I only desire you shall tell me what you prefer.'"[55]

Susan's typical school day began before daybreak. Since practical electrical lighting was still more than a decade in the future, savoring every moment of daylight was essential. She rose daily at 6:30, ate breakfast at 7:15, then began her trek to the university at 7:45. Dissecting occurred from 8:00 to 10:00 a.m., followed by an hour-long anatomy lecture, "which is made perfectly fascinating by having every thing that is lectured about right before me." The next class, chemistry, was "in another beautiful building at some distance, so we have a nice five-minutes' walk in the fresh air."[56]

Neither dormitories nor dining halls were provided for the students, so Susan and her peers walked to and from their landlords' or host families' homes morning, midday, and night. "At 12 I run home with an appetite for my dinner, and at 1 o'clock I saunter out to get the air and sun for an hour; go to the 'Hoch Promenade,' a beautiful walk on a high hill, in the middle of the town, and overlooking the lake and the mountains."

Following her mid-day dinner break, Susan returned to anatomy class from 2:00 to 3:00. Three more hour-long classes followed: microscopical anatomy, osteology, and zoology. "Then home to supper, and then study: so pass the days. Saturday morning, I dissect all the morning; and in the afternoon I do a little sewing and go for a long walk; and Saturday night I sleep soundly, I can tell you."[57]

In Susan's detailed letters about her schooling to friends and family in America, there is no sense of frustration—perhaps surprising, since all her lectures were in German. "I am all well settled, and fairly started to work, and exceedingly happy," she wrote to her mother, noting that her German-language comprehension was better than she had expected. "[W]hereas I expected to understand nothing for two weeks, I find I can follow most of the lectures right along."[58] Though Dimock's peers were impressed with her language comprehension, she was modest about her abilities, even two years into her studies. "German is now very easy,— that is, to understand; but I believe I make very laughable mistakes still in speaking and writing. The students laugh at me very often, but politely and kindly, so that it is not unpleasant."[59]

Susan's professors were an eclectic group of personalities and talents. The venerable Adolf Gusserow, a noted gynecologist and Susan's thesis director, was also president of the School of Medicine from the summer of 1870 to winter term, 1871. The liberal-minded internist Anton Biermer, who had originally written Susan's letter of acceptance to the medical school, was both a professor and Dean of the Medical Faculty. Georg Hermann von Meyer, a famed anatomist described as both "fatherly" and "well-disposed," came to praise Susan for her energetic striving, dedication, strong character, and for proving, once and for all, that "it was possible for women to dedicate themselves to the medical profession without sacrificing their femininity."[60]

It was under von Meyer that Susan dissected each morning between eight and ten o'clock. "In the parlor," the professor reflected, "I am probably the most favored [by all the students], where there is something interesting to be seen, I am summoned and all is explained to me in detail. Miss Dimock the American is my faithful companion."[61] His "faithful companion" was clearly enchanted by her experiences in von Meyer's classroom. "The professor, whom I like very much, is in the dissecting-room most of the time, and the students are as quiet and polite as possible. They smoke, and I dare say they joke, as I used to be told with a horrified air that they did; but the smoke is pleasant, and the jokes I cannot understand even if I could hear, which I do not, my table being at the other side of the room."

"It is too funny to see Professor Myer come up, look at my work, and remark, with a pleased look, '*Ganz schön!*'—quite beautiful."[62]

Susan's favorite professors were Oswald Heer and Arnold Escher von

Linth. Professor Heer was a former student of theology who had always been fascinated by the natural sciences. A handsome man with long sideburns, a fine chiseled face, and strong chin, Heer taught both botany and entomology.[63] Susan's classmate and close friend Marie Vögtlin, wrote, "There are very few people that I admire as much as Professor Heer; it is a pleasure for me only to see him at a distance. He is of an indestructible goodness and friendliness to every man, and as unpretentious and simple as a great scholar."[64] Maria saw Susan's other esteemed professor in a quite different light. Professor Arnold Escher von der Linth was, in her view, "the most comical, old-fatherly man you can think of, but in his comportment, very courteous and good."[65]

Awash in all these fine professors and exceptional learning experiences, Susan never lost sight of her good fortune—as a medical student, of course, but especially as a woman studying side-by-side with men in one of the world's best medical colleges.

"My lectures grow more and more delightful the better I understand them. It is so nice to have good professors, and to have them kind to one! I think I shall all my life feel the advantages of having come here, where I am admitted on an equal footing with men-students, where professors are kind and interested in one's improvement; and I am sure I shall be a better doctor, for I am learning all the foundation studies so thoroughly, and I never was so well and strong, it seems to me, in my life."

"I hardly know what fatigue means, either of mind or body."[66]

As vital as medical studies and learned professors were to Susan Dimock's extraordinary experience, so too were her medical school peers, her other acquaintances, and the places she travelled when not bound by books, lectures, and surgical instruments.

Preeminent among Dimock's peers was the Swiss student, Marie Vögtlin, the only member of The Zurich Seven without any previous medical training before entering medical college. Two years Susan's senior, Marie was a minister's daughter from a pretty little farming town named Brugg in the canton of Aargau, who had spent her childhood years in the much poorer village of Bözen. Like young Susan, Marie had grown up in a supportive family that loved education and books. While Susan had long devoured every medical tome within reach, Marie's avid reading had grown to include liberal thinkers like British political economist John Stuart Mill and the Italian revolutionary activist Giuseppe Mazzini. Unlike Susan, Marie's desire to become a physician didn't emerge until later in her teens, after the breakup of her engagement to Friedrich Erismann. As it turned out, Erismann married the first of The Zurich Seven, Nadezhda Suslova, in April of 1868.

Susan and Marie became fast friends the first month of their schooling together and maintained that connection throughout and beyond their academic years. It was, in Marie's opinion, a mutually beneficial camaraderie. Marie knew the Swiss people, the land, and the German language, all of which helped Susan acculturate in this foreign setting.

"I have made an arrangement with the American" wrote Marie, "to study together each evening. She is not very knowledgeable in German, but she has already completed two and a half semesters in Boston [at the New England Hospital] and has a firm grasp of material that is still new to me. She told me that she was poor and struggles to make ends meet; she would have to look for an English [-speaking] student to help her with her studies, and that would be financially difficult for her. I was happy to ask her to take me on instead of the student and now we have an association which works to our mutual benefit; I will have the opportunity to really learn English."[67]

As a member of the bourgeoisie, Marie had already studied English and French. But young Susan, of course, knew infinitely more of the English language—including complex medical terms—as well as a great deal of biology. And just as Marie could introduce Susan to her Swiss friends and family, Susan could arrange for Marie to meet the Americans she knew in Zurich. "I'm getting to know many Americans through Miss Dimock, whose friends here invite me," Marie explained. "[T]oday I was with the American consul and his family, and then I went with other Americans to the Üetliberg [a panoramic high-altitude hike on Zurich's 'own' mountain]—already for the second time since I arrived. English is always spoken and I'm hoping to learn it properly. I even think in English and am learning all the technical terms for Anatomy and Chemistry in English."[68]

Among the Americans in Susan's ever-growing circle was her host family that resided at Brandschenkestrasse 30 in Zurich. "The D______ family, with whom I have lived for a year now, are delightful people to be with," she wrote to Dr. Zakrzewska in Boston, "and Mrs. D_____ has made her house a real home for me."[69] "[They] have been four years in Europe," she explained to Dr. Samuel Cabot, "and ... are so kind and pleasant that it is like home to be with them. Altogether I have everything to make me happy and content."[70]

It was common in nineteenth-century letter-writing to protect the privacy of a person's name by using the first letter of that name followed by a long dash, in part because such letters were frequently shared with friends and neighbors. But why Susan chose to obscure the surname of her Zurich landlord and not the names of others mentioned in the letter is unclear. The "D_______" family was, in fact, the wealthy and well-known Dennisons of Waltham, Massachusetts. Aaron Lufkin Dennison, his wife Charlotte Ware Foster, and their children—Charlotte Elizabeth, Edward Boardman, Ethie Gilbert, and Franklin—were a highly respected Massachusetts family who played a pioneering role in America's industrial revolution.

Father Aaron was a businessman and watchmaker who founded, and sometimes lost to bankruptcy, a number of businesses ranging from jewelry sales and paper box manufacturing to watch repair, watch cases, and the creation of fine affordable timepieces.[71] In 1850, Dennison and his partners David Davis and Edward Howard created the business that would eventually become the Waltham Watch Company. The trio did not manufacture America's first watches or clocks. Instead, their plan was to design and manufacture movement parts of watches that were precision-made and fully interchangeable, thereby precluding the need to craft each individual watch by hand. The system they eventually perfected and patented became known as "The American System of Watch Manufacturing."

The Dennison family's sojourn in Zurich was to accommodate one of Aaron's constantly-evolving watch manufacturing ventures. Because of the higher skills and lower wages of Swiss journeymen relative to their American counterparts, Dennison and family relocated to Zurich in order to organize and oversee the fabrication and export of fine watch parts to his new Tremont Watch Company, formed with partner A.O. Bigelow. When that project failed and the company folded, Dennison moved to England where he helped organize the Anglo-American Watch Company in Birmingham.

The upshot for Susan was twofold. First, she was able to enjoy the fascinating company and comfortable surroundings of the welcoming Dennison family when they lived in Zurich. But secondly, she too had to relocate once she learned of their plans to move to England. Luckily, Susan had the help of Marie Vögtlin to fill that void.

In 1870, Susan Dimock moved out of the Dennisons' and into the Heims' at Zeltweg 57—a 15-minute uphill walk to the Polytechnikum and the medical college. Susan couldn't have found a happier place for the last year of her Zurich studies. "I go to the friends whom I like most of all," she confessed to Dr. Zakrzewska, "most kind, happy, fresh and learned people. There are two sons and one daughter, who is of my age and one of my best friends."[72]

Businessman and banker Johann Konrad Heim, his wife Sophie Elisabeth Fries, and their three children Sophie, Albert, and Ernst were those "most kind, happy, fresh, and learned people." Susan's closest school classmate, Marie Vögtlin, had met the young Italian teacher, Sophie Heim, during the beginning of Marie's medical studies. Through Sophie, Marie eased into a friendship with the Heim family, including her brother Albert, whom Marie married in 1875. Brother Albert became both a personal friend and professional connection. His teacher and sponsor at the university was Arnold Escher von der Linth, a beloved geologist and one of Susan's favorite professors. In 1872, a year after Susan's departure, 23-year-old Albert was made Escher von der Linth's successor as professor of technical and general geology at the Polytechnikum.

The new lodging agreement with the Heim family thrilled Marie Vögtlin, both for Susan and for herself. "She is so happy and I'm so glad that she has a home once more and is so close by."[73] Being close by meant that Marie, her "faithful companion" Susan—and often Sophie Heim as well—could spend even more time together. Sometimes that meant enjoying the rich cultural life in the Heim house itself: Sophie's brother Ernst was a professional violinist; Marie played the piano; and Sophie's aunt Nanette was a painter, an art school director, and a close friend of Johanna Spyri, the woman who would write the best-selling children's novel, *Heidi*.[74] As for Susan, "She had no technical skill, but her keen appreciation and enjoyment of art was a source of great delight both to herself and to her friends."[75]

Other times Susan and her friends would attend cultural events in and around Zurich, including concerts, plays, dance performances, operas, lectures, and art exhibits. Wandering through town, they would pass by small shops vending everything from sewing machines, sunglasses, stylish French gloves, and sturdy leather shoes to body oils and soaps, writing and drawing supplies, endless beer varietals, and that perennial Zurich favorite—fancy infused mineral waters. Among the wonderfully odd array of events available to them during Susan's last year of school were an endlessly hyped masked ball (*Grosser Maskenball*); an animal trainer showcasing his exotic "African Menagerie"; the sensational "Siamese Twins" at Hartopff's Museum; a panorama of a famous Swiss mountain, the Rigi; and even one spectacular concert of music and singing by the Blechschmidt family, performed in a gazebo overlooking the Wolfbach canal and illuminated by fireworks.[76]

Since they were bright and curious sophisticates, it's likely that the discerning young ladies frequented the popular Café Literaire, enjoyed photo exhibits at the Café du Nord, or attended organ concerts at the Fraumünster Church or performances of Mozart and Schumann at Tonhalle. Equally enticing to Susan, Marie, and their peers would have been the ballet and opera held at the Aktien or Stadt (City) Theaters, and vocal and instrumental works at the Kronenhalle or the café at the Hotel du

Cheval Blanc. Great choirs and their musical conductors were exceptionally popular at the time, as was the work and enduring influence of Richard Wagner, who had been a regular presence in Zurich from 1849 to 1858.[77]

"I have also plenty of pleasure beside my work," admitted Susan to Dr. Zakrzewska. "I go to-morrow for instance, to Locher-Balbus,' the Professor of *Materia Medica*, to coffee and wine with the class of gentlemen. On Tuesday evening, I am invited to a grand concert. I have many more invitations this winter than I can with pleasure and profit accept, and so I decline."[78]

Marie Vögtlin's interest in the Italian nationalist hero, Giuseppe Mazzini, must have also rubbed off on the curious Susan. Susan noted that "I go on Saturday afternoons to an Italian lecture from the Italian professor on Italian literature, which is very pleasant. I do not know whether Dr. Sewall told you that I had the great fortune to make friends with Mazzini last summer. He has since sent me his letter *Ai Nemici*. I am only learning Italian a little, so that I may fully enjoy my Italian journey when it comes."[79] Studying Italian in preparation for a summer excursion to Italy was typical of Susan. She had, after all, already learned German in order to take classes and write papers at Zurich's medical school.

Sometimes Susan's Italian literature study was followed by more physical pursuits. "Tomorrow in the morning I will be with Miss Dimock at Miss Heim's for Italian literature," recalled Marie Vögtlin, "then we lunch together and go to an ice skating station and conduct experiments there. Miss Heim and Ernst, Sophie's youngest brother, want to teach me and I am very enthusiastic—it is one of the healthiest forms of exercise—and after I have learned how to move in water, I now want to conquer the ice too. I am so delighted!"[80]

The most physically ambitious of the outings shared by the young women were the mountain hikes they undertook, often accompanied by their professors or male friends. Just a few weeks after the start of their first semester together—during the Pentecost holiday following Easter—the classmates planned a trip to one of Marie's favorite landscapes in Glarnerland, a narrow valley in the majestic mountains of eastern Switzerland.[81] It was the first of many such excursions, inspiring a bemused Susan to later admit, "I have seen a large part of Switzerland and chiefly on my feet."[82] One such excursion, in May of 1869, included Marie, Susan, and a new friend, the young male medical student, August Forel. "The Excursions usually last five hours or six in the same day. We [Marie and Susan] have seen with delight the fact that we are among the better pedestrians of the whole band, and in any case, endure thirst and heat much more easily than the gentlemen."[83]

Time and again, it was proven that Susan and Marie were more athletically adept than their male colleagues might have imagined. Marie observed that no one had to make special allowances for the young women. "I can't begin to tell you how well everything is going.... On excursions it was a real pleasure to see the comradely way that the students treated us. Sometimes it's funny when we have to climb down a cliff or cross a stream—then everyone is waiting to see if we can do it alone. So far there is nothing that we couldn't honorably accomplish."[84]

Economics professor Karl Victor Böhmert recalled an eye-opening trek he took with the "young ladies" in July of 1869. "I accepted an invitation to take part in a four-days' botanico-geologico excursion," Böhmert recounted, "which my colleagues, Professors Heer and Escher von der Linth, the most competent botanists for Swiss and mountain plants, undertook with their assistants, and more than thirty students of the High and Polytechnic schools."

"At the assigned hour of starting from Zurich, I was not a little astonished to find among the members of the excursion, armed with alpenstaffs, botanical boxes, and travelling bags, two young ladies. Professor Heer told me that these two ladies were regular attendants of his lectures; and that, so far from producing any disturbance in the class, their modest and discreet behavior had such a good influence on the manners and behavior of the students as to make their presence in the longer excursion very desirable."[85]

The group hopped the train to Zug, then from Lake Zug took a steamer to Arth. After Arth, they proceeded on foot by Goldau and the Lowerzer See to Brunnen. "It was a fabulous night," recounted Marie of one special evening in Brunnen, "right in front of our window the lake with the reflection of the silver moon. We started off at 4 a.m., as we had both agreed to a private visit to the Grütli [a mountain pasture heralded as the site of a legendary oath in Swiss history] with the clergyman Pfister. I don't think I could have stood it if I hadn't visited this much-loved site ... [J]ust as we landed, the sun rose all golden. I can't describe the impression that this morning hour made on me—I've never experienced anything more beautiful and I will never forget it. That quiet place seemed like the holiest temple I have ever entered."[86]

The trio of Marie, Susan, and clergyman Pfister from Wiedikon rejoined the rest of the group at Axenstrasse, a famously scenic winding road in central Switzerland, some forty miles from Zurich. More strenuous hiking—sometimes up to ten hours a day—was interspersed with taking in breathtaking Alpine views and collecting botanical samples. "It was a picturesque group," mused Marie, "the wine jug in the middle and leather-clad glasses on all sides and great hunks of ham everywhere."[87]

Despite heavy downpours as they descended the mountain on the last day, the women mountaineers pulled sturdy rain hoods over their heads and fared better than their soggy male companions. The result, in the view of Professor Böhmert, was rather revolutionary: "On the whole tour, the ladies have shown themselves equal to the majority of the men, not only in scientific zeal and mental energy, but in endurance of the difficult labors of the two passes. They were always among the first to reach the end of the journey.... Professors and students alike felt that they had witnessed a triumph of womanly work and endurance."[88]

Susan Dimock and Marie Vögtlin had again become role models—first inside the classroom, and now in the rugged out-of-doors—inspiring Professor Heer to remind the young men on the trek, "what a high duty it was for them to help women to overcome the obstacles with which they have yet to contend." They clearly had not yet absorbed that Susan and Marie were quite adept at overcoming obstacles on their own.

As the semesters rolled on, Susan Dimock and the rest of The Zurich Seven were enchanted and challenged by new courses and new experiences, both in and out of the classroom. Susan wrote home about how she relished the medical school's "clinical advantages," delighted in receiving sturdy new surgical cases and containers from European manufacturers, and was fascinated by the fact that "Zurich is unhealthy enough in the poor quarters to keep the medical wards full.... The lying-in hospital is also quite full generally."[89]

Susan and her classmates knew that medical wards were full outside their city limits as well, due largely to the Franco-Prussian War, which began raging just beyond Switzerland's northern border in the summer of 1870. Intrigued and inspired by the Swiss government's non-partisan involvement in the new International Committee of the Red Cross, Zurich's medical students and citizens-at-large were kept keenly aware of the battles, prisoners, and casualties of war thanks to newspaper reports, letters, and street conversations.[90] Classmate August Forel recalled how he personally "followed events in the Oberstrass beer-garden, and meditated on the tragic history of the nations."

August Forel eventually joined an 1871 trip to the Franco-Prussian battlefields near Belfort, France, with a group that Zurich medical school professor Edmund Rose organized to aid injured soldiers from either army. Appalled by the brutality and suffering he witnessed on and off the battlefields, Forel was haunted by gruesome scenes, including "discovering some severely wounded Frenchmen ... with frostbitten feet, who were lying wretched and forsaken in various cold, dark cellars." Forel empathized with the French and was unimpressed with Professor Rose and his male medical students, many of whom were pro–German and "felt very important, … the first thing they did in their exalted mood was to begin drinking with Rose."[91]

Despite their medical training and desire to help the Red Cross efforts, Susan and most of the Zurich Seven did not join Professor Rose, his assistants, and the senior male medical students who accompanied him to the war. Only the eldest and the sole married member of the Seven, the Russian Mariia Bokova, volunteered and was accepted, making her the lone woman expeditionary on that 1871 trip. She was later singled out by Rose, who praised Bokova for winning everyone's hearts "by her steady and self-sacrificing efforts on behalf of the wounded."[92]

Meanwhile, Susan had her schooling to fill every waking hour. "I do not find that the work is one bit hard," she wrote to her mother, "but the contrary. Eight hours slip by like beads, and then between every hour there is a change, nearly always, from one building to another; and night comes, and I can sit down cosily and study, and can be sure of sleeping all night."

"I am often asked if I am not doing too much, but I can't think that I am."[93]

Susan's persistence, patience, and ever-increasing skills produced both excellent grades and admiration from her peers and her professors. Those skills didn't escape the notice of her closest comrade, Marie Vögtlin, who bragged to a friend, "Miss Dimock and I are probably the best in the entire anatomy class."[94]

Though anatomy and several of the other courses Susan and her classmates tackled would be familiar to modern medical students, many of their classes would not. In an age when antiseptic surgical methods were new and revolutionary, when penicillin and aspirin were unknown, and when the germ theory of disease was still in its infancy (and widely doubted), it was far more appropriate for Susan to learn about the healing properties of plants and to value natural history. Such knowledge was taught in mandatory courses through a discipline known as "Natural Philosophy."[95]

"Next summer I shall spend nearly all the day in the Clinik [sic], and shall review the natural sciences; at any rate, botany and zoology," she explained in a letter to Dr. Zakrzewska. "With physics, mineralogy, and chemistry, I shall have quite finished this winter. I have enjoyed these things very, very much. I have been very much interested in geology this winter, because I have some friends who are geologists."[96]

Work was, as ever, periodically interspersed with play. During the summer of 1870, Susan enjoyed "six weeks of uninterrupted rest and pleasure in Italy." And while she was always concerned with thrift—conscious of the school loans she planned to repay to both friends and family—she fully understood that such journeys could be as healing as the plants she studied in botany class. "Travelling expenses might have been avoided," she admitted in a letter to Dr. Zakrzewska, "but my mother authorized this expenditure. In fact, you see [the costs are] little, while the pleasure and advantages which I have thus enjoyed have been very great." As proof of her financial prudence, Susan dutifully provided Dr. Zak a list of her previous schoolyear's expenses.[97]

Board, washing, and lights	*frs.*	*884.91*
College expenses	*"*	*689.10*
Travelling	*"*	*262.75*
Clothes	*"*	*263.51*
Sundries	*"*	*30.00*

Following her Italian travels, Susan returned "fresh and happy" to an intense schedule of non-stop "clinical work, microscopy, autopsy, the surgical course upon the dead body, &c.; in short, work in which my hands rested my head." Those studies segued into classes on midwifery, medicine, surgery, "topographical anatomy," percussion and auscultation—tapping on, and listening to, specific parts of the body as part of clinical examination—as well as forensic medicine.[98]

At this point in her studies, to even the most casual observer of her academic and personal life, one thing was undeniable: Susan Dimock was receiving a far more thorough, scientific, hands-on medical education—and having more varied life experiences—than if she had stayed in Boston and attended Harvard Medical College.

In part because each had started schooling at a different time and with varying degrees of prior medical experience, Susan and her eclectic band of female classmates graduated over a period of several years.

In 1867, Russian student Nadezhda Suslova, the first of The Zurich Seven to matriculate, was also the first to graduate. At the end of her well-received dissertation defense, and after some forceful questioning by the group of examining professors, surgeon Edmund Rose observed, "Soon we are coming to the end of slavery for women, and soon we will have the practical emancipation of women in every country and with it the right to work."[99] The second Russian, Mariia Bokova, graduated four years later. Some xenophobic observers, both in the city and the student body, were wary of these "radical" emigrees and the dozens of other Russian and Eastern European women who swept into Zurich, inspired by Suslova and Bokova's successes. Russian women were sometimes lumped together as nihilists and radical feminists who huddled in rooming houses separate from other nationalities, and who brandished the strange habits and "uniforms" of political dissidents—round blue spectacles, sailor caps, and short-cropped hair. They were surely guilty of all sorts of "immoral" behavior, not the least of which was smoking in public.

Susan was initially worried by the dozens of Russian women who poured in following Suslova and Bokova. Since a number of them were too young and obviously unqualified, she and several of her female classmates were concerned that new tensions between the male students and the flood of female Russian students might endanger future possibilities for all women at the university.[100] In time, however, Susan rejected the negative stereotypes being circulated and expressed her appreciation of, and compassion for, the Russians' unusual circumstances in a letter to her mentor, Dr. Samuel Cabot in Boston.

"These two women [Suslova and Bokova], the only Russians who have graduated at Zurich, showed through the years of my acquaintance with them the greatest nobility, goodness and rectitude of character. After [their] graduation ... the number of Russian students rapidly increased, and although of course among 100 women a few must be found whose aims are not so high, yet very many showed a nobleness of purpose and unselfishness of life which cannot be overlooked. Many were very rich, but ready to sacrifice in order to help the poor...."

"That some of these young girls have [been] food for scandal by the utterance of many wild and foolish tenets is certainly true, but it must be remembered that they were almost children, and so deserving of the pity and protection of every generous and strong man and woman. And in no case have I heard of one immodest look or word or act on the part of any of them."[101]

The second of The Zurich Seven to graduate—after Suslova and before Bokova—was the attractive and arguably "legendary" Englishwoman from Wales, Frances Elizabeth Morgan. Described by her contemporaries as cool, regal, self-possessed, crisp, and authoritarian, she astonished her professors and fellow students by tackling sixty hours of university work per week, taking a side course in Sanskrit, then completing her medical degree in only three years, rather than the standard five. A favorite anecdote about Morgan's strong personality involved a dissection demonstration, during which anatomy professor Hermann von Meyer suggested excluding the female students from this potentially shocking sight. Morgan's classic retort: "Herr Professor, it is much more shocking and improper to make exceptions here. We wish to study the subject without restrictions of any kind."[102]

Though some were amused or miffed by Frances Morgan's royal

demeanor, fellow student August Forel—a close friend of both Susan Dimock and Marie Vögtlin—noted that "the seriousness, the aristocratic calm, and the queenly superiority of this remarkable girl exacted such respect from us all that none of us would have dared to make a tactless or sarcastic remark."[103]

When Morgan defended her dissertation on March 12, 1870, interest in the marvelous medical women of Zurich had grown so intense—and the crowd of onlookers and supporters grown so large—that the event had to be relocated to the university's most spacious auditorium, the classically grand "Aula" in the Semper Building of the Polytechnikum. The same was true when Susan Dimock was examined on Thursday, October 26, 1871, as the fourth woman doctor from Zürich. For both Morgan's and Dimock's appearances, the crowds were estimated at well over four hundred.

On the day of Susan's defense, an academic procession entered the Aula, led by the rector of the University of Zurich. Members of the medical faculty came next, resplendent in their colorful robes, followed by Susan herself. The calm, attractive, twenty-four-year-old American was prompted to take a seat next to the rector at the head of a long, narrow table, formally draped in green felt.[104] With scores of intrigued students, professors, women friends, and physicians looking on, Susan proceeded to answer questions about her dissertation on "The Different Forms of Puerperal Fever," which she wrote entirely in German.

Susan's elaborate essay on what was popularly known as childbirth or childbed fever was, as described by memoirist Ednah Dow Cheney, "illustrated not only by a report of the cases occurring in the Zurich Hospital, but also by diagrams of the fever curves during the recovery of the patients." Susan's treatise chronicled and evaluated the latest knowledge on puerperal fever, including the then-novel idea of using clinical thermometers and daily temperature charts to accurately observe the constitutional disturbance of the fever on the patient. "This treatise, which is admirably written," added Cheney, "received high encomiums from her instructors, and justified the expectations of her American friends." Rather than cite specifics from Susan's well-received thesis, Cheney acknowledged, "It is too long and too purely technical to be of interest to the general reader."[105]

After a lengthy period of questioning by professors and audience members, Susan's anatomy professor, Georg Hermann von Meyer, stood up and directly faced his student. Von Meyer beamed with pride while explaining the high esteem in which Susan was held by himself and his colleagues and emphasizing the "energetic striving and dedication that speaks for her strong character." Before finishing, von Meyer added, "You have shown by your example that it is possible for women to devote themselves to the medical profession without sacrificing your femininity."[106]

It was true that von Meyer, popularly known as "Knochenmeyer" or "the Bone-merchant" due to his intense interest in the human skeleton, had long been an advocate of higher education for women. Still, many of his peers found it hard to absorb the fact that a woman could be skilled, smart, womanly, lovely, and kind—all in the same package.

The last three members of The Zurich Seven graduated after Susan's departure from the university in the late fall of 1871. First came Eliza Walker, who was the youngest of the seven when she arrived in Zurich at age nineteen. Hailing from Edinburgh and dubbed "la très jolie Ecossaise" by August Forel,[107] Walker balanced her medical studies with working as an assistant in the woman's ward of the Zurich cantonal hospital—the first female to hold that position—yet took only four years to complete her medical coursework. She graduated with honors in 1872.

Next came Louisa Atkins of England, a widow whose husband had died in service to India, and who took the standard five years to finish her degree. Part of the reason she required a longer period of study than the rest of The Zurich Seven was her general lack of experience in medicine and the challenges she experienced in scientific study. While known to be hard-working, self-disciplined, gentle, and friendly, Atkins had, in the words of Forel, "a much less elevated sense of herself" than her peers.[108] Like Eliza Walker, she graduated in 1872.

The last of the seven to finish her medical degree was Susan's closest friend, Marie Vögtlin of Switzerland. Though she completed her coursework in 1872, a year after Susan's departure, Marie had no previous medical training before enrolling in Zurich. To help bridge that experiential gap,

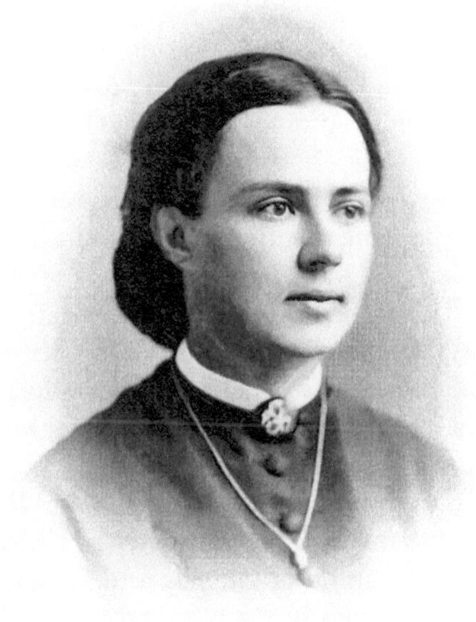

The last of The Zurich Seven to finish her medical degree was Susan's closest friend, Marie Vögtlin (1845–1916) of Switzerland. After completing her coursework in 1872, she sought further studies in Leipzig and Dresden, Germany, before returning to Zurich and passing her doctoral examination in 1874. She was the first woman in Switzerland to earn a medical degree and practice medicine (image via Wikimedia Commons).

she sought further studies in both Leipzig and Dresden, Germany, before returning to Zurich and passing her doctoral examination on July 11, 1874.[109]

In the end, "the Zurich experiment" in medical education proved eminently successful. Given the years of hard work Susan Dimock and her six female colleagues committed to medical schooling—and the training many of them had pursued even before upending their lives and traveling to Zurich—it was perhaps no surprise that all members of The Zurich Seven went on to become medical pioneers in their respective countries.

Nadezhda Suslova was both Russia's first female physician and the first modern woman to receive a medical degree from a recognized university of high academic standards. She became a feminist legend in her homeland through her medical work, writings, and philanthropy. Her fellow Russian, Mariia Bokova, earned two doctoral degrees, first in Zürich and next in in Vienna, then joined the Russian Academy of Medicine as a researcher. She, too, became a Russian hero as well as a model for the Vera Pavlovna character—a woman who fights convention to pursue economic independence and study science and medicine—in Nikolai Chernyshevsky's novel, *What Is to Be Done*?

Frances Elizabeth Morgan left to work at St. Mary's Dispensary for Women and Children in London and become the first female doctor registered in Wales. After marrying George Hoggan, she was half of the first husband-and-wife medical practice in Britain. Eliza Walker gained renown as a Scottish physician and as the first women in the United Kingdom to qualify and work as a doctor. Walker established both the Read Dispensary for Women and Children in Bristol and, later, the Bristol Private Hospital for Women and Children. The third British student, Louisa Atkins was appointed to the Birmingham and Midland Hospital for Women in 1872 and officially admitted to medical practice five years later. She became a resident at the Women's Hospital of Queens and General Hospitals. Marie Vögtlin was the first women in Switzerland to earn a medical degree and practice medicine. She married geologist Albert Heim in 1876, raised three children, and was heralded for her pioneering work in gynecology and as director of the Swiss Nurses' School pediatric division.[110] One of Switzerland's best-known citizens, Vögtlin-Heim's many honors included a commemorative postage stamp in 2016.

The sole American in the group, Susan Dimock, pursued further medical instruction in Vienna and Paris before returning to Boston to become resident physician at the New England Hospital for Women and Children. There, in the facility eventually renamed the Dimock Center, she garnered praise for her leadership, her exceptional surgical skills, and for professionalizing the first nurses training program in the nation.

The successes of The Zurich Seven, both in school and in their sub-sequent professional careers, placed Switzerland at the forefront of medical education for women during the last quarter of the nineteenth and first part of the twentieth century. Initially dozens, then eventually hundreds, of women enrolled in Zurich's medical school in the decades following Susan and her colleagues' graduations. Until the onset of the First World War in 1914, Zurich matriculated more female medical students than any university in the world, with Paris running a strong second.[111]

The United States trailed its European counterparts during this era. "I am sorry to be forced to say that it is not the Republic of America which has given the proof that 'science has no sex,'" admitted Dr. Marie Zakrzewska back in Boston. "But it is the Republic of Switzerland which has verified this maxim. Our best women physicians have been educated there as well as in Germany and in France."[112]

The "Republic of America" had tried. In 1873, for example, the fledgling Boston University merged with Samuel Gregory's old New England Female Medical College—the mediocre facility that Dr. Zak had abandoned in 1862—making it the first accredited coeducational medical school in the nation. The resulting Boston University School of Medicine, however, was initially homeopathic, not part of the allopathic mainstream medical establishment supported by powerful groups like the American Medical Association and the Massachusetts Medical Society. Other coed medical schools followed, though largely outside staid New England.

It wasn't until 1892 that an elite eastern American medical school comparable to the great European Universities—Johns Hopkins in Baltimore, Maryland—began accepting women on an equal footing with its male students. Their reasoning was practical, inspired by a $500,000 grant that a group of wealthy, influential women were able to offer in return for the access.[113] Still, the elite eastern school that Susan Dimock had once wanted to attend, the hallowed medical college at Harvard University, was more resistant to inclusiveness than much of the rest of the nation.

Harvard Medical School admitted its first freshman class of twelve women in September of 1945.[114] Had Susan Dimock waited to enter with that inaugural class, she would have been 98.

Before returning to Boston and assuming her new role as resident physician at the New England Hospital, Susan Dimock, MD, had two more European stops to make: Vienna, the City of Music, and Paris, the City of Light.

For the twenty-four-year-old Susan, Vienna, already a classical music mecca, had two special allures. By the early 1870s, the capital of the Austro-Hungarian Empire had secured its position as the international center of medical innovation and surgical excellence. It was also the home of Theodor Billroth, who, at the age of forty-two, was acknowledged worldwide as "the surgeon's surgeon."[115] Like Vienna, Paris was a magnet for culture and art—both adored by Susan—but also the location of La Maternité, one of the world's oldest and most prestigious lying-in hospitals. Because the newly graduated Dr. Dimock was committed both to serving women patients and becoming the best surgeon possible, and because her hard-working mother was willing to continue sending her money, she opted to extend her European sojourn nine months longer. This was a voluntary extension of her studies. At the time, medical school graduates were not required to pursue internships before opening a practice.

Despite the difficulty of leaving her Swiss home and friends, Susan looked forward to reconnecting with two of her old classmates once reaching Vienna, almost four hundred miles away. Both Mariia Bokova of Russia and August Forel of Switzerland had moved to Vienna from Zurich to work with specialists in their chosen fields. Bokova and Forel had bonded earlier, both in medical school and on the Belfort battlefront of the Franco-Prussian War, where they had volunteered for a school-sponsored medical expedition. Now in Vienna, Bokova was pursing her love of ophthalmology and Forel was working in the laboratory of Theodor Hermann Meynert, an influential psychiatrist whose future students would include an ambitious young Austrian named Sigmund Freud.

With several letters of introduction in hand, Forel and Bokova's former classmate reached Vienna the first week of November 1871. "One of the students from Zurich (Miss Dimock, the American) must have arrived here, I haven't seen her yet," Forel wrote to his mother on November 6.[116] As in Zurich, the University of Vienna had no dormitories of its own. Hence, to be as close as possible to all the activities at the Vienna General Hospital and the Viennese Medical School, Susan found lodging essentially next door, *Im Thurm, Ally-Krankenhaus* ("In the tower, Hospital Alley").[117] Though university records indicate that she never enrolled as a student, that was not unusual—women were not admitted to Vienna's medical college until 1900. Instead, Susan's goal was to buy tickets for medical lectures and to observe or participate in every clinical experience possible.

The man Susan Dimock most wanted to meet in Vienna was Theodor Billroth. She had known of the eminent surgeon for years and even referenced him in her Zurich dissertation. One of the reasons young Susan was initially drawn to study medicine in Switzerland—aside from her rejection by Harvard—was that Billroth taught at the University of Zurich. By

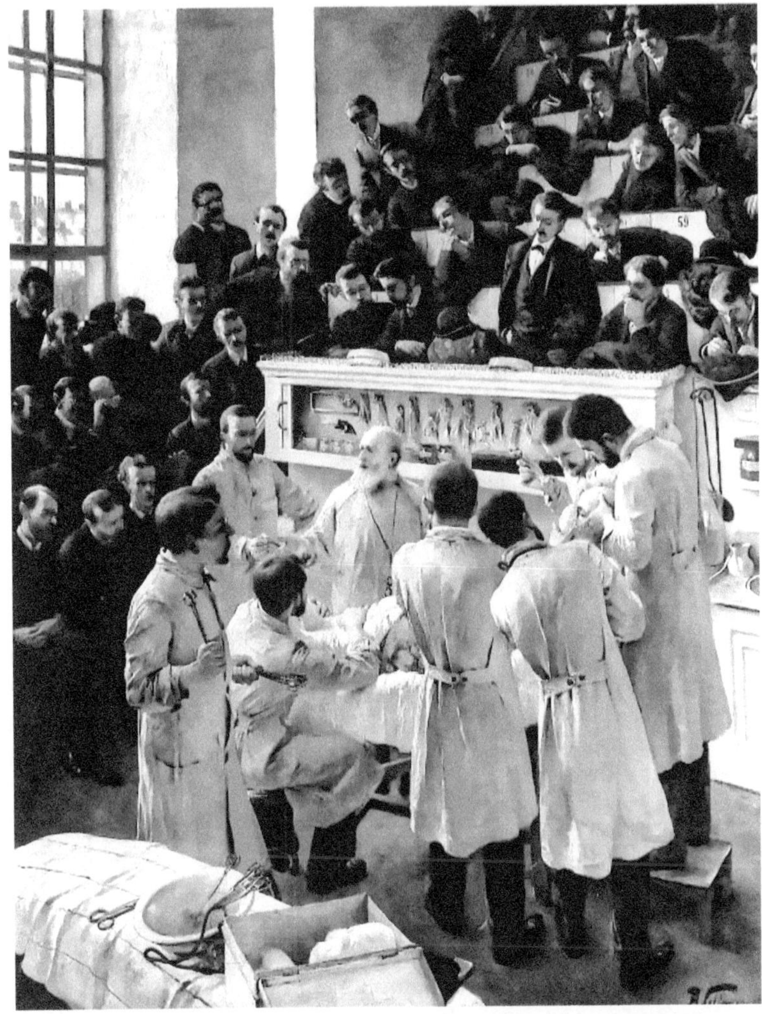

One reason Susan Dimock traveled to Vienna following graduation was to observe Theodor Billroth (1829–94), the legendary "surgeon's surgeon." Billroth inspired Dimock's meticulous medical records, her use of thermometers, her daily charts to track patient wellness, her careful descriptions of operations, and her intense interest in diagnosis (oil painting of Billroth operating by Adalbert Seligman; image via Wikimedia Commons).

the time Susan arrived in Zurich in 1868, however, Dr. Billroth had relocated to Vienna where he had been appointed professor of surgery at the University and chief of surgery at the General Hospital. Now, three years later, the two doctors, Billroth and Dimock, were finally in the same town. It clearly mattered to Susan Dimock. Given Theodor Billroth's well-known discomfort with women entering the field of medicine, the feeling was probably not reciprocated.[118]

After purchasing the appropriate course tickets at what was known as the "Second Viennese Medical School," Susan joined the scores of eager students who regularly packed into Dr. Billroth's popular lectures and demonstrations. Because of Billroth's brilliance, as well as his "surgical flair, his sense of the dramatic and his kindly philosophy," more than four hundred students were often seen vying for some three hundred seats. At the lecture hall's center stage stood the stocky professor, with blue eyes, bushy eyebrows, a thick reddish beard, and an inimitable sense of humor.[119] Above and around him, three distinct groups crowded in together—undergraduates, graduate assistant surgeons, and postgraduate visiting surgeons, most of whom hailed from other countries. According to Billroth biographer Karel Absolon, it was those visiting surgeons, like Susan Dimock, who "learned most from the material presented in lectures and by observing in the operating room, the wards, and the autopsy room."[120] The reason was undoubtedly that while the undergraduate and graduate students were required to be there, the visiting surgeons felt privileged to be there.

What Susan absorbed from her extended exposure to Theodor Billroth in Vienna can only be deduced from her subsequent medical practices in Boston. Billroth's great attention to detail in surgery may well have inspired Susan's meticulous record-keeping, her careful descriptions of operations, and her intense interest in diagnosis. Billroth was among the first surgeons to use thermometers and keep daily temperature charts to track patient wellness—practices that Susan subsequently initiated at the New England Hospital. Billroth stressed the significance of well-trained nurses in surgical settings. Over the next decade, Susan professionalized the first formal nurses' training program in America and Billroth co-founded a school of nursing in Germany. Billroth sometimes worked himself to the point of exhaustion and was as demanding on his students as he was on himself—traits that, for better or worse, Susan later repeated in her own workplace. And while Billroth was known as a pioneer in the field of esophageal resection during the period when Susan attended his classes, it may have been his successful work on large tumors of the neck that inspired an ambitious neck tumor surgery Susan executed in Boston two years later.[121]

The instructor to whom Susan Dimock was formally attached at the Vienna General Hospital (*Allgemeines Krankenhaus der Stadt Wein*) was not Billroth, however, but Dr. Marcus Funk, who taught in the departments of obstetrics and gynecology. Susan regularly attended Funk's lectures in the General Hospital and accompanied him on clinical rounds. After working in tandem over a period of several months, Funk found his young American protégé to be exceptionally talented, industrious, charming, and skilled—and, perhaps most impressively, unafraid to offer an independent opinion. Years later, Dr. Funk recalled that Susan regularly "stepped into the sick-room, full of propriety and modesty, and as though she were treading on holy ground." He was struck by how "she listened with rapt attention to my every word, ... examined the patient tenderly and with merciful hand, ... thoroughly and completely; [and] how she handled any and all instruments with skill, clearly comprehending all phases of a disease, accurately distinguishing the essential from the incidental (a rare gift in women)."

Like his fellow colleagues at the Vienna General Hospital, Dr. Funk was frankly surprised to find all these qualities in a female doctor. But his conclusion was straightforward. "The question, whether a woman can be fit for the study and practice of medicine, has been definitely answered by the appearance of Dr. Susan Dimock." Funk's greatest compliment was a succinct recommendation. When asked for advice to aspiring young doctors, he replied simply, "Make yourself to be like Miss Dimock."[122]

Meanwhile, twenty-four-year-old Susan was as eager to explore cultural life in Vienna as she had been in Boston and Zurich. "You, who are interested not only in my medical but also in my social relations," she wrote to Dr. Zakrzewska, "will be glad to hear that both are extremely pleasant and gratifying."[123] To her delight, Susan discovered that costs in Vienna were not much more than those in Zurich, which allowed her to purchase medical equipment for Dr. Zak's hospital as well as to enjoy the many pleasures the city had to offer.

Adding to that delight was the little posse that shared the young American's Viennese adventures. Soon after settling in, Susan joined forces with her former Zurich classmates Mariia Bokova and Auguste Forel, as well as Forel's friend, Carl Eugen Hoestermann, an assistant at the Meynertschen Klinik. Calling themselves the "Wiener Quartet," the foreign foursome must have been a curious sight: two independent, strong-willed women marching through downtown Vienna with two young male doctors who—with their slicked-back hair, drooping mustaches, and short, bushy beards—could have passed for brothers.

There was, of course, much for them to explore, including the sparkling, "beautiful Blue Danube"—romanticized in composer Johann Strauss's 1867 waltz—which flowed through the city *en route* to the Black Sea. Though the Wiener Quartet's reactions were not recorded, Professor Billroth was duly unimpressed with Herr Strauss's vision of the iconic waterway, noting that, in reality, the river was, "just like the medical faculty, ... a mixture of yellows and browns."[124] Far more colorful were the carnivals, dances, and music that permeated the environs.

Walking from the hospital and medical school towards city center, Susan and her colleagues may have passed the stables of the Spanish Riding School or watched its famed white Lipizzaner stallions in classic dressage. They surely wandered through the Ringstrasse, the newly opened circular boulevard that surrounded the heart of the city and was lined with parks, monuments, and the grand buildings of the Hofburg Imperial Palace. Their vanity must have been fed by getting individual portraits taken at a local photo studio—images that Forel later conserved in a cherished photo scrapbook. And their artistic appetites may have been whetted by magnificent edifices like the ancient St. Stephens cathedral, the beloved *Burgtheatre* (then called the *K.K. Hoftheater nächst der Burg*), renowned as the most important German-language theater in the world, and the State Opera House (*Wiener Staatsoper*), which had opened just two years earlier with a performance of Mozart's *Don Giovanni*.

Sometimes paired off and sometimes as the full quartet, the young doctors probably explored Vienna's many coffee-houses, savored her pastries and brews, attended her theaters, and investigated her museums throughout the chilly winter of 1871–72. August Forel wrote his mother that "For three days it has been snowing and freezing to split stone. Yesterday the weather was wonderful; a clear sky, but it was freezing hard. I went to see the Belvédère gallery with Miss Dimock. The building is magnificent; and the paintings too; there is a mass of originals by Rubens, Van Dyck, Rembrandts, etc."[125]

Forel, a proud Swiss citizen, loved his comrades, but was open about his personal disdain for the native Viennese. "You have to see this population," he exclaimed, "it is something curious; they only think about having fun and making money; the rest matters little to them."[126] It's doubtful that Forel, Dimock, *et al* were similarly disappointed by one of the city's newest permanent residents, a gentleman named Johannes Brahms. During the Christmas season of 1871, the beloved German composer, pianist, and conductor moved into an apartment at Karlsgasse 4, at the behest of his good friend Theodor Billroth, himself an amateur violinist and pianist. Brahms kept the apartment and the friendship for the rest of his life. The result, in the words of biographer Karel Absolon, was that "Brahms stimulated the musical life in Vienna as Billroth stimulated the medical life…. Their reputations were established."[127]

Quite possibly the oddest person Susan Dimock and friends may have encountered during their Vienna sojourn was Captain George Costentenus, an exotic Greek Albanian visitor popularly known as "The Tattoo Man." Moritz Kaposi, a graduate of the University of Vienna medical school, invited the thirty-eight-year-old Costentenus to appear before the Vienna Medical Society in the midst of the Weiner Quartet's stay. As a trained dermatologist, Kaposi was curious about Costentenus, who was covered head-to-toe with 388 closely interwoven, symmetrically arranged tattoos, allegedly inked on his body during his three-month imprisonment by Chinese Tartars in a region later known as Burma (now Myanmar). As the Tattoo Man, Costentenus was a medical marvel and the talk of Vienna—explored and analyzed by Kaposi and exhibited on numerous occasions to other professors of dermatology and university faculty. In an article published in 1872, Dr. Kaposi described Costentenus as being "of middle height, handsome, powerfully built and well-nourished ... [His] skin is covered with dark blue tattooed figures among which are strewn smaller figures in red." The gracefully artistic figures that filled every bodily nook and cranny, including his "private parts," ranged from crowned sphinxes, snakes, elephants, swans and dragons to "all kinds of other subjects such as bows, quivers, arrows, fruits, leaves, and flowers."[128]

Following Susan Dimock's departure from Vienna in the spring of 1872, Dr. Kaposi continued his dermatological research, which included publishing a paper describing a cancer of the skin he had recently identified. More than a century later, Kaposi's sarcoma (KS) would become widely known when it appeared in young gay men with immune deficiencies from HIV or AIDS. In 1875, Kaposi was appointed professor at the medical school, then, five years later, chair of the Vienna School of Dermatology. Meanwhile, The Tattoo Man traveled to the United States, where he contracted with P.T. Barnum to tour with "The Greatest Showman's" traveling extravaganzas.[129]

Paris was the next stop on Dr. Susan Dimock's international agenda. Susan had long dreamed of traveling to the City of Light while in Europe. "Whether I go ... or not will, of course, depend upon the state of affairs in Paris," she wrote to Dr. Zakrzewska, acknowledging the possible dangers there after France's defeat in the Franco-Prussian War, the establishment and destruction of the Paris Commune, and the ruins left in the wake of this chaotic time. But by the spring of 1872, calm had clearly settled into Paris and rebuilding had begun. "That I am able to spend a fourth year in Europe I owe to my mother," Dimock acknowledged, "as indeed I owe most of the good things which I have had in my life."[130]

As it turned out, Susan's Paris visit lasted for only a few weeks. Since she arrived in April, her timing was ideal. The flurry of broad boulevards, parks, squares, and fountains developed in the 1850s and '60s, when Baron George-Eugene Haussmann famously restructured the cityscape, were slowly returning to their former bloom, as were the plantings in iconic public gardens like the Luxembourg and Tuileries. Though the city was continuing to suffer economic distress, Parisians' hopes and dreams were starting to rebound as well. And though no one was yet quite aware of it, the era later known as La Belle Époque had just begun.

The institutions of most interest to a young American doctor in 1872, however, were some of Paris's oldest medical facilities: L'École de Médecine, l'Hôtel-Dieu, and La Maternité. Though the school of medicine and the city's largest hospital—the 1400-bed, five-storyHôtel-Dieu, diagonally across from Notre Dame Cathedral on Îsle de la Cité—were essential stops, it's likely that La Maternité at Port-Royal, the lying-in hospital for the poor women of Paris, held the greatest intrigue. Susan may have first heard about La Maternité from Dr. Solomon Satchwell in North Carolina, since her beloved hometown doctor had once studied in Paris. She most certainly knew of its fame from Dr. Zak in Boston. Dr. Elizabeth Blackwell, the pioneering female doctor whom Marie Zakrzewska helped open the New York Infirmary for Women and Children in 1857, had taken courses at La Maternité in 1849, following her graduation from Geneva Medical College in New York. Blackwell recalled the curious old hospital fondly. "Imagine a large square of old buildings, formerly a convent, set down in the center of a great court with a wood and garden behind, and many little separate buildings all around, the whole enclosed by very high walls...," Dr. Blackwell later wrote. "The inner court is surrounded by *les cloîtres*, a most convenient arched passage which gives covered communication to the whole building, and which I suppose was formerly traversed by shaven monks on their way to the church...."[131]

Little had changed from Blackwell's description by the time of Susan's Parisian sojourn. In 1872, patients were still treated free of charge at La Maternité, as they were in all of Paris's hospitals. Doctors from around the world specializing in obstetrics still eagerly sought clinical visits there, anxious to view an institution that exclusively served women in labor and that offered first-hand views of as many as a dozen deliveries each day. And though the hospital was staffed by and set up to teach midwives, it was a mecca for those seeking experience in the child-birthing process, whether midwives, nurses, or physicians.

It's likely that while in Paris, Susan at least stopped by one other medical institution, the grisly sideshow known as the Paris Morgue. Located not far behind Notre Dame Cathedral since 1864, the morgue was conveniently lodged on the edge of the Seine. When dead bodies were found floating in the river or abandoned on dark back streets, they were brought to the morgue and displayed in glass cases, with the hope of identifying the deceased. Though set up as a practical way to get the corpses recognized and claimed—which it often did—the Paris Morgue also became one of nineteenth-century Paris's most popular and macabre tourist attractions, drawing curiosity seekers by the thousands. Starting in the last two decades of the century, it was even listed in travel guidebooks, including those published by the prestigious Thomas Cook & Son of London.[132]

During that same spring of 1872, Susan Dimock was also able to meet one last time with her "dear companion" from Zurich medical school days, Marie Vögtlin. The two met some 250 miles east of Paris, in Alsace-Lorraine, a border region ceded from France to the German Empire in the wake of the Franco-Prussian War. Though the weather was miserably cold and snowy, the two women spent three days together in the picturesque, medieval city of Strasbourg. Lodging in local inns, cooking for themselves, and chatting endlessly by the fireside, Marie and Susan shared a delightful final visit, speaking "at very great length about all kinds of things." Of Susan, Marie wrote, "she looks great, has round red cheeks, so different from last fall. She has changed a bit in her opinions and in some nuances of her character. Just as we all change according to our circumstances." As for herself, Marie had already admitted, "You know, a great part of the changes I have undergone, my new positive outlook, has to do with the company of Miss Dimock.... I feel ten years younger than a year ago."

When it was time to say goodbye, Marie compared their parting to dying, worrying that "we will probably never see each other again."[133] As it turned out, Marie was more prescient than either of the two friends would have imagined.

After all her European farewells, Susan Dimock sailed across the Atlantic. The young doctor's last major visit before returning to the New England Hospital in Boston was her hometown of Washington, North Carolina, and her reasons were both personal and professional. The personal excuse was to see friends and especially her mother, who had worked tirelessly to help finance Susan's medical studies abroad. Susan was finally able to view first-hand how the ever-resourceful Mary Malvina had supplemented monies made through her teaching with two especially creative endeavors: using her backyard to breed mockingbirds as well as to grow lavish beds of lavender, which were sold to urban markets and Northern shops. Decades later, a local historian observed that Washingtonians still marveled at how Mary Malvina had sent daughter Susan "every penny she could scrape together."[134]

Equally important as visiting her mother, however, were Susan's professional aspirations. During her final months in Europe, the ambitious Dr. Dimock had sent a petition to her old friend and mentor, Dr. Solomon Satchwell, requesting that the all-male North Carolina Medical Society consider granting her membership. Satchwell proudly presented Susan's formal request at the Society's annual meeting in New Bern on May 17, 1872, followed by a letter from Susan's mother, several recommendations from prominent men of Boston, and some of Susan's medical papers from her Zurich days. The papers were written in German, which all present admitted they could not decipher. Dr. Edmund Burke Haywood of Raleigh heartily supported Satchwell's proposal to accept Susan in a "strong and telling" fifteen-minute speech, noting that "the day was upon us that this and all other societies were compelled to recognize female Physicians." Haywood's clear wish was that North Carolina would take the lead in this important tribute to women's accomplishments. Following some heated discussions, Society members narrowly approved accepting Dr. Susan Dimock as an honorary member, by a vote of 17 ayes to 15 nays.[135]

When Susan arrived in Washington in June of 1872, her friends, family, and neighbors were anxious to greet her and congratulate her for becoming the first female member of the North Carolina Medical Society. An article in *The Washington Echo* noted that despite some disgruntlement by those still dubious of women entering male professions like medicine, Susan's "modesty and lovely demeanor, while it silenced all cavils, won all hearts."[136]

Though buoyed by the honors and appreciation, Dr. Susan Dimock knew that the hour had finally come. It was time to return to Boston.

CHAPTER 4

Medical Practice

The year was 1872. Susan Dimock, freshly returned from her European medical studies, was now twenty-five years old. In the eyes of her Boston contemporaries, she was a *woman* now, "of medium size, with a clear, fresh complexion, a full but not very high forehead, gray eyes and dark hair." Her mode of dress was in the professional fashion of the day, generally black, and "neither remarked for display nor singularity." Her mouth was of particular curiosity to some, "expressing as much gentleness as firmness." And her voice—born in the South, molded in the North, and matured in Europe—was consistently described as soft and sweet. When Susan Dimock spoke, her articulation was clear, her delivery deliberately slow, and her vocal tones soothingly low.[1]

It was, one could argue, the perfect voice for a doctor determined to calm and comfort her ailing patients.

Eighteen seventy-two was also a leap year. And for Susan, a more perfect metaphor could not be found.

First came the advances in her professional life—which began soon after landing in Boston. "One of the pleasantest events of the year," announced Dr. Lucy Sewall in the New England Hospital's 1872 *Annual Report*, "has been the return from Europe of Dr. DIMOCK ... to take charge of the Hospital."[2] Sewall fairly reveled in her description of this momentous changing of the guard: as of August 20, 1872, Susan Dimock, M.D., honors graduate of the University of Zurich School of Medicine and a highly skilled surgeon, was replacing Annette Buckel, M.D., as the hospital's official resident physician.

The second leap Susan experienced that summer involved the demographic and topographic changes in the city of Boston itself. Since her departure four years earlier, the population of the "Hub of the Solar System" had expanded by almost thirty percent, topping off at more than 250,000 residents. Part of that growth was due to the annexation of the town of Dorchester and the area now known as Mattapan. Part was the continued influx of European immigrants—mostly Irish, but also

Germans, Scots, Russian and Polish Jews, and Swedes.[3] Part was the desire of more and more workers to relocate from rural Massachusetts into the city, to partake of its rich job opportunities. And part was the ongoing process of land-making necessitated by that ever-growing population. During Susan's absence, the newly created *terra firma* in the marshy old "Back Bay" had steadily inched westward, spawning new building construction along the way; Fort Hill had been levelled and used to create yet more land for development; and much of Boston's inner harbor had been filled and molded into a stretch of acreage now called Atlantic Avenue. In the course of 1872, Susan and her friends could watch railroad tracks being laid down that new harborside avenue, connecting the city's bustling northern and southern freight train terminals, near today's North and South Stations.

Attitudes in Boston had changed as well. By the time of Susan's return, mourning the casualties and costs of the Civil War and the subsequent Franco-Prussian War had largely been replaced by prayers for, and celebrations of, peace. The World's Peace Jubilee and International Music Festival, which ran for eighteen days in the early summer, was still the talk of the town. A mammoth Peace Jubilee Coliseum, temporarily erected in the recently filled Back Bay, had hosted tens of thousands of guests who thrilled to performances by talents like the African American Fisk University Jubilee Singers and the bands of London's Grenadier Guards. The *pièce de résistance* of the Peace Jubilee had been a 1,000-member orchestra and 20,000-voice chorus led by visiting Viennese composer and waltz-king, Johann Strauss. Having studied, lived in, and attended concerts in Vienna earlier that same year, Susan must have been delighted at the coincidence of her two worlds.

Susan encountered a quieter but equally powerful invocation of peace in Julia Ward Howe's newly created holiday, the "Mother's Day for Peace," now being celebrated every June 2 in Boston and beyond. It was the first official Mother's Day observed in America, and another feather in the cap of the illustrious Mrs. Howe.[4]

Still basking in fame for writing the popular "Battle Hymn of the Republic," Julia Ward Howe was one of dozens of strong women Susan now observed emerging as veritable forces of nature in Boston. During Susan's four-year absence, Louisa May Alcott had grown from a promising local short-story writer to an international literary star, thanks to the extraordinary success of *Little Women*. Ellen Swallow had become the first woman admitted to the new Massachusetts Institute of Technology. Lucy Stone had begun publishing the influential feminist *Woman's Journal*, buoyed by a powerful writing and editing staff that included Howe, Alcott, Mary Livermore, William Lloyd Garrison, and Stone's husband, Henry

—— THE ——
WOMAN'S JOURNAL.

A Weekly Newspaper, published every Saturday in Boston, devoted to the interests of women — to their educational, industrial, legal and political Equality, and especially to their right of Suffrage.

EDITORS:

LUCY STONE,
H. B. BLACKWELL,
ALICE STONE BLACKWELL.

Occasional Contributors:

JULIA WARD HOWE,   LOUISA M. ALCOTT,
MARY A. LIVERMORE,   MRS. H. M. T. CUTLER,
ELIZABETH STUART PHELPS.

SUSAN C. VOGL, Business Manager.

TERMS, $2.50 A YEAR.

$1.25 for six months, 50c. for three months, in advance, 5 cents for single copy. Half price to Libraries and Reading Rooms.

CLUB RATES:—Five copies one year, $10.00

BOSTON OFFICE: 3 PARK STREET,

WHERE COPIES ARE FOR SALE AND SUBSCRIPTIONS RECEIVED.

WOMAN SUFFRAGE TRACTS.

Thirty different woman suffrage tracts (sample copies) sent post paid for 10 cents. Address,

WOMAN'S JOURNAL, BOSTON, MASS.

When she returned to Boston in 1872, Susan joined the dozens of strong women who were then emerging as veritable forces of nature. Among them was Lucy Stone, whose influential feminist *Woman's Journal* was buoyed by powerful contributing writers like Julia Ward Howe, Louisa May Alcott, and Mary Livermore (image via Wikimedia Commons).

Blackwell. Numerous other women who had previously sharpened their skills fighting for the abolition of slavery or volunteering their services during the Civil War had now moved full-force into the cause of women's rights in general and into "woman suffrage" in particular.

As a result, Susan Dimock—now a pioneer as well, and arguably the best-educated, most skilled woman surgeon in the nation—found herself in exceptionally fine and eminently supportive female company.

Surely the most important leap forward in the summer of 1872—at least from Susan's perspective—was made by the New England Hospital itself, in its move from downtown Boston to the hills of Roxbury. "[T]he hospital was much changed since [Susan] left it," explained Ednah Dow Cheney, "for it was now established in a new and commodious building, in a high and airy situation, offering ample accommodations for an increased number both of students and patients."[5]

When Susan departed Boston for Zurich in 1868, the hospital and its dispensary had been packed with patients in a cluster of small chambers on Warrenton and Pleasant streets, near today's Charles Playhouse. During Susan's four years of study abroad, however, Dr. Zakrzewska, Dr. Sewall, Ednah Dow Cheney, and their colleagues had been fundraising and planning, with the goal of expanding and relocating their busy downtown medical facility. Thanks to a series of state-funded grants, several fundraising fairs, as well as benefits, subscriptions, and the kindness of strangers, the estimated cost of $100,000 for a new hospital seemed an attainable goal. The bulk of those dollars were contributed by women eager to help other women move out of the domestic sphere and into the male-dominated public sphere. Some of the female donors were professionals who earned their own money, while others gifted funds from husbands or family inheritances.

Collecting $100,000—a sum comparable to more than two million dollars today—was no easy task. If there was any doubt that the huge financial burden of building a new hospital could be met, however, it was quelled by two exceptionally large donations: bequests from Mrs. Robert Gould Shaw, and the estate of an eccentric Boston heiress known as Miss Nabby Joy.[6] Mrs. Shaw's gift was not surprising, since her wealthy and socially progressive family had long supported the work of the New England Hospital. Less predictable was the money from the late Miss Joy, who had simply instructed the executors of her will to distribute her sizeable fortune among several dozen different Boston charities and institutions, of which the New England Hospital was one. Coupled with a $40,000 mortgage and the impending sale of their old Warrenton Street property for $35,000, these two women's gifts enabled the hospital to move to a newly constructed permanent home in the "Boston Highlands" in 1872.[7]

"At the time the new location was considered quite out in the country," remembered Dr. Emma Call years later.[8] Indeed, the Boston Highlands were part of the old town of Roxbury, which Boston had annexed in 1868. Though some argued that location was too lengthy a horsecar or train ride from Boston's central district, others insisted that the benefits of the site far outweighed the distance. Land, of course, was much cheaper in Roxbury. A wealthier clientele lived nearby, which the doctors hoped might buoy the hospital's ever-struggling finances. But equally important to the women doctors was the Roxbury setting: wide open spaces, gently rolling hillsides, abundant trees, soothing country breezes, and plentiful sunlight were simply not available in the dirty, congested, overbuilt streets of downtown Boston.

Since the physicians believed that air, sunlight, natural surroundings, and open space were vital for healing their female patients, they sought those elements both in the hospital's new site and in the design and construction of its buildings. Medical science in the 1870s had not yet outgrown the notion that "miasmas"—easily transmitted, particle-laden clouds of noxious, foul-smelling "bad air"—could be mitigated if such poisonous vapors were regularly replaced by clean, fresh air.[9] (Even when germ theory finally prevailed in the 1890s, it was found that ridding rooms of bad odors often eliminated bacteria as well.)

Assisted by the visions of Building Committee chair George Bond, Committee treasurer Samuel May, and the prestigious architectural firm of Cummings and Sears,[10] the women doctors had finally met the major needs they had outlined together back in 1870: more grounds for the hospital campus, private rooms and a parlor for their patients, more space for every department, an appropriate and separate Children's Ward, and an opportunity to house and teach more students. The New England Hospital still was, after all, "the only place in New England where practical experience for medical women could be obtained."[11]

Wandering through the gently sloping Roxbury campus in the summer of 1872, Susan Dimock could observe first-hand the results of such thoughtful planning by her medical colleagues.

Most visually striking was the campus' central edifice, an imposing red-brick structure set regally on the edge of Codman Street. Resting on a craggy Roxbury Puddingstone foundation, this picturesque medical and administration building was designed in the popular High Victorian Gothic style of the day, with contrasting stone stringcourses, arched window heads, multi-colored roof slates, and a flurry of turrets and dormers. Open air porches wrapped around parts of the exterior on all three floors. Windows were plentiful and large, and the hallways wide. Each of the hospital's spacious, well-ventilated, sun-filled wards had its own open

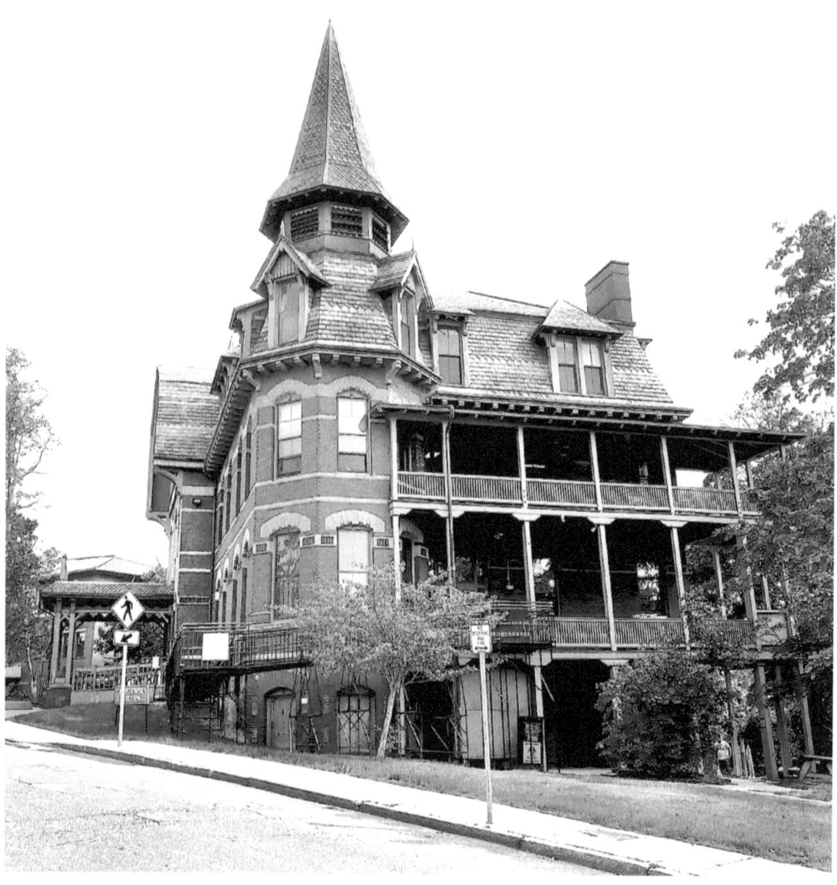

Resting on a craggy Roxbury Puddingstone foundation, the New England Hospital's picturesque medical and administration building was designed in the popular High Victorian Gothic style of the day, with contrasting stone stringcourses, arched window heads, multi-colored roof slates, and a flurry of turrets and dormers. Today it is known as The Z Building (photograph © the author)

fireplace, replete with wood or marble mantels. As a result, the chambers seemed more "like the rooms of a private home" than bleak hospital wards.[12] Especially exciting, both to the doctors and the patients, was the inclusion of a Children's Ward in the upper story of the main building—a ward that the old downtown hospital never had room to accommodate.

Despite those homey elements, Susan could easily see that the building's interior was as simple as the exterior was ornate. In an effort to avoid dust, dirt, and that infectious miasmic air, the women doctors had made a deliberate effort to avoid rugs, ornamentation, and filth-collecting crevices.[13] An optimum healing environment was foremost in their minds. When Susan arrived, many of the rooms were also still quite bare—lacking all the beds, chairs, tables, cabinets, and other necessities required. Lucy Stone's *Woman's Journal*—the Boston-based suffragist paper that regularly reported on and supported the hospital's efforts—announced that this void would soon be filled, since, "[s]undry benevolent individuals and various churches have undertaken a greater part of [the New England Hospital's] required furnishing."[14]

In addition, the layout and design of the new hospital's inside space was distinctly different from other hospitals Susan had frequented. The architects had used the "pavilion plan" popular in mid–nineteenth-century French and English hospitals—designs that used sunlight and open spaces to ward off miasma—but added much more privacy. "The excellence of the interior arrangements," explained Alice Crosby, "especially of the wards and the nurses' rooms, which differ from those of any hospital known to the committee, is due to the Women Physicians,—who having learned from long experience the needs of their patients, have striven to meet them by arrangements at once simple and ingenious."[15] The hospital's 1872 Annual Report, for example, boasted that "each [medical] ward consists of two rooms, one for two beds and one for four, with a nurse's room between them. The nurse can thus often have the benefit of the solitude and quiet of her own room, and yet be in such close neighborhood to her patients, that nothing can escape her notice."[16]

Being a medical facility that put the needs of women and children first, the New England Hospital placed a special emphasis on helping maternity patients. Susan had learned in her student days, both in Boston and abroad, that the scourge of maternity wards worldwide was puerperal, or childbirth, fever. She had even written her Zurich graduation thesis on the topic. As early as 1843, the medical community in Boston had been warned by their own Dr. Oliver Wendell Holmes that doctors themselves might be playing a part in spreading the disease as they moved, unsterilized, from patient to patient. Many local doctors were also aware that, in 1860, Louis Pasteur had convincingly argued that not miasmas, but microbial chains of streptococci were the culprit behind childbirth fever—and that women injured in labor were particularly susceptible to infection.[17]

While some accepted and many others rejected those new theories, they were all handed a reality check with the crisis at Boston Lying-In, a competitor of the New England Hospital that also specialized in maternity patients. The term "lying-in" originally referred to the practice of patients resting in bed for an extended period of time following childbirth; it later came to mean "childbirth" in general. The catastrophe at hand: Boston Lying-In was forced to close its doors for sixteen years, from 1856

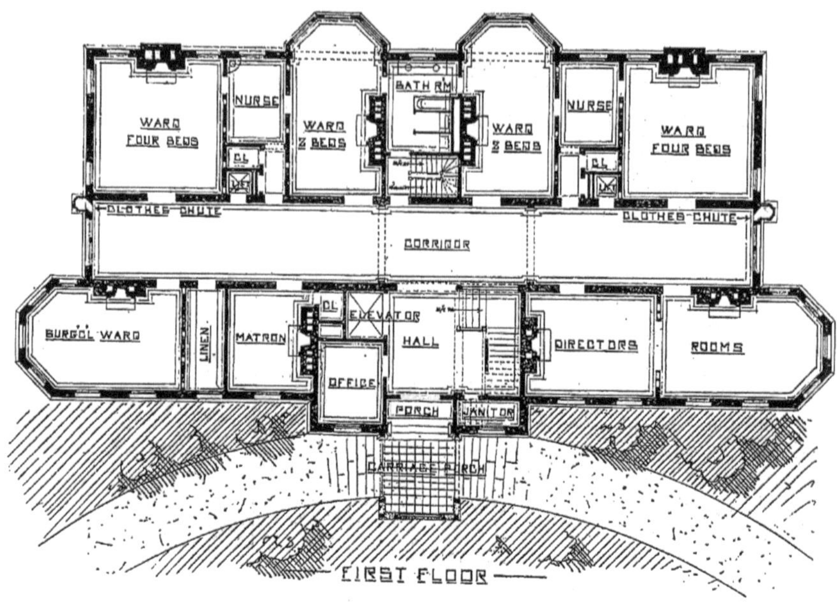

At the 1876 Philadelphia World's Fair, the Boston-based architectural team of Cummings & Sears were honored for the New England Hospital's "well-studied design, securing economy of service, good distribution of various parts, good ventilation, and cheerful accommodation" (New England Hospital for Women and Children Records, Sophia Smith Collection, Smith College, Northampton, Massachusetts; used by permission of the Dimock Center, Roxbury, Massachusetts).

to 1872, because it simply could not contain recurring epidemics of childbirth fever. The New England Hospital's founder, Dr. Marie Zakrzewska, was sobered by the news. As a result, she had often recommended that her patients deliver their babies at home rather than in the dangerous confines of a hospital, where such fevers were known to spread with alarming and deadly speed. "The humblest home," Dr. Zak warned, "is safer than the best hospital."[18]

In her first campus tour, Susan Dimock must have been delighted to discover that the threat of puerperal fever had been considered in the hospital's accommodations. The Maternity Cottage was built as a separate, two-story frame structure, deliberately set away from and behind the main red-brick Victorian building. That location in itself protected patients in the central hospital from possible exposure to the fever. To avoid contagion within the Maternity Cottage itself, the building was designed with two identical floors, allowing one to be actively used should the other become contaminated and require cleansing and airing. Both floors had multiple chambers—separate rooms for labor, delivery, and patient recovery.[19] And while the Maternity Cottage offered just twelve beds, the much larger central building was built to accommodate seventy.

As Susan finished her exploration of the Roxbury campus, she passed by and over the foundations of a well-equipped, self-sufficient, modern community: there was a sturdy horse shed to house the veteran doctors' four-legged transportation, a web of underground drainage systems, a large cistern for water storage, as well as pumps and pipes leading in from Lake Cochituate in Natick, the source of Boston's public water supply since 1848.[20]

What she did not find in the Roxbury complex was a replacement for the hospital's downtown Dispensary. The women doctors knew that their poorest and neediest patients lived not in the rambling meadows of pastoral Roxbury, but in the overcrowded slums of Boston's inner city. "A most important part of the work of the New England Hospital has always been the Dispensary, where medical advice and medicines are given to the poor within the city limits," read a souvenir booklet for one of the hospital's fundraising fairs. Knowing that their Dispensary was considered "one of the most beneficent charities for suffering women and their children,"[21] the doctors balked at making these people travel such a distance. In-town patients would have been forced to walk for hours, or to pay to board horse-cars on the Forest Hills and Egleston line or trains on the Providence Railroad.[22]

As a result, the hospital's primary Dispensary stayed where it was needed, in a rented house at 315 Tremont Street, on the corner of Tremont and Pleasant. Susan would soon know it well, and commute from Roxbury to work there every Tuesday and Friday.[23]

All in all, Susan must have been pleased with the giant leap forward made by her colleagues, mentors, and friends. Now it was time for Dr. Dimock, resident physician and chief surgeon of the New England Hospital for Women and Children, to get to work.

Though the official "opening day" for the New England Hospital in Roxbury was October 29, 1872, Susan Dimock had much to accomplish from the moment she officially joined the staff, a full nine weeks before that formal dedication.

First in order was understanding the new hospital's chain of command and division of labor. As resident physician and chief surgeon, Susan was expected to oversee the hospital's daily operations, following the direction of the attending physicians, doctors Marie Zakrzewska and Lucy Sewall. In addition to carrying out medical directives from the attendings, Susan was charged with performing surgeries, monitoring patients, supervising interns, training nursing students, and contacting the attendings in the case of emergency.

Susan was also scheduled to work at the hospital's downtown dispensary twice a week, as one of four rotating dispensary physicians.[24] If she needed medical advice in either of those locations, she had access to the wisdom and experience of the hospital's official Consulting Physicians—Walter Channing, Henry Bowditch, Edward Jarvis, and Samuel Cabot. All four of these men were well-respected, highly educated, and Harvard-affiliated Boston doctors who actively supported the cause of women in medicine in general and the New England Hospital in particular.

Unlike the attending physicians, Susan was required to actually *live* at the hospital. Her private parlor, tucked between the hospital wards, saved her the expense of outside accommodations. More importantly, it enabled her to tend to her professional duties both day and night. Because the hospital was far from a money-making enterprise, the resident physician was the only paid member of the medical staff. Her monetary compensation, however, was nominal by any standard: the yearly salary paid to Dr. Susan Dimock, then the best-trained female surgeon in America, was $300 a year. During that same period, the *lowest* paid female teacher in the Boston public schools earned $600 per academic year, while the Mayor of Boston and the *chef de cuisine* at the Parker House hotel—both, of course, men—were paid a whopping $5,000 per annum each.[25]

Susan Dimock was both a pragmatist and an overachiever. Wanting to pay off her medical school loans as quickly as possible, she opened her own medical practice in downtown Boston. Susan's arrangement was hardly unique: in the nineteenth century, it was standard for physicians, both male and female, to donate their professional services to charity hospitals, then make their real living though private medical offices and home visits, where they catered to a more affluent clientele.

For Susan, the medical formula was simple: most afternoons, after finishing her multitudinous hospital duties in Roxbury or the downtown Dispensary, she would run off to her office at 8 Park Square to use her medical skills with patients of far more substantial means than those at the New England Hospital. The financial result was fairly astonishing: she was able to liquidate her educational loans in under three years. Her hometown North Carolina newspaper, *The Washington Echo*, bragged that the town's favorite daughter was not only saving lives in the New England Hospital, but—thanks to her private practice—"was rapidly making a fortune."[26]

Given that exhausting, round-the-clock schedule, it was a good thing that peers characterized Susan as "a young woman of energy, enthusiasm, and attractive presence."[27] She would need all those traits, and more, to keep up her pace—and her penchant for perfection.

Susan Dimock's first physical assignment was actually "moving" the hospital, including every*thing* and every person in it. Along with colleagues and a crew of volunteers, the young doctor spent much of the late summer of 1872 relocating equipment, furnishings, and patients from downtown Boston to the Roxbury highlands. The number of patients to be transplanted, however, turned out to be smaller than expected. Susan learned that a late spring epidemic of puerperal fever had claimed the lives of four of the New England Hospital's maternity patients and forced administrators to shutter their lying-in wards. To compensate for the loss of space, the doctors and their interns had opted to visit many of the patients in their homes instead.[28] Moreover, the Roxbury hospital had been near enough to completion that physicians were able to relocate some of their downtown patients into the new, unfinished, and sparsely furnished facility as early as the spring. With the aid of Susan and others, that three-mile move—presumably done with horsecars, trains, and horse-drawn wagons and carriages—was completed by mid–September.

At the same time, Susan was tasked with reorganizing and professionalizing the hospital's Training School for Nurses. Though Dr. Marie Zakrzewska had initiated some education for nurses soon after founding the hospital in 1862, the regimen she instituted was too short, too superficial, and too inconsistent to produce quality results. Susan Dimock vowed to change all that. While studying and traveling in Europe, she had met the legendary Florence Nightingale, observed Nightingale's pioneering nursing school in London, and visited the Protestant Deaconesses in Kaiserswerth, Germany, who had introduced a young Nightingale to both theology and nursing skills. Firmly believing that "favorable surgical outcomes rested largely on the patient's postoperative nursing care,"[29] and inspired by the European models she had witnessed, Susan immediately began designing a lengthier and more demanding nursing program for what was to become America's First Professional Nurses Training School.

What she needed, of course, were students on whom to test her ideas.

Part of Susan's challenge was convincing a doubting populace that nursing in America could become an honorable profession, rather than what many saw as undesirable, menial work, and "a trade of last resort for middle-aged spinsters and impecunious widows."[30] The negative image was not helped by Bellevue Hospital in New York City, where imprisoned prostitutes were given the option of becoming nurses or remaining in jail.

Dr. Alfred Worcester, a physician at the Boston-Lying-in Hospital, recalled Dimock's first efforts at enticing a higher level of student into her school. "Forty years ago, I remember a charming visitor at our [Waltham] home, Dr. Susan Dimock, trying to persuade my mother to allow one of my older sisters to enter her training school for nurses, which she was about to start at the New England Hospital for Women and Children. This was the earliest American school for nurses. My mother's objections were emphatic," continued Worcester. "Contrary to Dr. Dimock's insistence that such a school and such a career was entirely suitable for well-educated young women, my mother maintained that nursing, excepting of course volunteer neighbor nursing, could properly be undertaken only by mature women who must in some way work for their living. To her the idea of a daughter leaving her parents' home for such a calling was intolerable...."

"I remember feeling at the time that Dr. Dimock somehow was right in her contentions," added Worcester. "And I shall never forget her earnestness and her disappointment as I drove off with her to the railroad station."[31]

As ever, Susan Dimock persisted. And her first applicant appeared shortly after the young doctor's official residency began. On September 1, 1872, a thirty-one-year-old woman named Linda Richards, discouraged by some less-than-stellar experiences at Boston City Hospital, appeared on the doorstep of the New England Hospital on Codman Street, Roxbury. Having heard that a serious nursing school was about to open, she had sent in an application weeks earlier, then been told to stop by that day.

"I was shown into the reception room by a maid who said, 'You are to wait here till the doctor comes to see you,'" remembered Richards years later. "I had not long to wait till a small, very dignified and very pleasant little lady appeared and introduced herself as Dr. Dimock, saying to me, 'You are Miss Richards, I suppose.'" Richards nervously confirmed her identity, then asked, "May I enroll now as a student nurse in this hospital?" Susan placed a chair near Richards, requested the applicant sit beside her, then proceeded to ask several questions. Within a short time, the doctor smiled warmly and offered, "In that case, you are my first student!" Susan finished the conversation by delineating the duties and qualifications of a good nurse, emphasizing "gentleness and kindness, earnestness and promptness."[32]

Decades later, Richards recalled that day in great detail. "When [Dr. Dimock] had ended her little talk, which left an impression on me which has followed me all these long years since that time, she went with me upstairs and spoke to a nurse who came to us. After introducing me she said, 'This is our first nurse to enter the training school.'" One of the Hospital's veteran nurses took Richards to her room, prepared her for duty, then led her into a ward as her assistant. "To say that the nurse greeted me cordially or kindly, would be stating an untruth," Richards politely recounted. "When has one ever seen old hospital nurses cordial to pupils entering the training schools? ... [T]he majority of old school nurses ... were very jealous of those who, they felt, would supplant them and who they, in their own hearts, knew would care much better for the sick under their care."[33]

The tensions between old-school and new-school nurses would not end anytime soon. But Susan, determined to improve, legitimize, and modernize the profession to European standards, forged ahead. When not assisting old-school nurses with incoming cases, Linda Richards also helped Susan move even more patients from downtown Boston to the Roxbury hills. Thankfully,

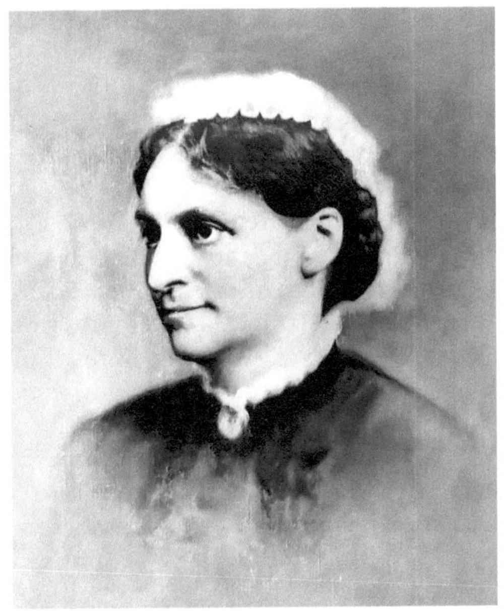

Linda Richards (1841–1930) was the first student to enroll in and graduate from Susan Dimock's pioneering nursing program at the NEHWC. Heralded as "America's First Trained Nurse" and the "American Florence Nightingale," Richards directed, established, or inspired high-quality nurses' training programs around the world (used by permission of the Dimock Center, Roxbury, Massachusetts).

over those first two weeks of September 1872, four more women entered the hospital's new nursing program.

With a full class of five, training began in earnest.

The year-long nursing program Susan Dimock instituted—which replaced Dr. Zak's six-month course—was divided into four periods. Her hope was that three months each spent in the medical, surgical, and maternity wards, then another dedicated to "night nursing," would qualify the students for every situation possible.[34] There were no textbooks and no exams. There were also no uniforms required—or even available—so students were asked to purchase and wear washable calico dresses and felt slippers. Rather than paying for their education, they were offered an allowance of one to four dollars per week, depending on how the hospital valued their services.[35]

When training began, the hospital had three active floors in the main building, housing seventy-five patients, with two to a room. The nurses were considered the lowest rung on the ladder—save, perhaps, for the maids and cleaning ladies—being outranked by the all-female medical students, the female resident physician, the female attending physicians, and the male consulting physicians. Like Susan Dimock, the nurses were expected to live, sleep, and eat at the hospital. Soon after training began, the New England Hospital's five novice nursing students realized that Susan, though inspired by Florence Nightingale, had instituted a system with a few significant differences from the Nightingale Method. Like Nightingale, Susan's students were given moral and character training. Unlike Nightingale, Susan's nursing students were trained by a physician rather than by a head nurse; they lived among their patients instead of in a separate nurses' building; and, perhaps most importantly, in Dr. Susan Dimock's world, nursing students were considered not simply to be students, but to be *both* students and workers.

The result was, at first, something short of disastrous.

As student Linda Richards recalled, "Our days were not eight hours; they were nearer twice eight. We rose at 5.30 a.m. and left the wards at 9 p.m. to go to our beds, which were in little rooms between the wards. Each nurse took care of her ward of six patients both day and night. Many a time I have got up nine times in the night; often I did not get to sleep before the next call came."[36] Richards and her fellow students had no evenings out, no Sundays off, and no down time for recreation or study. Every other week they were given one afternoon off, but only from 2:00 to 5:00 p.m.

Surely, the nursing students respected Susan and acknowledged that she "acted from conviction and principle rather than from impulse or theory." And they were charmed by her personality, which was generally described as "very winning, and ... personally agreeable to all." But Susan's honorable principles, winning personality, ladylike habits, "dainty freshness," and her slow, distinct speech, "which gave an impression ... of almost childlike simplicity,"[37] belied a fact that the students learned all too soon: since Susan Dimock was accustomed to laboring day and night, she expected the same from her nursing students—her *de facto* "workers." Their beloved resident physician, one observer mused, "ruled her hospital like a Napoleon."[38]

Predictably, the nursing students became stressed beyond measure.

Knowing that fatigue among her fellow nursing students had become dangerously acute—and that it adversely affected patient care—Linda Richards approached Susan directly. Susan clearly heard the complaint and began to make changes. "After the first six months a night nurse [one of the pupil nurses] was employed, and the day nurses were allowed to go to bed and to sleep," explained a much-relieved Richards. With a new, workable rotation plan in place, life improved for everyone at the hospital. "We soon had a second class of nurses also," added Richards, "and when I came away at the end of the year we had seventeen nurses in the school, instead of the five when the school opened."[39]

Determined to improve the nurses' training program even further, Susan Dimock began organizing formal lectures for her five original students. Set to begin in January of 1873, the talks were designed to be practical, plain, and filled with valuable information about "the care to be used by the nurse in the treatment of surgical cases, and in the minor accidents which do not call for the attendance of a professional surgeon."[40] Three of the lectures were to be given by Susan herself, while other hospital physicians agreed to deliver the remaining nine. Lecture topics ranged from Dr. Dimock speaking about "Surgical Nursing" and Dr. Emma Call discussing "The Use of Disinfectants to Prevent Contagion" to Dr. Marie Zakrzewska on the "Position and Manners of Nurses in Families."[41]

While all the lectures were appreciated, apparently Susan's were particularly memorable. Susan's manner in the lecture-room was described as "quiet, simple, and self-sustained … her thought was clear and her language appropriate, and she illustrated her subject very plainly and forcibly."[42] Though part of Susan's appeal was those easily digestible deliveries, part was surely due to the innovative ideas she introduced to her Boston audiences. Inspired by her years of study in Europe, the young doctor presented new implements and methodologies to both her students and colleagues. Prominent among the instruments she brought back to Boston were foot-long thermometers, which tucked under the armpit and were the first clinical gauges for measuring patient temperature ever used in the hospital. Susan also initiated—and fiercely advocated—the creation of daily temperature charts. Her nursing students would soon be up every night, hand-drawing grids onto sheets of blank paper, to be used as fever charts the following day. According to Dr. Emma Call, "The use of the thermometer and keeping of the charts, may be considered one of the most important steps toward solving the problem of puerperal infection, since before then there had been no accurate means of estimating the amount of constitutional disturbance in such cases."[43]

Perhaps to fill the room, and certainly to fill a need, the decision was made to open Susan's nursing lecture series to outsiders—to nurses not attending the school, to area hospital directors, as well as to other interested women. "The attendance was very large," remembered Alice Crosby, "many young girls coming to benefit by the freely offered instruction." As it turned out, Susan's lecture series became so popular that the following year it was agreed to issue tickets in advance.[44] "I attended those,"

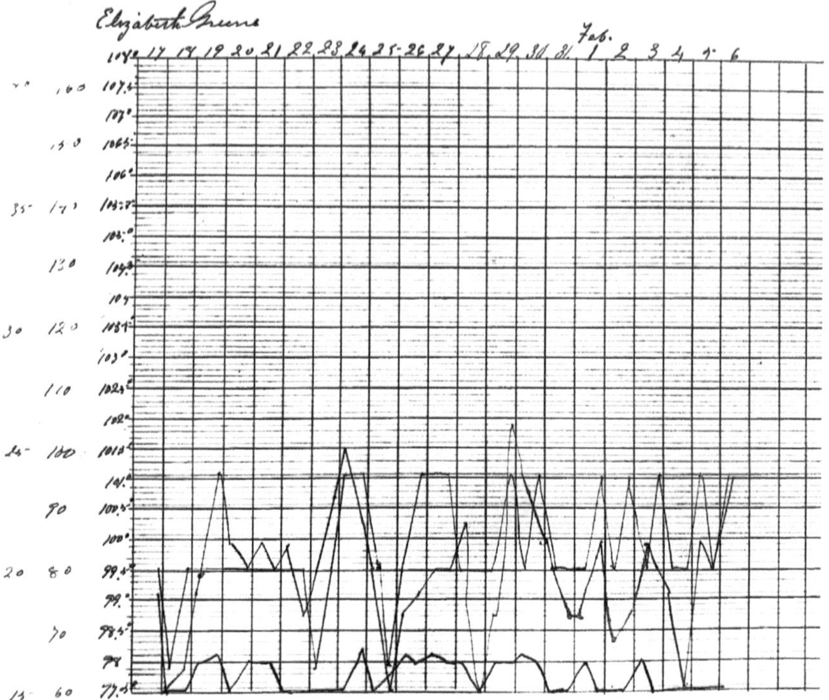

Susan Dimock ushered in the first year of using thermometers to keep regular temperature charts at the New England Hospital. The daily graphs—hand-drawn by her students every night after evening rounds—tracked patient wellness and had an immediate impact on the scourge of maternity wards worldwide: the dreaded puerperal fever (New England Hospital for Women and Children, Records of Medical Wards and Surgical Wards, Boston Medical Library in the Francis A. Countway Library of Medicine, Harvard University, Boston, Massachusetts; used by permission of the Dimock Center, Roxbury, Massachusetts).

recalled Susan Dimock's friend Lilian Freeman Clarke, "and a sentence which closed one lecture made a strong impression on me. With earnestness which came from deep and strong feeling, [Dr. Dimock] said: 'Think that every patient is your sister. Imagine that you see your *own sister* in that bed before you; and treat her in every respect as you would like your own sister to be treated.'"[45]

Exactly a year after the Nurses Training School made its debut, Susan's first student, Linda Richards, graduated from the New England Hospital's pioneering program. Heralded to this day as "America's First Trained Nurse" and the "American Florence Nightingale," Richards went on to become an iconic figure who directed, established, or inspired high-quality nurses' training programs around the world, from Boston, Philadelphia, and New York to Michigan, Connecticut, and even Kyoto, Japan. Richards' graduation, unfortunately, was not one of Dr. Susan Dimock's finest moments. As the story is told, Richards was called to Susan's office without the slightest notion why. When she entered the room, Susan reached into her desk drawer, grabbed a document, then handed Richards a scroll of white paper with black script and an embossed golden seal. "What is it?" Richards asked. "Your diploma," the physician replied. The pair shook hands, and Richards returned to her patients, not quite realizing what had just transpired.[46] Richards' diploma is now in the collections of the Smithsonian Institution.

Though the nurses training program was up and running by the late summer of 1872, the New England Hospital for Women and Children had not yet celebrated its formal dedication and opening. The long-scheduled date for that gala was October 29, 1872, coinciding with the hospital's annual meeting. But sadly, that highly anticipated and widely publicized event had to be postponed.

Because two weeks before the Roxbury hospital's dedication, the city of Boston ground to an unexpected halt.

The troubles started with the horses.

No one would have guessed that an outbreak of equine influenza reported in Canada on October 1, 1872, would affect the city of Boston only two weeks later. But it did. In 1872, horses were the lifeblood of America's transportation systems. Moreover, city-dwellers were as dependent on horsepower as their country cousins. In cities, horses were mounted as individual steeds and employed to tow everything from modest work carts, carriages, and wagons to large streetcars, canal boats, and firetrucks. Now, with hundreds upon thousands of these horses starting to develop flu symptoms—fever, coughing, weakness, depression, loss of appetite, and sometimes even death—both rural and urban populations became quickly immobilized. And with an incubation period of no more than three days, the equine influenza spread swiftly southward from Canada, eventually affecting some seventy-five percent of America's horse population.

By the middle of October 1872, what came to be called "The Great Epizootic" had overrun much of New England. In Boston, freight sat idly on the docks, mail and groceries went undelivered, and the web of inlaid metal tracks crisscrossing downtown streets fell quiet, since the city's trolleys were all pulled by horses. As a result, Bostonians took to their bricked, cobblestoned, and packed-earth roads on foot, and the city's doctors—accustomed to taking their horse-drawn rigs to visit patients near and far—followed suit. A reporter for *The Boston Transcript* did see a medical upside to this lack of transportation: "The streets and stores are … quite full, … gay with the prevailing colors of feminine apparel.… Doubtless the compulsory exercise will prove beneficial to the health of the majority of the fair pedestrians, as well as to that of the men."[47]

With transportation at a standstill—and the new hospital so far from the city center—Dr. Zak, Dr. Dimock, and the other women of the New England Hospital for Women and Children agreed to postpone the October 29 dedication of their Roxbury campus for "a fortnight," due to "the absolute impossibility of conveying our friends to the spot."[48] Two weeks, after all, was the time authorities predicted it would take for many individual horses to recover from their worst flu symptoms.

What the doctors didn't count on was another "trouble" on the heels of this one. And it proved to be a far bigger calamity than they could ever have imagined.

"The Great Fire of 1872" wasn't the first to devastate large segments of Boston, or even the first Boston blaze to merit the title of "great." But it was, as it turned out, the largest and most destructive conflagration in the city's history. The infamous fire began on the evening of Saturday, November 9, presumably sparked by the basement boiler of a dry goods store and hoop-skirt factory on the corner of Summer and Kingston streets. By 7:24 p.m., when the first alarm was turned in by a passerby at firebox 52 on Summer Street, it was too late. Flames had already leapt across Summer to Otis Street, charring roofs, exploding windows, and sending off sheets of flame. From there, as the wind-fueled destruction swept northeast and east, fiery flashes and meteor-like granite blocks sailed from mansard roof to mansard roof, undaunted by the firefighters and fire engines that came in from neighboring towns and states. Previous troubles, of course, compounded current troubles: many of the heavy fire engines had to be hand-hauled by teams of men, since their horses were still disabled with the equine flu.[49]

From the elevated slopes of Roxbury, Susan Dimock and her colleagues could easily hear the booming explosions and watch flames shooting into the billowing smoke-clouds above the cityscape throughout the night. A rosy glow could reportedly be spotted ninety miles away at sea, and as far north as Portland, Maine.[50] Though undoubtedly relieved that their new hospital was far from the line of fire, the doctors were less confident about their vulnerable downtown Dispensary. Happily, when the embers cooled, it turned out that the New England Hospital's Dispensary on Tremont Street was more than four blocks from the southernmost edge of the fire.

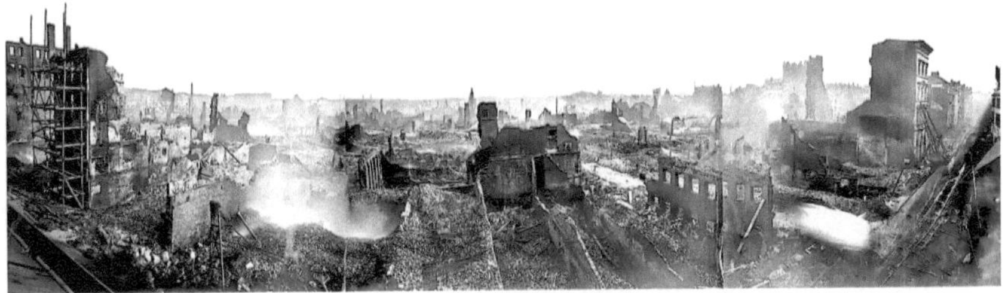

Among the troubles encountered by the New England Hospital as it began its move to a new location was the Great Fire of 1872, the largest and most destructive conflagration in the city's history. The blaze consumed some 65 acres and 776 buildings in downtown Boston, causing an estimated $60 to $75 million in damage, comparable to $1.4 to $1.7 billion today (Boston Fire from Washington & Bromfield, panoramic by John Adams Whipple, 1872; image via Wikimedia Commons).

Though the bulk of downtown Boston was saved, the devastation was astonishing: most of the city blocks from Washington Street down to Boston Harbor, and from Summer Street to the backside of State Street had been scorched into an unrecognizable skeletal mass of melted granite and mounds of rubble. Beloved Boston physician and poet Oliver Wendell Holmes was driven to verse as he viewed the aftermath:

> *The cloud still hovers overhead,*
> *And still the midnight sky is red;*
> *As the lost wanderer strays alone*
> *To seek the place he called his own,*
> *His devious footprints sadly tell*
> *How changed the pathways known so well;*
> *The scene, how new! The tale, how old*
> *Ere yet the ashes have grown cold!*[51]

Dazed citizen-survivors scattered throughout the area ranged from firefighters, armed guards, and volunteers to curious crowds and pilfering opportunists. In the end, the Great Boston Fire of 1872 consumed some 65 acres and 776 buildings, causing an estimated $60 to $75 million in damage, comparable to $1.4 to $1.7 billion today. Though thousands of workers—mostly women—were left jobless by the blaze, only a merciful handful were left homeless or dead.[52]

Susan Dimock had experienced terrible town fires before, and at a much closer range. Only eight years earlier, shortly before her seventeenth birthday, her North Carolina hometown had suffered two devastating blazes in as many weeks. During the second conflagration, the horror must have been palpable as she lost her entire neighborhood and, even worse, the Dimock family business and home. Moreover, the periodic booms she heard during the Boston fire—as windows exploded outward and fire-fighters blew up buildings—sounded much like the cannon balls that had ricocheted through her hometown when Confederate and Union troops clashed during the war. If such recollections flashed in Susan Dimock's mind in November of 1872, there was little time to dwell on nightmares. She and the rest of the hospital staff were confronting more immediate issues.

First, of course, was ascertaining if there were any women needing medical assistance in the aftermath of the Boston fire. Second was deciding whether or not to postpone, yet again, the formal dedication of the new hospital in Roxbury. Third was dealing with the discovery that "[t]he great fire of November destroyed a part of our [Annual] Report which was already in type." When that Annual Report of 1872 was finally published, it acknowledged that the Great Fire had completely destroyed the downtown office of their Building Committee chair, Mr. George W. Bond, including numerous bills and papers from his committee. "The confusion and hindrance consequent," they concluded, "has much delayed this Report. The same fire subjects us to heavy expense in repaying lost insurance and in paying assessments, the extent of which is not yet known."[53]

Once assured that their downtown patients had been cared for, New England Hospital officials decided to carry on with their Roxbury dedication as scheduled. "We hesitated to go on with our simple services," the women reasoned, "but we felt as if it were one of those truly holy occasions in which we could unite with thankfulness of heart, however deep was our sadness. The very pressure of the times, tending to throw so many women out of employment and to bring on sickness and want where it was not known before, made us feel how precious might become the house of refuge which we were opening for the suffering and needy."[54]

Hence, on November 12, 1872, "under the shadow" of the Boston fire, the New England Hospital for Women and Children finally held the formal rituals for their new Roxbury facility. The hospital's resident physician, Dr. Susan Dimock, apparently charmed the crowds with what was described as "a graceful and beautiful address." "She appeared so attractive and winning while speaking," one observer noted, "that she won her way into many hearts."[55]

Meanwhile, pundits were surveying the devastating remains of Boston's downtown. "Talk of the ruins of Pompeii and Palmyra!" wrote veteran abolitionist William Lloyd Garrison, "You should see those of our city. I wander among them awe-stricken and overwhelmed, as though they were a thousand years old, and beyond all hope of a reconstruction of those magnificent buildings which seemed to have been built to endure for many generations." Others disagreed with Garrison's grim analysis.

"Boston will build itself up better than before," predicted suffragist leader Lucy Stone in *The Woman's Journal* only a week after the fire. "Its crooked ways will be made straight, and a new tide of sympathy will set towards it, because it has suffered."[56]

As it turned out, Lucy Stone was right. Within weeks, rubble from the gutted and shattered structures was starting to be plowed, consolidated, and dumped into Boston Harbor, to serve as fill under the new Atlantic Avenue. New roads were laid, both straighter and wider than the colonial ones they replaced. In the meantime, numerous business owners found they had enough insurance to begin the rebuilding process straight away. Moreover, some of the buildings lost—like the old Trinity Church on Summer Street—were soon replaced by gems like the architecturally exquisite *new* Trinity Church that architect H.H. Richardson built in what came to be called Art Square, today's Copley Square.

As the city of Boston dove into the work of recovery, the women of the New England Hospital focused on fundraising. Though the Roxbury campus was now formally open and operative, they knew that much remained to be done. And since the hospital had always depended on fundraising fairs as an important means of support, December of 1872 initially seemed a perfect time to hold another such public event. The venue they chose was Horticultural Hall on Tremont Street, a convenient downtown location for holiday shoppers.

Although the women assumed they would raise money "for the completion and support of the Hospital" through the sale of innumerable Christmas gifts, the results were ultimately disappointing.[57] One reason for their relative lack of success may have been the unusually stormy weather that week and the record cold temperatures that plagued Boston all that winter. But much more likely a culprit was the Great Fire itself. "[T]he repeated disasters of the time rendered the collection of funds a much more trying and difficult labor than usual," they admitted. "[I]t was not easy to go to men whose warehouses and offices were in ashes, or to women who had lost their investments…, and ask them to give us the money that we needed to complete our building and to carry on our work." Though the fair's attendance seemed low compared to previous ventures, the group was able to net $5,300—comparable to $122,000 in 2022 dollars.[58]

Having survived the Great Epizootic and the Great Fire, Susan Dimock and her colleagues at the hospital found themselves facing yet another challenge, this one all too familiar. The problem: a small, yet irritatingly vocal, coterie of male doctors who disapproved of women studying or practicing medicine. And curiously, two of the most notorious enemies actually *worked at or consulted for* the New England Hospital for Women and Children.

The first was Dr. Horatio Robinson Storer, in many ways the quintessential Boston-born and -bred male physician. After attending the classic Brahmin triumvirate—Boston Latin School, Harvard College, and Harvard Medical School—he studied abroad for a year, then returned home to open his own practice, specializing in obstetrics and gynecology. During the 1860s, he also founded the first medical society and first medical journal devoted exclusively to gynecology. With such female-centered medical experience and interests, Dr. Storer seemed a perfect match for the fledgling New England Hospital for Women and Children; and indeed, he had willingly become the first male doctor on their staff, due to the lack of any female gynecologists to fill the position. The appointment was undoubtedly a dream come true for Storer, guaranteeing him an unlimited number of women on whom to practice his skills.

Susan Dimock had briefly crossed paths with Dr. Storer back in 1866, when she first became a student at the hospital. That year, however, Susan's friend and mentor, Dr. Lucy Sewall, concluded that three patient deaths in the New England Hospital's surgical wards had been the result of "hazardous operations" performed by Dr. Storer.[59] A subsequent hospital ruling—that surgeons clear high-risk operations in advance with their female physician colleagues—clearly offended the gynecologist. Storer severed ties with the hospital shortly thereafter.

After leaving the New England Hospital in 1866—on the heels of his dismissal from a teaching position at Harvard Medical School—Storer's negative attitudes and comments about women physicians became increasingly vitriolic. "We may grant, and grant it freely," Storer explained in a widely quoted theory, "that in some matters, women intellectually, are as completely mistresses of their subject as we are master of ours. But beyond this there is a point that is fundamental to the whole matter … and that is, this inherent quality in their sex, that uncertain equilibrium, that varying from month to month according to the time of the month in each woman that unfits her for taking these responsibilities of judgment which are to control the question often of life and death…."[60]

In 1872, Horatio Storer was forced out of medical practice altogether, after one of his risky operations caused his female patient a near-fatal infection. One medical historian surmised that with Storer's withdrawal from the profession, "the opponents of women in medicine lost a vigorous spokesman."[61] Since Storer also successfully fought to criminalize abortion in the nineteenth century, he continues to be invoked and revered by anti-abortion activists in the twenty-first century.[62]

Though Horatio Storer was pushed to the sidelines in 1872, the "opponents of women in medicine" soon gained yet another vocal spokesman in Dr. Edward Hammond Clarke. In 1873, Dr. Clarke, recently retired from seventeen years of teaching at Harvard Medical School, joined the consulting staff of the New England Hospital. Such a move might suggest that he wanted to help educate women in medicine. But that same year, Clarke published *Sex in Education; or, A Fair Chance for the Girls,* which swiftly became both the most popular, and the most notorious, anti-feminist book of the era. The first edition sold out in one week.[63]

The underlying premise in *Sex in Education* was that although women could indeed delve into disciplines like medicine, they ought not to engage in intellectual activity with the same rigor—or in the same setting—as men. Coeducation, in Clarke's opinion, was unthinkable. Like many other male physicians of his time, he supported women studying medicine, as long as they did it at a modest, feminine pace and at a modest, much less demanding, all-female institution. Clarke firmly believed that women who studied excessively and overdeveloped their brains were depriving their sexual organs of energy and growth, thereby threatening the wellbeing of future generations.

In *Sex in Education*, he illustrated his theories with seven case studies of female students gone awry, each story overflowing with impressively technical, though patently absurd, medical arguments. Typical of Clarke's statements: "There have been instances, and I have seen such, of females in whom the special mechanism we are speaking of remained germinal,—undeveloped. It seemed to have been aborted. They graduated from school or college excellent scholars, but with undeveloped ovaries. Later they married, and were sterile."[64]

Women's rights advocates in Boston were appalled and went swiftly on the attack. A literary campaign was launched against *Sex in Education*, with heavy-hitters like Lucy Stone, Julia Ward Howe, and Ednah Dow Cheney on the frontlines.[65] Arguably the most eloquent offensive was taken by Dr. Mary Putnam Jacobi, a former intern at the New England Hospital and recent honors graduate of *L'École de Médecine* at the Sorbonne in Paris. Her first published treatise on the rights of women in education and the facts of female physiology was "Mental Action and Physical Health," which appeared in a large volume of essays called *The Education of American Girls*. In her essay Jacobi "picked apart Clarke's arguments, attacking his reasoning about disease causation, his knowledge of physiology, and his lack of experimental evidence."[66]

Despite the uproar, the New England Hospital's founder and chief officer, Dr. Marie Zakrzewska, elected to remain silent. Rather than criticize Storer's and Clarke's offensive writings and opinions, she thanked both men for their service to the hospital. It appears that Susan Dimock, well known for her "admirable tact,"[67] followed suit, since no record exists of her either writing or speaking publicly against these blatant affronts to women physicians. Both women were used to employing their intelligence and grit to navigate adverse circumstances, tame obstinate adversaries, and accomplish their own purposes. And Dr. Zak knew that Susan's mere presence as a strong, independent, and eminently talented surgeon and resident physician—as well as a notably attractive, charming woman— spoke volumes in itself.

In the hospital's annual report for 1873, taking the high road remained the operative theme. All of the women and men who had shepherded the facility from its humble buildings to this grand new hospital realized the responsibility of their mission. They saw the New England Hospital for Women and Children as "a beacon set on a hill where all may see it."

"[N]ow that we have achieved so much, have gained the confidence of a large public, have shown that we meet the needs of the sufferers of our community, and have builded [sic] our house, ... any failure to make the work as good on this larger scale as it was in its humbler beginnings, would put back the great cause of Woman's Medical Education everywhere...."[68]

So Dr. Dimock, Dr. Zak, and their colleagues opted to move beyond the troubles and simply continued performing the best possible medical services for women around. Perhaps they even sensed then what later generations would confirm: that they were in the process of making women's medical history.

The newest home for the New England Hospital for Women and Children was a beacon set on a hill in more ways than one. In addition to being lodged on a Roxbury hillside and serving as a model for women's medical education, it was now acknowledged as one of Greater Boston's largest hospital facilities. With full departments of obstetrics, gynecology, and pediatrics, it was also the only Boston hospital to care for all the medical needs of women and children under a single roof.[69]

As the resident physician of this medical beacon, twenty-five-year-old Dr. Susan Dimock, anxious to set a stellar example, sought perfection in all she could control. And as virtual overseer of the hospital, she controlled a great deal—from personnel training and patient care to many of the details of daily operations.

As Susan began morning hospital rounds each day, she was simply dressed in light garments—and invariably trailed by her students. While those students stood respectfully at a slight distance, she approached each bed and engaged the patient in conversation. The rights of those patients—poor or rich, Black or white—were uppermost in Susan's mind.

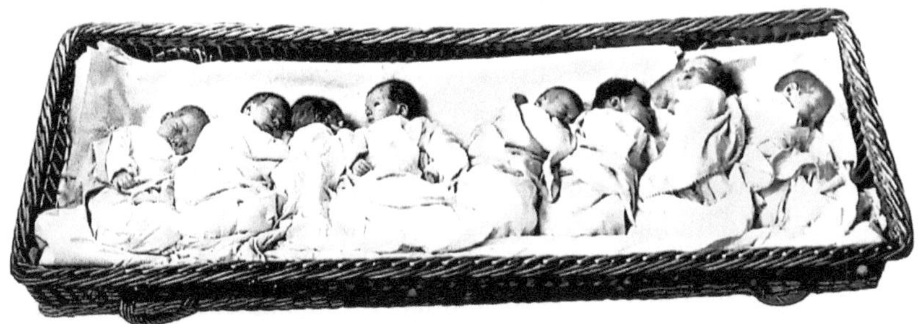

A basket of babies delivered at the New England Hospital for Women and Children. By 1872, NEHWC was one of Greater Boston's largest hospital facilities. With full departments of obstetrics, gynecology, and pediatrics, it was also the only Boston hospital to care for all the medical needs of women and children under a single roof (used by permission of the Dimock Center, Roxbury, Massachusetts).

"Her manner was very kind, but dignified and quiet," observed Ednah Dow Cheney. "[Dr. Dimock] never entered into any conversation with the patient which was not strictly professional."[70]

As admirable as Dimock's demeanor and distance appeared to some, these traits were viewed critically by others. "Her manners had a slight flavor of aristocratic coolness," admitted Cheney, "which accounted, perhaps, for the few cases in which she failed to please."[71] It's likely that the young doctor was trying to embody her vision of a professional woman—or, at least, a woman with more years of medical experience than she had yet acquired. Susan's friend Lilian Freeman Clarke saw the doctor's slight distancing as "a certain grave sweetness combined with reserved force; an earnestness and dignity which commanded respect and even cause an involuntary sense of awe."[72]

Whatever the reason, it's doubtful that Susan allowed any negative opinions about her carriage to hurt her deeply. If they did, she hid her pain well. Contemporary accounts suggest that the young doctor had neither the time nor the volition to worry about what others thought of her, whether negative or positive. "With an unbounded desire for attainment," reasoned Cheney, "she was almost contemptuously regardless of popular applause."[73]

Her desire for attainment, however—the determination to practice the best medicine possible—was quite another matter. Susan Dimock's drive for personal achievement and skill had been with her since childhood, when she consistently ranked at the top of her school classes and perused Latin medical texts in her free time. Her love, or perhaps her need, for excellence had manifested most recently in the medical knowledge she eagerly brought back to Boston from her European sojourns. Stimulated by her studies with many of Zurich's finest scientific minds, and inspired by the renowned Dr. Theodor Billroth in Vienna, she had grown especially fond of the physical tools of modern medicine. During her last months in Europe, she wrote enthusiastically about purchasing a new microscope for the hospital with monies forwarded by Dr. Zakrzewska.[74]

Arguably more important than the microscopes or various surgical tools she collected abroad were the clinical thermometers she transported stateside. Close to a foot in length, these axillary temperature gauges were initially awkward to use. Since they were not self-registering, they could only be read while tucked under the patient's armpit, "a feat not easy to accomplish in poor light," remembered Dr. Emma Call. Nurse Linda Richards expressed her own frustration that "the thermometers were large, clumsy things which bent at right angles which had to be left in the axilla [armpit] fifteen minutes before the temperature must be read before removing the thermometer. ... These were very precious articles, costing five dollars [$100 in 2022 dollars], and nurses when unfortunate enough to break one had half the price to pay."[75]

Thanks to those new thermometers, however, Susan ushered in the first year of keeping regular temperature charts at the New England Hospital. The daily graphs—hand-drawn by her students every night after evening rounds—had an immediate impact on the scourge of maternity wards worldwide: the dreaded puerperal fever.[76] As a result, by the end of Susan's first year as resident physician, the *Annual Report* proudly boasted that "notwithstanding the prevalence in Boston and vicinity of puerperal fever," the hospital had cared for 95 maternity patients without a single death.[77]

In an era when many American doctors failed even to wash their hands between autopsies, patient visitations, and surgeries, Susan—again, inspired by her German-trained medical mentors abroad—stressed the importance of hygienic habits. While in Zurich and Vienna, she had heard about pioneering doctor Ignaz Semmelweis' studies demonstrating that hand disinfection could drastically cut the incidence of puerperal fever in obstetrical clinics. As noted earlier, Semmelweis' findings were not widely accepted by the medical community until long after his death.[78] A colleague noted that Susan's "greatest anxiety was to maintain the purity and wholesome condition of [the] wards, so that recovery should be safe."[79] Given that antibiotics were still a thing of the distant future—Sir Alexander Fleming didn't discover penicillin until 1928—it's fair to say that the best any doctor could do in the 1870s was provide sunlight and cleanliness for her wards. To that end, Susan fully utilized the large, sun-filled windows and wraparound porches of the new hospital building, since "the sun-bath was one of her favorite methods of restoring the health and vigor of … her patients."[80] Understanding that emotional comfort was also part of the recovery process, Susan must have been pleased with other amenities the new facilities provided, including a spacious, sunny dining room for patients, complete with a piano where they could gather to sing or enjoy entertainment.[81]

During that inaugural year in Roxbury, Susan Dimock and her colleagues at the New England Hospital served a total of 3,544 women and children from Boston and beyond: 244 were admitted to the hospital on the Roxbury campus, 395 were treated in their homes, and 2,905 were cared for at the downtown Boston Dispensary at 315 Tremont Street.[82]

Despite all the initial troubles—the Great Fire and the Great Epizootic of 1872, and the verbal attacks by disgruntled male physicians—it was, they agreed, an auspicious start.

Moving their primary care facility from downtown Boston to the "Boston Highlands" began a demographic shift that challenged Susan Dimock's commitment to serving women and children of all classes and races. During the hospital's first decade on Warrenton Street, near the site of today's Charles Playhouse, two blocks from Boston Common and the Public Garden, the patients hailed largely from poorer socio-economic classes who lived nearby. Wealthier patients "whose means enabled them to pay for superior accommodations," could not easily be housed in the small hospital space on Warrenton, since rich, entitled women often demanded private rooms and more personal supervision.

With the spacious new Roxbury hospital in full operation, that began to change. "We have now rooms on the first floor, which will accommodate a few patients of this class," announced the *Annual Report* of 1872. "Ladies can thus have a good room, in a good healthy situation, and be sure of faithful care and nursing, at a price much less than it would cost them at a good boarding-house, with the services of a physician and nurse."[83] The fee was a $10 per week, comparable to more than $200 in 2022 dollars. One of Susan's colleagues, Dr. Emma Call, was blunt in her recollections of the shift. "At the time the new location was considered quite out in the country, and … only accessible from the city by slow and infrequent horse cars … [As a result] the class of patients … was a much better one, and we have never had any considerable number of the most undesirable cases, which inevitably gravitate to an institution located in the midst of a dense population."[84] The "most undesirable cases," decried by some and unmentionable by name in polite Victorian society, included unwed mothers, poor immigrant women, prostitutes, alcoholics, formerly enslaved African Americans, and victims of physical and sexual abuse or rape.

The ability to cater to wealthier, paying patients was an obvious boon to a hospital that was in constant need of financial aid and forever holding fundraising fairs and contribution campaigns to that end. But the gradual shift in the hospital's patient population was also consistent with the emerging new era of medical care that was in its infancy across the nation. In the analysis of historian Virginia Drachman, "During the last quarter of the nineteenth century and the first quarter of the twentieth, American hospitals evolved from institutions of medical charity and social control into institutions of medical science."[85]

It would be safe to assume that Dr. Susan Dimock was fully committed to both ends of that spectrum—to medical charity *and* to medical science. To its credit, and despite Emma Call's elitist recollection, the New England Hospital *did* continue to help the poor, the immigrant, and the unwed, even while moving forward with wealthier patrons and new scientific trends in medicine. The downtown Dispensary, where Susan worked every Tuesday and Friday, serviced the bulk of the hospital's patients, many of them charity cases, albeit with "ambulatory," or outpatient, care. Moreover, some of the impoverished and the needy still frequented the Roxbury hospital, despite its distant location. The caveat: a patient with money could always find a room on the Roxbury campus, but those requesting one of the Free Beds had to apply and be evaluated by the resident physician before being admitted. Free Beds, endowed by benefactors for $5,000 each, provided the patient with complimentary care.

The New England Hospital's Free Bed system clearly appealed to Susan. "For years this has been the only lying-in hospital of Boston and vicinity," she observed in her 1873 year-end report, "and although during the past year the Boston Lying-In Hospital has opened a small hospital for such patients on McLean Street still the need remains great. Wives of poor men who cannot afford to pay for the services of a nurse, wives more unfortunate whose husbands have deserted them,—these come to us and are welcome." Susan went on to describe a group that was even more destitute, "girls often not yet seventeen years of age, who have been betrayed and abandoned, but whose greatest desire is still to lead virtuous and respectable lives; these find here a refuge in their hour of greatest need. If we refuse them this refuge we thrust them only too surely to suicide or a life of infamy."[86]

If Susan Dimock's own writings don't suggest an overly condescending attitude towards the less fortunate women she was helping, some of her colleagues' writings do. "Dr. Dimock was very wise and very tender towards the erring sufferers," observed Ednah Dow Cheney. "[S]he never believed that one fault sunk a woman below redemption, or that even sin places a fellow-being out of the range of human charity. Her charity was calm, wise, and discriminating, and she was deeply grieved if an opportunity for succoring a woman of this class failed her." What neither Cheney nor Susan openly verbalized was that the New England Hospital shared a bias that pervaded most public hospitals of the era: in order to be admitted, their female patients had to be deemed "worthy" of care. Prostitutes, for example, had chosen an unacceptable lifestyle, as had chronic alcoholics. Their cases might only be considered if pleaded by a clergyman or some compassionate, upstanding citizen. Unwed mothers may have been taken in by the hospital as charitable cases, but not if they were having a second "illegitimate" pregnancy. That, apparently, was one fault too many.[87]

It was perhaps a perfect circumstance that Susan's very first maternity patient was a woman of color—and of limited means as well. When the woman gave birth to a daughter at the New England Hospital for Women and Children, she asked Susan to become the child's godmother. Honored by the request, Susan accepted, thereafter taking "a strong personal interest" in the child, who became a regular visitor to her physician godmother. During one of those visits, Susan gifted her godchild "the only doll which Susan Dimock ever played with, and which had been carefully preserved."[88] The act was especially poignant, since Susan had been born into a North Carolina family, in an antebellum society that willingly enslaved African Americans. Though Susan remembered acknowledging the evils of slavery by the age of eight, the fact that her own mother's family condoned ownership of other humans, and that her parents kept "house slaves" in their hotel, may have still weighed heavily on Susan's bright and questioning mind.[89]

That same year, Susan recalled that a "poor woman from.... Cape [Cod], came to me one Sunday, in the pouring rain." The woman's once well-to-do husband was out of work, and the woman herself was sick, destitute, and many months pregnant. After two weeks of medical care, solitary rest, and nourishing food provided by the hospital, the patient's spirits and health improved and her child was born safely. Following a month's stay—at the time, the average "lying-in" patient at the hospital remained for twenty-two days—the Cape Codder returned happily to the home her husband had managed to set up in her absence. After completing a follow-up visit with the patient four weeks later, a city missionary stopped by Susan's office and reported that "the poor woman declared that she had never been in a place which seemed so like heaven as the Hospital did."

"Such cases," acknowledged Susan, "are very numerous."[90]

An oddly fortuitous occurrence, both for Susan and the hospital, came early in 1873, when the doctor's long-time companion and closest confidante, Bessie Greene, arrived at the Roxbury campus in a horse-drawn carriage. Susan had first met Bessie nine years earlier, in Sterling, Massachusetts, shortly after the Dimock family's arrival from the war-torn South. As their teenage friendship blossomed, Bessie had heard Susan's avid interest in medicine, and had introduced Susan to Dr. Marie Zakrzewska, founder of the New England Hospital for Women and Children. Dr. Zak loaned medical books to Susan, took her in as a student for two years, then helped finance her formal medical school training in Zurich.

As noted in earlier chapters, the thread that linked these three women was an old abolitionist connection. Susan's aunt's house in Sterling had been a stop on the Underground Railroad, and both her aunt's family and Dr. Zak were friends with William Lloyd Garrison and his children. Bessie Greene, in turn, was the daughter of a prominent Boston abolitionist and cousin of the late Robert Gould Shaw, the white colonel who led the all-Black 54th Massachusetts Regiment. Though the anti-slavery mission ended after the war, many of these progressive families had worked and socialized together for years. Susan's abolitionist uncle, for example, was William Lloyd Garrison's dentist.

On February 9, 1873, Bessie Greene's visit to Susan Dimock at the New England Hospital was not a social call, though it ended with a profound social benefit. Described by her contemporaries as fair-skinned, light-haired, beautiful, and "all sunshine and brilliancy,"[91] twenty-six-year-old Bessie was seeking care for her knee. Three months earlier, Bessie had been vaccinated in five areas below her left patella, most likely for smallpox. The vaccination marks healed poorly and began to ulcerate, forcing her into six weeks of bed rest. "[S]he had scarcely recovered her strength," read Susan's report, when the generally graceful Bessie "fell over a hassock in the parlor … and struck upon her left knee. It immediately commenced to swell, and soon there was a large protrusion just beneath the patella to the inner side of the ligamentum patella."

Bessie was admitted to the New England Hospital, and over the next four months, Susan, her students, and her nursing staff nurtured her with a panoply of the era's most reliable homeopathic salves and scientific interventions. The knee was alternately measured, splinted, wrapped in bandages, painted with iodine, rubbed and bathed in camphor, and submitted to physical therapy. Derived from an Asian tree, camphor was a traditional medicine with antibacterial, antifungal, and anti-inflammatory properties, often used to treat skin conditions as well as joint pain. Tincture of iodine had long been employed as an antiseptic. At the end of Bessie's lengthy stay, Susan wrote, "knee quite comfortable. Can walk with ease. Discharged well."[92]

As important as these and other medications were considered in the healing process, Susan Dimock did not regard them as the most vital part of a doctor's or nurse's job. "If I were obliged in my practice to do without sympathy or medicine," she often told students in her lectures, "I should prefer to do without medicine."[93] In the 1870s, however, medicines and medical practices were notably different from what they would become even two decades later. During Susan's tenure, treatment often consisted of tender loving care, nutritious foods, prolonged stays at the hospital, and an abundance of "botanicals." There was no systematic use of antiseptics, no knowledge of germ theory or bacteriology, no use of sterile rubber gloves, and no notion of boiling to sterilize surgical instruments, partly because many of the steel devices were glued to rubber or wooden handles that would have deteriorated in boiling water.[94]

Meanwhile, more than Bessie Greene's knee had a happy ending. Bessie's four-month medical sojourn produced two benefits. First, she was able to regularly see Susan Dimock. In the words of many of their contemporaries, the two were bonded with a trust and intimacy that recalled the Biblical duo of David and Jonathan.[95] Secondly, in the course of her stay at the New England Hospital, Bessie came to share Susan's concern for her neediest maternity patients. "[I]nstead of being afraid to attack a difficult problem and feeling excused by youth and inexperience from handling it," observed Bessie's friend Lilian Freeman Clarke, "she determined courageously that something should be done."[96]

In the fall of 1873, Lilian joined forces with Bessie to establish what came to be known as "The Invisible Institution." Lilian explained it was so-named "because although doing the work of an institution, it was found better to aid each patient as a personal friend; not founding a 'Home,' and so avoiding the heavy expenses and cumbrous methods of institutional charity."[97] The two women devoted themselves to assisting married and unwed mothers in their last months of pregnancy and early months of motherhood, visiting them while in the hospital, then helping them avoid placement in asylums or having to give up their infants for adoption. In many cases, Bessie and Lilian were able to find these women employment where they could keep their children with them—albeit for decreased wages. Bessie and Lilian's successful mission of finding women "situations where they could keep their babies with them, giving sympathy, advice, and material aid," made the Invisible Institution, which offered all of its assistance pro bono, one of the first social services in the nation.[98]

Coincidentally, another young woman who was to become a close friend to both Susan and Bessie followed a path similar to Bessie's. She came to the hospital for personal help in 1873, only to become an active advocate and participant in the hospital's medical mission. Caroline

Marsh Crane, a twenty-eight-year-old woman of "great physical beauty, fine literary tastes, and rare accomplishments,"[99] approached Dr. Zakrzewska while suffering from what was alternately described as failing health and a nervous breakdown. Since her mother had died of puerperal fever when Carrie was only two, and her father had remarried and fathered several more children, she spent much time with her aunt and uncle, who lived and served at the U.S. Consulate in Turin, Italy. When Dr. Zak recommended that Carrie take a year off for "some physical labor and rest of mind," Carrie decided to enroll in Susan Dimock's nursing school and devote her time to helping the hospital. Though she left the New England Hospital late in 1874 to return to her arts education in Italy, she had found some new friends and improved health during her mission.

Together and separately, the three friends—Susan, Bessie, and Carrie—helped maintain the light of the "beacon set on a hill" that the New England Hospital for Women and Children had clearly become.

Dr. Susan Dimock was remembered as a woman of many talents. For some, it was her teaching that shone most brightly. "There are few who possess an equal power of imparting knowledge," recalled her medical student Mary E. Little. "This was done, not by lectures of pouring out her own ideas, but by adroit questions, rousing the latent thoughts in other minds. … Students were [also] exhorted to listen carefully to every thing [*sic*] a patient wished to tell them, and to make her feel that all she told was of interest to her physician."[100]

Others saw her relationship to her patients as her greatest strength. "Her very entrance into the ward seemed to throw a halo of joy around us," recalled a long-term patient, who described Susan as tender, kind, sympathetic, and, most importantly, empathetic. "How many times have the soft caresses of her fingers upon my forehead, or gentle pressure on my hands, speaking more than words, sent a thrill through my body, that at once soothed my weary frame!"[101]

Medical colleagues, in turn, were impressed by Susan's diagnostic capabilities. "I have never known a physician, man or woman, whose diagnosis and judgement, in regard to a case, I valued more than I did hers," commented one such associate, adding, "It is a mistake to consider her pre-eminently as a surgeon; it was her reasoning powers which gave her such marked superiority."[102]

Despite those accolades, the skill that clearly set Susan Dimock apart from other women doctors of her era—and from multitudes of male doctors as well—was her exceptional work in the field of surgery. As Ednah

Dow Cheney noted, "anyone who saw Dr. Dimock at the operating table, where she was as calm and self-possessed as in the morning visit; who watched the extreme delicacy and skill with which she handled the tools, and the loving care with which she guarded the sensibilities of the patient,—must have recognized the eternal fitness of things, and seen that she was in her rightful place."[103]

During Susan's inaugural year at the New England Hospital for Women and Children, the surgical wards were full and the results excellent: "In these Wards … no death has occurred," she proudly announced in her first annual report. Her second year was also successful. A total of 252 patients were treated in the hospital, including 57 surgeries—three more than the previous year. "In the Surgical Wards we have lost only one patient," wrote Susan, "a little child who was brought in almost dying, with multiple abscesses affecting the joints." Still, she added proudly, "No patient has died after an operation."[104]

Surgical theaters in the 1870s were a far cry from their twenty-first-century counterparts. None of the standard modern-day operating attire was in use at the time: not gowns, caps, masks, nor protective gloves. Outfitted in her simple black cotton dress, probably partly covered by a rubber apron, Susan was generally surrounded by a curious coterie: her medical students in street clothes, a surgical nurse or two in calico dresses and slippers, and—if the operation was unusually complex—a consulting surgeon like her old friend and mentor, Dr. Samuel Cabot, dressed in a dark, three-piece business suit. Based on images from the era, it's likely that they all crowded around the operating table, with no barrier between them and the surgical patient. Unlike many of her male contemporaries, however, especially those in the over-packed amphitheaters of medical schools, Susan never allowed the curiosity of her students or peers to take precedence over the needs of her patients. Surgery was not a "show," but a way to gently, swiftly, and effectively aid the ailing.

Lighting, too, was far different in Susan's day. In the 1870s, Boston homes and businesses were illuminated by gas lamps, candles, and fireplaces. During that era, the anesthetic of choice for surgical patients was ether, as it had been for almost three decades. The problem: though diethyl ether could now be safely administered to patients going under the knife for relatively long periods of time, it was also extremely flammable.[105] Since electricity would not be introduced into the city until the 1880s, and not widely used until much later, and since gaslight was too dangerous for the surgical wards, sunlight played an indispensable role in the art of surgery, with well-placed mirrors and glass-encased candles filling in the gaps. Fortunately, Susan Dimock was working in the airy, clean, sun-filled wards of the new Roxbury facility rather than the hospital's dark, old, cramped quarters in downtown Boston. Sunshine was good for the patients' health and spirits—and vital for the surgeon's vision.

The tools of her trade had grown some since Susan's student days at the hospital. More specialized medical instruments had been gradually added to the traditional microscopes, scalpels, forceps, scissors, surgical needles, and cautery irons of the 1860s. Sadly, as noted before, many of these metal implements still had wooden and rubber handles that would have disintegrated if regularly boiled in water following surgery. Since Joseph Lister's work on antiseptic techniques was not yet widely accepted, all-metal "antiseptic" instruments—ones that could be effectively sterilized—would not come into wider use until the 1880s. Similarly, Louis Pasteur's germ theory, extended by Robert Koch's work on bacteriology, was not fully recognized until the 1890s. Susan Dimock's colleague, Dr. Emma Call, later admitted, "In the period from 1872 to 1877, I find very little to indicate any systematic use of antiseptics [at the New England Hospital]."[106]

What Dr. Susan Dimock might have accomplished had she begun practice ten or twenty years later—when "modern medical technique" was rapidly evolving—is a matter of conjecture. But what she did achieve from 1872 to 1875 was nevertheless notable.

In two of her most significant surgeries, she safely removed unwanted objects from inside female patients. In the first, executed in January of 1873, a fifty-two-year-old housewife with an unusually large bladder stone was brought to the New England Hospital's resident physician, and Susan's small team went to work. An ether anesthesia was administered, probably by placing a cone-shaped towel with a sponge inside over the patient's mouth and nose, then dripping ether onto the "mask." It was an inexact science, at best. Next, Susan began a surgical procedure known as lithotrity, which involved crushing the stone with a specialized instrument passed through the urethra to the bladder. The instrument she used, called a lithotrite, had been introduced in France and Britain to replace the older process of lithotomy, an invasive, slicing process that sometimes ruptured the peritoneum—the membrane lining the cavity of the abdomen—or displaced the bowel.

Discovering that the woman's bladder stone was some two-and-a-half inches in circumference, Susan chose to dismember it in stages. First, the young surgeon probably used a double-current catheter to draw out the patient's urine and fill the bladder with tepid water. That liquid provided a buffer of sorts, preventing Susan from accidentally grasping the mucous membrane with her tool. Holding the long, slim metal lithotrite in her bare hands, she slid it gently up through the urethra. The curved tip of the instrument had mechanical jaws that, with the turn of a small wheel at the other end, grasped and chewed one segment of the stone into smaller particles that were easier to pass. After crushing and flushing one segment of the stone, Susan repeated the process. According to the case record, the patient "recovered from the effect of the ether with very little vomiting, and was comfortable the remainder of the day."[107]

"The favorable patient outcome of the lithotrity performed by Dr. Dimock easily ranks her among the [male] surgeons of her era, especially with so large a stone!" wrote medical student William Randall King in his 1997 doctoral thesis. King was particularly impressed by the technical difficulty of blindly approaching a bladder stone, then grasping and breaking it several times in such a brief operative period.[108]

The hospital's Consulting Surgeon and longtime ally, Dr. Samuel Cabot, agreed with that assessment. "It was not merely her skill, though, that was remarkable, but also *her nerve,* that qualified her to become a great surgeon. I have seldom known one at once so determined and so self-possessed. ... [Dr. Dimock is] sure to stand, in time, among those at the head of her profession."[109]

Over the next month, Susan repeated the lithotrity several times with equal success. When the final chunk refused to budge, she went in with metal forceps, ultimately dislodging and withdrawing the remaining stone. The resulting pain in the patient's bladder was alternately treated with subcutaneous injections of morphine. Naturopathic remedies followed: teaspoons of citrate of magnesia were given as a laxative, while a flax seed poultice was applied to the vulva to reduce inflammation. Curiously all three of those treatments—morphine, citrate of magnesia, and flax seed poultice—still exist in the twenty-first century, though the latter two would be considered alternative, rather than mainstream, medicine. Morphine was such a popular painkiller in the nineteenth century that opium addiction became epidemic.

Arguably more impressive than Dr. Susan Dimock's bladder stone removal was a neck tumor operation she performed in September of 1873. That month, seven-year-old Sarah from Nantucket was admitted to the New England Hospital for Women and Children. Two years earlier, she had been struck by a hand cart just below and behind the lobe of her right ear. Though her neck had originally just swelled, there was now an enormous tumor on the side of her neck.[110]

Surrounded again by her team of medical students, nurses, and Dr. Cabot, Susan began the process of surgical removal. After the patient was etherized, the doctor made two incisions over the tumor, then cut the sternocleidomastoid, a large muscle that allows the head to rotate and the neck to flex. With the tumor thus exposed, Susan observed that it was composed of "lobules" varying in size "from a pea to a goose egg." Since each

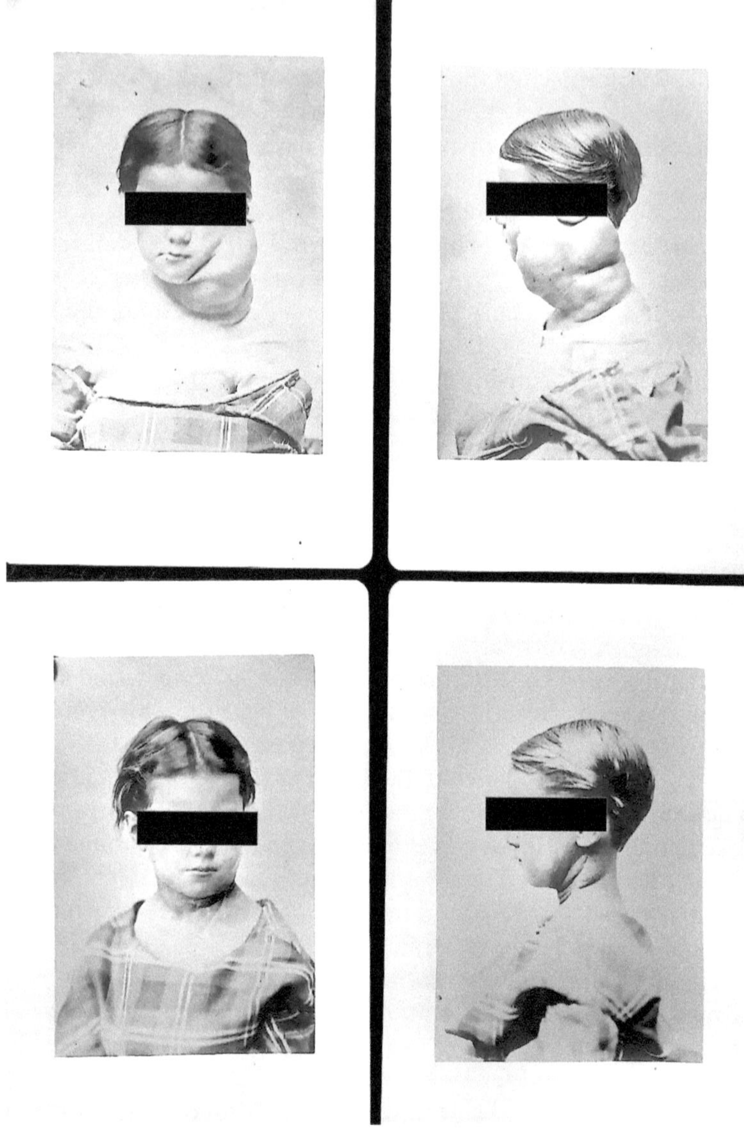

One of Susan Dimock's most exceptional surgeries involved removing an enormous tumor filled with 71 individual lobules from the neck of seven-year-old Sarah from Nantucket. Hiring a photographer to take Before and After images was not standard practice at the time and a testament to the significance of the operation (New England Hospital for Women and Children, Records of Medical Wards and Surgical Wards, Boston Medical Library in the Francis A. Countway Library of Medicine, Harvard University, Boston, Massachusetts; used by permission of the Dimock Center, Roxbury, Massachusetts).

mass was enclosed in a separate capsule, she tore each capsule open and removed the contents. In total, seventy-one "tumors" were removed with relatively little bleeding. Using wire sutures, Susan first closed the edges of the wound, then did the same with the sternocleidomastoid muscle—the former with fifteen sutures and the latter with just two.

Following the operation, Susan and her team placed a wooden splint along the back of Sarah's head, then rolled cotton bandages around her forehead and chest to immobilize the area, control bleeding, and absorb any drainage. Just two days later, the sutures were removed and replaced by strips of adhesive plaster, which were switched every two days thereafter. The medications given Sarah during recovery were, again, what might be called alternative, holistic, or "natural" in the twenty-first century. To control her post-surgery vomiting, Sarah was offered a "drachm" of brandy and a teaspoon of water over ice every half hour. Every two hours thereafter the nursing team alternated between beef tea, milk, brandy, and water, while hot water bottles were placed by her body. Though hospital reports noted that Sarah cried a lot and was homesick, she was successfully released at the end of December 1873, after more than three months of rest and treatment.[111]

While visiting Boston almost a year later, Dr. Mary Putnam Jacobi— an advocate for women's medical education and the second woman to receive a medical degree from the University of Paris—was shown photographs of the neck tumor operation by Susan. The fact that a photographer was hired to take pre- and post-operative images was unusual in the 1870s, and a testament to the significance of the surgery. After reading the case record, Putnam Jacobi recalled that she had watched the renowned Dr. Charles Richet perform a similar operation in the Paris Clinique and attended his subsequent lecture, "in which he described the great difficulty of removing a tumor so deeply embedded in so dangerous a locality." While Putnam Jacobi observed that Richet both bragged about his success "and had taken care that a numerous auditorium should witness his triumph," she found that her old friend Susan Dimock was far more modest about her accomplishments. Putnam Jacobi remembered that after hearing about Richet's self-aggrandizement, "Dr. Dimock laughed, and said, 'I was asked why I had issued no invitations, but I had forgotten all about them.' She added, 'Indeed I have too little personal ambition to care who sees, when I am once assured my work is well done.'"[112]

During her contracted three-year tenure as resident physician at the New England Hospital, Susan successfully executed surgeries with a broad range of complexity. Some were considered relatively standard in the 1870s, like removing a tonsil from a nine-year-old boy or cutting out a non-cancerous fibrous tumor from a 38-year-old woman's uterus. The

<u>Treatment & Course.</u>

Sept 9th

10 ct. M.   Ether was administered and two in-
-cisions were made over the tumor, one
extending from a point half way between
the mastoid process and angle of the
jaw to the sterno clavicular articula-
-tion following the course of the Sterno.
cleido- mastoid muscle, the other ~~extend~~
~~-ing from the~~ middle of the first incision
and at a right angle to within half an
inch of median line. Sterno-cleido-mas.
-toid muscle was then cut and tumor
laid bare.   The tumor was composed of
lobules, varying in size from a pea to a
goose-egg each lobule being inclosed in
~~its~~ separate capsule The capsules being
torn open their contents were taken out
     Seventy-one (71) separate tumors were.
thus removed with very little bleeding
and the edges of the wound brought into
apposition by fifteen (15) superficial wire
sutures, the Sterno-cleido-mastoid muscle by
two (2) A wooden splint along back of head
& spine was applied, to keep head in proper
position, a roller bandage passing around
the forehead, another around the chest.
     She vomited three times: nausea con-
tinued four hours during which time brandy,
a drachm to a tablespoonful of water, and

Dr. Dimock wrote extensive notes on the "Treatment & Course" of the difficult 1873 neck tumor surgery. Presenting such detailed observations was standard practice for the young resident physician (New England Hospital for Women and Children, Records of Medical Wards and Surgical Wards, Boston Medical Library in the Francis A. Countway Library of Medicine, Harvard University, Boston, Massachusetts; used by permission of the Dimock Center, Roxbury, Massachusetts).

latter surgery was done with a now-obsolete surgical instrument called an *ecraseur*, which featured a handle at one end and a chain loop at the other that was used to encircle and sever a tissue mass.[113] A few of Susan's surgeries were of such clinical interest that she wrote papers on them for *The Medical Record*, a weekly journal of medicine and surgery that had been published in New York since 1866. One such procedure was her successful operation for a recto-vaginal fistula—an abnormal connection between the rectum and the vagina. In that paper, Susan explained her case, illustrating a new method that involved splitting and turning outward both rectal and vaginal layers of mucous membrane. Another of her surgeries described in *The Medical Record* was designed to correct fecal incontinence.[114]

In 1874, an eleven-year-old schoolgirl named Ednorah entered the New England Hospital for examination of her imperforate anus. It was Ednorah's aunt, a suffragist and prominent social figure in Boston's African American community, who brought the young girl to Dr. Dimock's attention. This was not Ednorah's first visit to a medical specialist. On the contrary: Susan's friend and mentor, the well-respected Dr. Samuel Cabot, had been treating Ednorah at the Massachusetts General Hospital since she was one week old, for what he initially deemed to be congenital constriction of the anus. Over the next decade, Dr. Cabot continued to operate on the youngster with no success. Her bowel movements remained irregular, and she remained incontinent.

When she met Susan in June of 1874, Ednorah was described as weighing 68 pounds and being poorly nourished, feverish, and incontinent of both feces and urine. During the physical examination, Susan found a false anus, apparently the original fistula, that was large enough to admit a forefinger as well as a true anus that could only "admit a quill." Following a prescribed regimen of castor oil, enemas, and Sitz baths, Ednorah was discharged and told to pursue good nutrition, exercise, and outdoor play for the rest of the summer. By September, Susan deemed Ednorah strong and healthy enough to undergo surgery.

During that September surgery, Susan observed that Ednorah's anus was so constricted that it would not admit the least dilation. When the anus was injected with water, liquid flowed freely through both openings. Susan began her surgery by dividing the bridge of tissue between the two openings, where she noted, "not much bleeding, the tissue cutting like a cicatrix." Once that procedure was completed, she observed that the opening formed was large enough to easily admit four fingers. In her report, the surgeon explained that "the cut surfaces ... to my surprise and great pleasure began to contract visibly and take on the folded appearance of a normal anus, so that after a lapse of ten minutes a quart of water being injected was retained perfectly, and only ejected with the use of a Sims speculum."

Immediately postoperatively, Ednorah was put to bed with dry heat applied to her abdomen. When she awakened later that afternoon, she was given "one teaspoonful of brandy and water and held small pieces of ice in her mouth" to allay the nausea caused by etherization. During her recovery, Ednorah slept satisfactorily and was able to eat meat and baked potato with no negative incidents. Meanwhile, she was given ginger tea and warm enemas to relieve her stomach aches. Soon she was sitting up, walking about, and eating fruit and vegetables. After just eight days of hospitalization, Ednorah was "discharged well." Susan wrote that the wounded surface healed rapidly and that there was neither a recurrence of fever nor involuntary defecation.

The operation proved a success for both surgeon and patient. Susan confirmed her independence of thought: she had carefully read Dr. Cabot's medical records based on his work of eleven years, respectfully consulted his notes, then made her own assessments, which resulted, finally, in a correct diagnosis. Ednorah, in turn, was given a new lease on life: later adopted by her suffragist aunt, she grew up to be a well-known elocutionist who performed on stages around the world.

In Susan's handwritten case report for Ednorah's surgery, she mentioned use of a surgical tool called the Sims speculum—a double-bladed, U-shaped instrument used to examine the cervix and vagina. Still part of the twenty-first-century surgical tool kit, the Sims speculum was developed by James Marion Sims, the South Carolina surgeon lauded as the father of modern surgical gynecology. Though Sims laid the foundation for much of the methodology and technology that Susan and her colleagues depended on in their daily work, the women might have had second thoughts had they known the full backstory. J. Marion Sims used enslaved Black females for what many twentieth-century critics decried as cruel gynecological experiments, executed without anesthesia. Working in Alabama in the late 1840s, Sims jeopardized the lives and well-being of enslaved Black women while developing techniques that would later save the lives and well-being of middle- and upper-class white women.[115]

Historical hindsight offers another interesting perspective on Susan's career. There is no question that by the 1870s, Susan Dimock and her female colleagues at the New England Hospital for Women and Children had medical expertise and skills equal to those of their male peers in Boston. To the casual observer, the surgeries, the care, the protocols, the methodology, and the chains of command were quite similar between, for example, the female-run New England Hospital and its male-run counterpart, Boston Lying-In. But there were significant, if subtle, differences.

The New England Hospital controlled sepsis among obstetrical patients far better than male-run hospitals of the era. The women doctors used forceps less frequently and had fewer complications with forceps patients than the men at Boston Lying-In. Lying-In kept their obstetrical patients for an average of two weeks, while the New England generally kept them for three.[116] And, according to statistics collected by former New England Hospital physician, Dr. Emma Call, obstetrical patients at the New England Hospital from 1872 to 1882, were six times more likely to survive than their counterparts at Boston Lying-In.[117]

It would be easy to assume that Dr. Susan Dimock dove into her taxing workload with such passion, persistence, and energy that she rarely had time for rest and relaxation. And it's true that every afternoon, when not running the hospital's Roxbury campus or working at its downtown dispensary, the young doctor also saw patients at her private Boston practice. She first rented a space at 8 Park Square in 1872, then moved to an office on Boylston Street, between Arlington and Berkeley streets. In 1874, her longtime friend and colleague Dr. Lucy Sewall purchased the building at 151 Boylston Street, just a stone's throw from Arlington Street Church. While it was Sewall's private home and medical office, she willingly shared the rooms—as well as several of her private clients—with Dr. Dimock. It's clear that 151 Boylston was a prestigious address at the time, since neighbors included numerous doctors and dentists, as well as famed hotelier Harvey Parker, Boston Museum founder Moses Kimball, and brewery magnate Jacob Pfaff.[118]

But between her professional duties, which began at dawn, and her preferred bedtime of nine o'clock, Susan Dimock did indeed carve out space for peace and pleasure. One of her favorite places to decompress was her private parlor at the Roxbury hospital. Scampering about the room or lolling on a warm windowsill were her pet spaniel, Dotty, and her kitten, Dainty. An inveterate lover of nature and art, the young doctor filled her sunniest window with plants and covered her walls with framed pictures. Ednah Dow Cheney fondly recalled that "beautiful little brackets adorned every appropriate place, on which stood vases holding waving grasses, graceful ferns, &c., with here and there a small bit of statuary or choice fancy article,—probably many of them treasured gifts from loving hearts."[119]

Susan also made time for friends, especially her dearest Bessie Greene, who could often be found in her home at Clarendon House, a hotel on Tremont Street near the site of today's Calderwood Pavilion, that served both short and long-term renters. "Susan Dimock comes to see me every day, almost, between four and five," wrote Bessie to a friend, adding realistically, "generally not till 5."[120] Susan and Bessie enjoyed taking in "heaps of music" in season. Once the regular performance season was over, Susan happily followed up with "amusing things—burlesque opera for instance, which my soul delights in."[121] During her last winter in the city, Susan—who lived at the hospital in Roxbury, four miles from downtown Boston—went to the theater twice a week, accompanied by Bessie, a student, or other young friends. Susan and company may well have slipped away to see one of actress Charlotte Cushman's many "farewell appearances," or enjoyed shows featuring Shakespearean actor Edwin Booth or Italian tragedienne Adelaide Ristori performing in popular downtown playhouses like the Globe or Boston Theatres, the Boston Museum, the Howard Athenaeum, or the Music Hall. Unlike the Boston theater district of today, which grew up after 1900, all those venues were close to Old City Hall and one of Boston's premier hotels, the Parker House—where famed actress Cushman actually resided, as did Bessie's parents, William Batchelder Greene and Anna Shaw Greene.

A longtime fan of walking and hiking, Susan may have spent some of her free time wandering in and around Boston Common, heralded as the nation's first "public green." On the Park Street side of the Common, she might well have stopped to visit the *Woman's Journal,* run by suffragist Lucy Stone, a perennial advocate for, and friend of, the New England Hospital. Facing the Tremont side of the Common were a wealth of cultural shops including the prestigious bookseller known as Osgood & Company, home of the *Atlantic Monthly.* Fond of both poetry and romance, Susan could have dropped in to purchase books by her favorite English poet (Browning), French novelist (Hugo), or German poet (Schiller).[122] Only one block to the east was a shop where Susan could satiate her musical curiosity, in the world-famous music store run by Oliver Ditson. And if she glanced up from the Common in the direction of Beacon Street, she would surely have marveled at the shining, newly gilded dome of the Massachusetts State House, while carefully skirting locals zipping by on those wonderfully strange two-wheeled bicycles, popularly called "flying velocipedes."

Susan and Bessie even managed to travel outside of Boston on several occasions, often to the seaside destinations Susan so loved. "We went to Plymouth, where the Pilgrim fathers first landed," she wrote to an old friend in Zurich in the late spring of 1874. "We stood on the rock to which they moored their boat that fearful, stormy day when the 'Mayflower' brought them to an unknown, desolate region, covered with snow. We had a lovely time in the woods and by the sea. The woods were sweet with the smell of the pines and of arbutus, all the fruit trees were just blossoming from our windows."[123]

Despite these relaxing outings and adventures, Dr. Susan Dimock—a woman of many talents and many responsibilities—was also a woman of profound weariness. In addition to her own intense work obligations, she had taken on Dr. Zakrzewska's patients and duties for several months, when the exhausted Dr. Zak left on her first vacation in years. Though Susan may have tried to mask her weakened state to her Boston peers, she confided to her Zurich friend, "I have grown very old with care and fatigue and want of health. Just think how I used to walk and now I can hardly walk a half hour without feeling the bad results."[124] Moreover, although her three-year contract as resident physician was set to terminate in the summer of 1875, the hospital board had already asked her to renew that agreement. "I can hardly make up my mind what to do," she admitted. "I want to stay since they want me, and yet do not know whether my strength will last so long for both my private work and the Hospital."[125] Still, she was convinced she would ultimately agree to continue her residency, "because I have become so much interested in the work, and I love it so much."[126]

Clearly, some compromise between work and play had to be found. That compromise would have unforeseen consequences.

CHAPTER 5

Death and Legacy

In 1875, Dr. Susan Dimock agreed to renew her three-year contract as resident physician with the New England Hospital for Women and Children. But she did so under one condition: that she be granted a five-month leave, allowing her some leisure time to travel back to Europe and visit medical colleagues and friends while perusing and purchasing state-of-the-art surgical instruments for use in her Boston practices.

On April 14, 1875, just ten days before her own twenty-eighth birthday, Susan wrote to Dr. Elizabeth Garrett Anderson, a pioneering London-based doctor. "I am just ready to go to Europe for five months," she began, adding regretfully that she could not stop in England, "so that I might see you, and express personally my great regard." Though separated by the Atlantic Ocean, the two doctors deeply admired one another. Both worked in hospitals where female doctors treated female patients and in societies where the concept of "woman doctor" was still unimaginable to many. While Susan was arguably America's finest woman surgeon, the 39-year-old Garrett Anderson was renowned as England's first qualified woman doctor and the founder of England's first hospital for women.

In addition to expressing her regrets, Susan shared with Garrett Anderson a wistful thought about her own life. "As for me, I have not one wish unfulfilled," she confessed. "Nay, I am so fortunate, that if I had a ring I would like Polycrates throw it into the sea. My practice is very large, and I have the utmost satisfaction of every kind in it."[1] Feeling gratitude for her good fortune, yet courting caution about the same, was a sentiment voiced by Susan more than once. On a visit to London five years earlier, she had admitted, "I do declare, I am in amazement. I do not know what it is that makes people so kind to me. It frightens me sometimes; I fear that I must have trouble, some time or other, to balance."[2]

Thirteen days after writing Garrett Anderson, Susan and two female friends were scheduled to board the S.S. *Schiller* in New York, beginning a transatlantic voyage that would dock at Plymouth, England, and Cherbourg, France, *en route* to its final destination in Hamburg, Germany.

On April 14, 1875, Susan wrote to Dr. Elizabeth Garrett Anderson in London. "As for me, I have not one wish unfulfilled," she began, "nay, I am so fortunate, that if I had a ring I would like Polycrates throw it into the sea. My practice is very large, and I have the utmost satisfaction of every kind in it" (Susan Dimock to Dr. Garrett Anderson, April 14, 1875; courtesy Kay Hicks, Lynchburg Virginia).

Ednah Dow Cheney recalled that the choice of that particular ship seemed auspicious, since Susan "was very fond both of poetry and romance, and … was pleased that the vessel in which she sailed bore the name of her favorite German poet, Schiller." Indeed, learning the name of her steamship may well have inspired Susan to re-read Friedrich Schiller's 1797 ballad, "Der Ring des Polykrates," and ponder hurling some beloved trinket into the sea to balance her good fortune.[3]

The friends who accompanied the youthful surgeon were her longtime companion Bessie Greene and their talented friend and former colleague, Caroline ("Carrie") Crane. By the time of their 1875 trip, Greene and Dimock had been bonded for a decade, both personally and professionally. Susan, of course, was on sabbatical from her work at the New England Hospital. So too was Bessie, since her "Invisible Institution," the charitable aid organization for needy young mothers that she ran with Lilian Freeman Clarke, had been working in tandem with the New England Hospital for the past two years. And though their mutual friend Carrie had most recently been living with her uncle's family in Vermont, she had worked closely with Susan and Bessie the previous year, helping out as a nursing volunteer at their Boston hospital.

It was Carrie's uncle, the powerful Senator Edmunds of Vermont, who arranged passage for Carrie, Bessie, and Susan on the S.S. *Schiller*. As might be expected from a man hoping to impress others with his wealth and prestige, Edmunds planned for the three young women to have the finest accommodations. The price for the tony First Cabin, or First Saloon, section where the women stayed was advertised as costing one hundred dollars per person, payable only in gold. Second Saloon, intended for middle class travelers, was a mere sixty dollars in gold, while the modest steerage section was only twenty-four dollars, payable in simple currency. Steerage was the crowded Third-Class section of the boat, couched in the lower decks and intended for immigrants and people of lesser means.[4]

Whether the three women were treated by Senator Edmunds, or repaid him for the luxury-class tickets, is unclear. Since her annual salary at the New England Hospital was $300, augmented by earnings from her private practice, it seems likely that Susan might have opted for something more affordable and less elitist than a $100 First Saloon stateroom.

It was more than the ticket expense, however, that made Susan appear out of her element on the *Schiller*—at least at first glance. It had been seven years since her first sea voyage to Europe, when she was an unknown, 21-year-old "experimental" student traveling to a far-away, foreign medical school. Her late father, Henry, had made his living as a newspaper editor and her mother, Mary Malvina, as a schoolteacher and hotel keeper. Now, in 1875 at the age of 28, Dr. Susan Dimock was traveling as an established and much-heralded Boston surgeon and resident physician, with prestigious friends and fans on both sides of the Atlantic. Still, Susan was not accustomed to the transatlantic cruise culture, which was filled—at least in the posh First Saloon section—with leisured women of means, traveling abroad with their well-bred offspring, in search of cultural enlightenment and spa treatments. Susan's norm, in contrast, was working around the clock while helping many of Boston's poorest and neediest women and children.

Bessie Greene's and Carrie Crane's family credentials were perhaps more in line with many of the First Cabin passengers on board the *Schiller*. Bessie herself was described as a "true lady by instinct, inheritance and breeding." On the other hand—and perhaps one element of her persona that deeply attracted Susan—was that Bessie was also "as entirely unsophisticated by culture, by society, and by foreign residence and travel, as the simplest country girl."[5]

The youngest of the three transatlantic travelers of 1875, twenty-six-year-old Carrie Marsh Crane, was described by Dr. Marie Zakrzewska as "possessed of great physical beauty, fine literary tastes, and rare accomplishments."[6] Born in Indiana to Thomas and Maria Andros Crane, Carrie lost her mother Maria to puerperal fever at the age of two. Though her father eventually remarried, Carrie spent many of her early years with her uncle and aunt, Ambassador George Perkins Marsh and his wife, Caroline Crane Marsh. Between 1861 and 1865, while the Civil War raged in America, young Carrie had lived in Turin, Italy, as a companion and writing assistant to her semi-invalid Aunt Caroline, meeting and greeting ambassadors, royalty, and prestigious world leaders on a weekly basis. As an early teen living in a foreign embassy, Carrie had attended all the best operas and ballets, while becoming fluent in Italian and beloved by all. In addition, Carrie's aunt Susan was married to Senator George Franklin Edmunds of Vermont—the gentleman who purchased the three friends their *Schiller* tickets.[7] Both the Marshes and the Edmunds were constants in Carrie's life. She had just spent the past winter lodging with Senator Edmunds' family in Vermont and was now on her way to Italy, where she planned to continue her literary studies while living at the embassy again with her beloved uncle and aunt.

S.S. *Schiller* was scheduled to depart from New York on Tuesday afternoon, April 27, 1875, only three days after Susan's twenty-eighth birthday. Though the German-owned Eagle Line (*Adler Linie*) vessel was advertised as traveling from New York to Hamburg, the pier where *Schiller* docked was actually in Hoboken, New Jersey, at the foot of First Street. But that pier was directly across the Hudson River from Manhattan, allowing Susan, Bessie, and Carrie a spectacular view of the rapidly growing city's vaulting spires and iconic buildings, including Trinity Church, Grand Central Depot, the brand-new *New York Tribune* building, and stores like Macy's and Alexander Turney Stewart's "Marble Palace." In the distance, they could also glimpse the still-under-construction East River Bridge (today's Brooklyn Bridge) linking New York and Brooklyn, and Castle Garden, American's first official immigration center.[8] The Hudson River itself was a marvelously colorful thoroughfare, teeming with four-masted schooners, sloops, ferries, and paddle steamers, interspersed with darting flocks of smaller boats and skiffs. It may well have pleased Susan to find herself in yet another city—like Washington, Zurich, and Boston—where a river played an integral part in that city's scenery and economic life.

As the three women passed through the Eagle Line's central pavilion, stood at pier's end, proffered their tickets, and strode up the gangplank, they could see that S.S. *Schiller* was an impressive vessel. The German Eagle Line had begun operations just three years earlier, at the end of the Franco-Prussian War, and had ordered the construction of two sister steamships—*Goethe* and *Schiller*, named for the German literary heroes—as their largest, sturdiest ocean liners. Though not the fastest ocean liner on the seas, *Schiller* was a sleek, 380-foot-long vessel with a modern iron-plated hull and fuel-efficient engines, brig-rigged with three

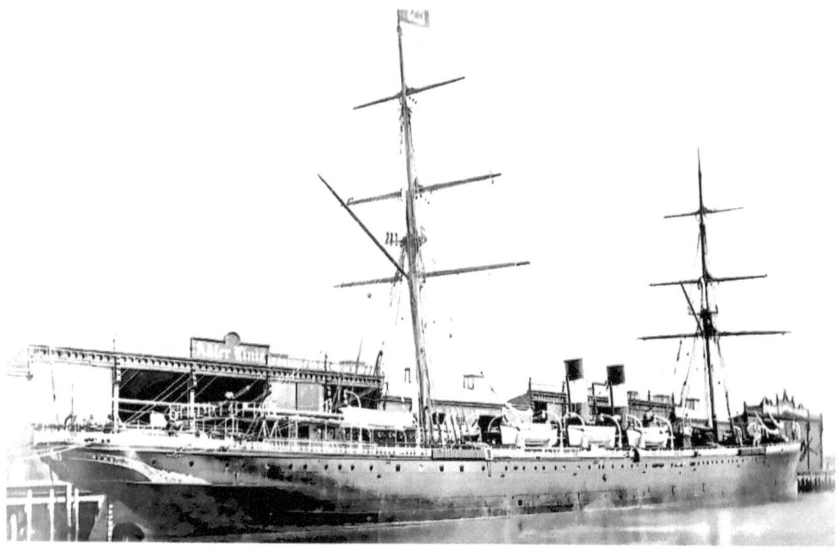

Susan Dimock, Bessie Greene and Carrie Crane boarded the S.S. *Schiller* from the Eagle Line pier in Hoboken, New Jersey, beginning a transatlantic voyage that would dock at Plymouth, England, and Cherbourg, France, *en route* to a final destination in Hamburg, Germany (Der Dampfer Schiller der Adler-Linie in Hoboken vor 1875; image via Wikimedia Commons).

square sails on the fore and main masts, enabling wind power to assist the engines or take over should those engines fail. With impressive dual smokestacks, 128-foot tall iron masts, and gleaming white sails and lifeboats, the vessel appeared as remarkable as the paperwork behind her construction claimed.[9]

Susan, Bessie, and Carrie boarded the steamship alongside an unusual number of women for the 1870s—a result, in part, of the absence of major wars on either side of the Atlantic. Some 100 of the 254 passengers booked on S.S. *Schiller* were female, ranging from numerous Americans and German-Americans of modest means visiting or returning to their homeland to wealthy, fashionably-dressed ladies planning their cultural season in Europe. Some of those ladies were determined to "improve their minds" by sampling the art and antiquities of the Old Country or visiting well-known Continental sites, while others were taking in the pleasures of health cures, spas, and resorts or the posh estates of relatives and friends.

Apart from some four dozen children, the rest of the seafarers were men, prominent among whom was German-born immigrant Joseph Schlitz of Wisconsin, whose commercial brew would later become known as "the beer that made Milwaukee famous." The nautically-minded were also impressed by the presence of thirty-four-year-old passenger Daniel

Webster Percival of Cape Cod, a sea captain and popular storyteller on his way to a new command in Liverpool for a vessel owned by Baker & Morrill. Adding to his charm was the fact that the convivial captain's family forebears included "Mad Jack" Percival, who famously circumnavigated the globe with U.S.S. *Constitution* ("Old Ironsides") thirty years earlier. Since "Old Ironsides" had been constructed in Boston, and since many distant branches of the Dimock family had long resided on Cape Cod, Susan may have been particularly delighted by Captain Percival's well-told tales.[10]

Running the whole *Schiller* operation was Captain George Thomas—a handsome, gregarious, bushily-mustached fellow of thirty-nine—and his crew of one hundred and eighteen. As the steamship prepared to depart, those crewmembers were on duty everywhere, and ranged from officers, sailors, engineers, and firemen to cooks, bakers, butchers, and both male and female stewards. A pair of marine artists, commissioned to paint seascapes and ship portraits for the Eagle Line, may well have aroused the cultured young women's curiosity. And while Susan Dimock was often interested in sharing stories with other physicians, it's unlikely that she gained any medical knowledge from the ship's two surgeons, Messrs Boll and Sanders. Medical personnel contracted to maritime travel were rarely of the same caliber or training as their land-based colleagues.[11]

More likely, Susan was simply relieved to breathe the fresh sea air and enjoy an unusual amount of leisure time, unencumbered by medical worries or work obligations.

As advertised, S.S. *Schiller* was prepared to depart at 3:00 p.m. on Tuesday, April 27. Once the gangplanks were pulled and the mooring ropes cast off, the ship's steam whistle blew and the ten-day voyage began—presumably a smooth, 3,577-mile transatlantic trip from Hoboken to Hamburg. In addition to the 372 passengers and crewmates on board, the vessel was fairly bursting with baggage: massive storage areas overflowed with passengers' trunks, dozens of mailbags, large pieces of agricultural equipment, sewing machines, $300,000 in twenty-dollar gold coins, and a plethora of other mercantile items, all destined for Europe and beyond. After slowly backing into the Hudson River from the Eagle Line pier, *Schiller* turned and forged ahead downriver, as well-wishers, family, and friends waved and shouted goodbye. As it turned out, "fare thee well" might have been a better wish than "goodbye," since a fishnet tangled in the rudder, the tide was receding, and the steamship was badly overloaded with cargo. As a result, *Schiller* was forced to anchor off Long Island, in Lower New York Bay, until the next morning's tide.[12]

No one aboard seemed dismayed over the false start, however, and socializing began at once, continuing in varied fashion over the next three, largely uneventful, and relatively clear, calm days. As delineated in an 1870

Harper's magazine article on "The Ocean Steamer," such socializing was the norm. "When the weather is tolerable," the article explained, the scenes onboard are "of a very active and incessant gossip—innocent because it is usually good-natured, and entertaining because it has the field entirely to itself. There is, in fact, nothing else to be done, and nothing to occupy the thoughts, for the mass of the company of passengers, but to inquire about, and talk about, their neighbors. ... In such a remarkably constituted society, consisting of a body of utter strangers to each other, but thrown by circumstances into the closest domestic intimacy, and exposed, moreover, as they all imagine, to common hardships and a common danger, it is very natural and very excusable that every body [*sic*] should wish to know who every body else is, and why and how they are crossing the Atlantic."[13]

Being in First Saloon lodgings, Susan, Bessie, and Carrie had the opportunity to wander the decks or lounge in the impressive forty-foot-square pavilion, with its overstuffed benches, raised skylight, and plush furnishings. Since most of the passengers had come in from New York, New Jersey, Pennsylvania, and the Midwest, the three friends may have enjoyed conversing with these strangers from afar as well as with the small number of fellow New Englanders on the voyage.

Through their ambassadorial and senatorial connections, Carrie and Bessie probably knew, or knew of, Mrs. Z.B. Caverly of Lowell, Massachusetts. Highly-esteemed in both New York and Washington, D.C., social circles, Rebecca Marquand Crosby Caverly was the daughter of powerful Lowell judge Nathan Crosby and the widow of Zechariah B. Caverly, who had served as Secretary of the U.S. Legation in Lima, Peru. Quite accomplished and fascinating in her own right, Mrs. Caverly was sharing a saloon-class stateroom with her sixteen-year-old daughter Amy and accompanying Mary Ridgway, the widow of Joseph Ridgway of Newburyport, Massachusetts, on the voyage.[14]

Poor Mrs. Ridgway had an unusually sad narrative to share. Over the previous six years, she had lost her husband and their two adult daughters in a cascade of unlikely and unfortunate travels.[15] Now, buoyed by the friendship of Mrs. Caverly—and the companionship of her own two motherless grandchildren, her widowed son-in-law, and a formerly enslaved female maid—Mary Ridgway was enjoying conversation with fascinating young women like Susan, Bessie, and Carrie. Still, the widow Ridgway had one goal in the forefront of her mind: her voyage on the *Schiller* was the first step on a prayerful pilgrimage to Nice and the Tyrolean Alps, the sites where her two adult daughters had died.

Though most of the *Schiller's* passengers did not share Mary Ridgway's sorrowful story, numerous other women onboard were similarly traveling with children. While the youngsters in First Saloon frolicked across the decks in the popular "sailor suits" of the day, the most proper ladies were decked out in onion-like layers of clothing, starting with corsets, followed by multiple petticoats, bustles, underskirts and overskirts, and topped off by fashionable apron-fronts. These already-bulky female outfits were often made even heavier, since many had cautiously sewed their valuables into the lining of their clothing.[16] Susan Dimock was likely attired more modestly than her comrades—often seen in her unadorned, simple black dress, a high collar fronted by a brooch or bow, a gold watch on a chain, and a dark bonnet.[17] Meanwhile, the first-class men were sporting substantially lighter Victorian fashions than their female counterparts, including short frock coats, full length trousers, upstanding shirt collars, four-in-hand neckties, and the inevitable top hat, derby, bowler, or Stetson.

With a southwesterly breeze filling the sails and engines at full steam, those opening days on the Atlantic must have seemed bucolic to Susan, Bessie, Carrie, and their new acquaintances. Outside, passengers walked, talked, lounged in deck chairs, or brandished their wooden cue-sticks while playing the quintessential cruise game of deck shuffleboard. Inside their private staterooms or in the shared, glass-ceilinged pavilion, they could play dominoes or card games, curl up and read in the ship's ample library, or join together in song around the saloon piano. At mealtimes, the women joined other First Saloon guests as they assembled around eight large tables in the pavilion, while their Second Class and steerage shipmates did the same in decidedly more modest settings below.[18]

All was good, so it seemed. But then April turned to May.

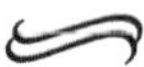

The first few days of May 1875 seemed dreary but hardly apocalyptic to the 372 adults and children aboard S.S. *Schiller*. Certainly, the skies had substantially darkened by Sunday, May 2, accompanied by heavy rains and a wildly churning sea. That sea kept Drs. Boll and Sanders—and perhaps Dr. Dimock as well—busy tending to wildly churning stomachs among the passenger list. As it turned out, the fourth of May was the last day the sun peeked out, enabling the ship's navigators to determine the vessel's exact location by taking accurate celestial readings with a sextant. As a result, save for a few hardy souls, the First Saloon guests opted to observe what they could from within the glass pavilion or return to their staterooms until clearer weather returned.

Over the following days, however, an ever-thickening cloud cover and a complete absence of sun forced the guests to remain inside and the sailors to fall back on "dead-reckoning" to determine their route and location. Captain Thomas and his skilled navigation crew were relatively sure their calculations were good. They could still track *Schiller*'s longitude with a chronometer, then estimate latitude by matching the ship's course with its speed—an impressive fourteen knots, with engine at full throttle and sails filled—for three days straight.[19] They were also fairly convinced they could accurately adapt the ship's compass readings, despite the fact that *Schiller* was one of those new iron-clads whose metal hulls threw "magnetic north" readings off by varying degrees, depending on the ship's location and direction.

There was yet another challenge to charting a course toward the English Channel, which transatlantic seafarers knew well. Essentially, the Duchy of Cornwall—located on England's rugged southwest tip—sits on a convergence of two seas. St. George's Channel comes down from the Irish Sea, north to south. Then Cape Cornwall meets the English Channel, where the prevailing currents run from east to west. Around the headland called Land's End and the Isles of Scilly, these two great ocean currents meet. The result is a real maelstrom of sea conditions, coupled with a quick movement from deep ocean to quite shallow seas. In addition, observers of the treacherous tides in the coastal town of Penzance still talk about the dangers of "pooks," a local term for very dense sea fogs. Those pooks can catch travelers unaware, completely disorienting even the most seasoned mariners as to their location and direction.

In sum, the hidden dangers ahead were many.[20]

Despite much experience and more than two decades at sea, Captain George Thomas' command of S.S. *Schiller* was his first. Perhaps partly for that reason, the captain was intent on arriving in Plymouth, England, on May 7, as scheduled. An on-time arrival would affirm his, the Eagle Line's, and the steamship's own reputation for punctuality—particularly significant in light of the *Schiller*'s delayed launch. The captain's *immediate* goal, however, was to locate Bishop Rock Lighthouse, on the western edge of the Isles of Scilly. Part of the Duchy of Cornwall, those Isles were a rocky, rugged archipelago—vestiges of one gargantuan mass of granite rock submerged in prehistoric times—situated twenty-eight miles southwest of Land's End. Made up of five main islands and more than 140 islets, the Isles of Scilly had long served as both a landmark and a vital first-landing point for transatlantic voyages. Of particular import was the tiny isle called Bishop Rock, where a lighthouse had perched since 1858.[21] Sighting a beam from that lighthouse, or even hearing its fog-bell warning, would confirm *Schiller*'s location for the captain and crew. Moreover, should the lighthouse keepers see that a passing ship was in danger, they could send out assistance or telegraph the mainland for help.

The Isles of Scilly themselves proved to be one more factor that played into the *Schiller*'s troubled journey. The larger, inhabited islands of St.

Mary's, Tresco, St. Agnes, St. Martin's, and Bryer were a welcome destination for many. But not so for some of the dozens of uninhabited islands and islets scattered around them. Like the jagged teeth of a submerged sea monster, many of these low-lying, sawtooth spikes of granite were largely invisible during high tide, only to ferociously appear hours later. Little wonder, then, that since 1700, more than 700 shipwrecks have been confirmed in and around these ancient Isles.[22]

By noon on Friday, May 7, Captain Thomas calculated that Bishop Rock Lighthouse was still 152 miles away but should become visible by 9:00 p.m. Susan Dimock and her friends may have been among the passengers who emerged onto the *Schiller*'s upper deck at 9:00 p.m.—in pitch-black night and impenetrable fog—to help crew members sight that first beam of light and hope. Everyone's combined efforts were in vain, as it turned out, since the dead-reckoning calculations were dead wrong. Rather than being on course to pass seven or eight miles south of Bishop Rock, S.S. *Schiller* was much farther north and currently sailing between that rock's lighthouse and the Great Crebawethen reef of the Western Rocks, heading straight toward the dreaded Retarrier Ledges.[23] Unaware of the imminent danger, many of the male passengers either returned to their staterooms by 9:45 or crowded into the saloon, drinking, talking, playing games, and listening to the piano. Many of the women and children had meanwhile retired to their beds.[24]

Despite *Schiller*'s proximity to the craggy shore, the fog-whistle and fog-bell from Bishop Rock Lighthouse went unheard amid the roaring wind and waves, while the powerful fresnel light went unnoticed. Then at 10:00 p.m. disaster struck: the vessel slammed into the Retarrier Ledges and soon began to list to starboard. Those not shocked by the first blow were rattled by the bumps, grinds, and rumbles that followed. Captain Thomas ordered the passengers to descend below, enabling the crew to gather and disseminate cork life vests and circular life buoys—and to prepare the ship's eight sturdy lifeboats, should conditions worsen. Though some passengers panicked immediately, others took a more optimistic view: if S.S. *Schiller* had lodged on a mammoth ledge at what seemed to be low tide, she would surely regain her stability and steam off those rocks into safe waters once the tides rose.[25]

What no one knew, at least at first, was that following Captain Thomas' effort to back *Schiller* off the ledge, the ship's iron hull ruptured. Seawater began to flow into her lower compartments, driving the steerage passengers to the middle and upper decks. Even worse, by 10:30 p.m., as the angry seas steadily rose, breakers began to wash over the tilting foredeck. Concerted efforts by the crew to cut free and lower the lifeboats were thwarted by throngs of panicking passengers and ever more furiously crashing waves. While some of the male passengers assisted the women and crying children, others resorted to heavy drinking in the pavilion, fighting the crew and each other, or rushing the decks and forcing their way into the half-prepped lifeboats. Captain Thomas tried to scare off the interlopers by firing his pistol several times, with minimal results. "The women and children had no chance," observed passenger Henry Sterne of New York.

Contrary to popular belief, the concept of saving "women and children first" was often quoted but rarely executed until well into the twentieth century. "Every man for himself" was more typically the norm, and male behavior on the *Schiller* proved no exception. Men tended to be physically stronger, more aggressive and competitive, more skilled at swimming, and less encumbered by attire than their female counterparts. Nineteenth-century women were less likely to jump into lifeboats and survive wrecks, due in part to their attachment to children, their relative immobility caused by bulky layers of clothing, and an inability to swim. Yet it was neither the male nor female passengers, but crew members, who had the highest survival rate in these shipwrecks, thanks to their familiarity with the vessel, survival training, and understanding impending maritime dangers sooner than the civilians onboard.[26]

Those *Schiller* crewmembers, when not wrangling with self-preserving men, began firing rockets, fireballs, and roman candles into the night sky, in the hope that Bishop Rock's lighthouse keepers, or even citizens of the inhabited Isles, would see or hear their desperate calls for help.

Despite all these efforts, the situation deteriorated minute by minute. Ultimately, only two of the eight lifeboats deployed, while the others sank, smashed, capsized, or drifted away. And as all classes of passengers were urged to move to the upper decks, groups and individuals were picked off by rising tidal waves, in a terrifying, repeating scenario. Women and children, urged for safety into the deck house, were swept into the sea, as the angry ocean ripped off the deck house roof and scattered all inside into the howling winds and churning waters. Leo Weste of Philadelphia, traveling with his wife Hermine and their daughter, witnessed the final moments of Susan and her friends: "They were all assembled in the pavilion; Miss Greene sat nearest the door, *[and by?]* her Miss Dimock, with their arms around each other, and their faces together. Then Miss Crane, Mrs. Caverly and her daughter. They sat calmly praying, till the waves rose. They then stood, holding on to each other till they were swept off together at 11 O.C."[27]

The frantic *Schiller* crew continued to fire guns into the night, hoping that someone, somewhere, would discern that the ship was in distress. But that too posed a problem. German steamers had traditionally fired guns to "report" their passage, allowing those within hearing distance to know that the ship would be arriving at port not long thereafter, and then telegraph that information ahead to prepare for their arrival. The international shipping community, however, had made recent efforts to codify signals, which dictated that guns should be fired *only* to indicate alarm and the need for immediate assistance. Because of these dueling traditions, *Schiller*'s distress signals, which were eventually heard at Bishop Rock Lighthouse and beyond, were assumed to be German "report" guns. Moreover, even had the listeners understood the signals, it would have proven impossible to launch rescue gigs—long, narrow, six-oared rowing boats—into the rough seas and dense fog until close to daybreak, when visibility and access began to improve.

As both *Schiller* and the ever-diminishing number of passengers on board continued to be shattered and scattered by the winds and waves, rescue ships began arriving—ranging from fishing luggers from the coastal Cornwall village of Sennen to swift and slim pilot gigs from St. Agnes.[28] Hour by hour, and day by day, valiant Scillonians scoured the rocks, waters, and nearby beaches both for survivors and victims. All those pulled from the seas, rocky ledges, shores, and lifeboats—some even clutching onto floating debris—were eventually brought back to the large island of St. Mary's and lodged either in Hugh Town's two hotels or the makeshift warehouse morgue at the end of the town's stone pier.[29] Despite all these efforts, the dreadful truth eventually became apparent: of the 372 passengers and crew aboard S.S. *Schiller*, only 37 survived. Most of the survivors were crew members, many of whom had lashed themselves to the rigging of the ship's iron masts. The sole woman saved was Christine Joens, whose husband John had forged through the crushing crowds on the main deck, lifted her in his arms, and thrown her into the Number Five lifeboat. That in itself didn't guarantee success, since only twelve of the thirty souls in that lifeboat survived.

The news of the disastrous wreck of S.S. *Schiller* broke on Saturday, May 8, by way of the telegraph cable laid half a dozen years earlier between the island of St. Mary's and Penzance, on the Cornwall mainland. The only trained telegrapher on the island was Alexander Gibson. According to popular legend, Gibson kept grinding out telegraph messages as the news trickled in, then collapsed after two weeks into a 30-hour sleep.[30] (The Gibson family later gained renown as photographers specializing in images of wrecked ships, with studios on both the islands and mainland.)

The *Schiller* wreck became the first disaster to be internationally publicized by telegraph. And the news grew grimmer by the day. Ever-changing details went first to London, then were dispatched worldwide by Lloyd's and the Reuters News Service. Thanks to the transatlantic

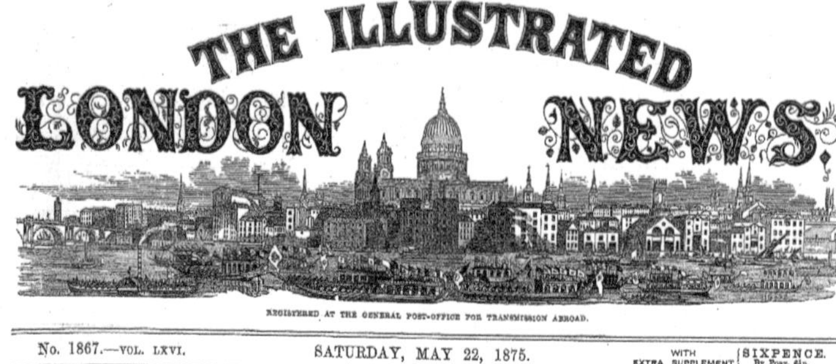

WRECK OF THE SCHILLER: THE RETARRIER LEDGES AND BISHOP ROCK LIGHTHOUSE, SCILLY ISLES.

The wreck of the *Schiller* made headlines in newspapers around the world. The cover of *The Illustrated London News* showed boatmen approaching the battered remnants of the ship on the deadly Retarrier Ledges, with Bishop Rock lighthouse in the background (The Wreck of the Schiller: The Retarrier Ledges and Bishop Rock Lighthouse, Scilly Isles; *Illustrated London News*, May 22, 1875; courtesy the Morrab Library, Penzance, Cornwall, UK).

cable, many readers on the eastern seaboard of the U.S. knew of the gloomy scenario before most of the inhabitants of the Isles of Scilly. The *New York Times*, which devoted its entire front page to details of the *Schiller* and its passengers, announced it thus:

> *Intelligence of shocking disaster has just reached this city. The Eagle Line steamship Schiller, Captain Thomas … has been wrecked off the Scilly Isles. It is believed that 200 persons have perished.*[31]

As the reported death tally rose from that initial 200 to some one hundred more, many around the world were duly pessimistic about the possible survival of their loved ones. Not so in Boston, where collective hope for Susan Dimock and Bessie Greene was stretched out for two more days. "Miss Dimock was a very good swimmer and was possessed of considerable courage," wrote the *Boston Evening Transcript* on May 10, "and it is possible that these companions may have survived the terrible disaster and landed on one of the islands."[32]

In fact, Susan's lifeless body had been found floating near the *Schiller* wreck the day before, pulled from the sea by one Stephen Jenkin on the large pilot gig *Queen*, based on St. Martin's island. As with the other victims retrieved from scattered sites, Susan's body was returned to St. Mary's and stored in the temporary morgue off Hugh Town pier, where her corpse was numbered, her body wrapped in calico cloth, and her belongings inventoried and bagged by the "Receiver of the Wreck." Her possessions were few: some coins, paper money, and bank notes; her gold watch on a chain; and two "cuffstuds," also referenced as "a pair of solitares."[33]

Friends, former schoolmates, and medical colleagues from both sides of the Atlantic reacted swiftly to the news of Susan's death. Lilian Freeman Clarke, the daughter of famed Boston minister James Freeman Clarke, sped to the Isles to retrieve both Susan's and Bessie's bodies. Once it was learned that Bessie's remains had not been recovered, her father, Colonel William Batchelder Greene, insisted on paying for Susan's return home. At the same time, Susan's English friends, Dr. Elizabeth Garrett Anderson and Frances Elizabeth Morgan (the latter, Susan's classmate from Zurich), had rapidly connected with Doctors Elizabeth Blackwell and Sophia Jex-Blake, as well as Anna Dahms, one of Susan's former students. This coterie of prominent female physicians and medical students agreed to immediately send Morgan's husband, Dr. George Hoggan, to the Isles of Scilly accompanied by Miss Dahms, who wanted to pay last respects to her former teacher and would be best qualified to identify the body.[34]

It soon became apparent that her body was easy to identify. Too many of the drowned were found badly decomposed, frozen in frantic gestures, or bearing facial expressions of fear or dismay. Not so Susan Dimock. In fact, word had spread rapidly that there was something unusual about Susan in death—something that set her apart from the other shipwreck victims. Lilian Freeman Clarke heard from the sailors and saviors that the doctor was found "floating on the water, with an expression of such peace and power on her face that it made a wonderful impression on all who saw it. Even the rough men who carried her to the shore were strongly influenced by it."[35]

Dr. George Hoggan, coming in from London, chronicled the experience with similar awe. "On our arrival at Scilly, the leading people, being advised of our coming, met us on the landing, introduced themselves by name, and offered to lend us every aid we might require." Dr. Hoggan and Miss Dahms were escorted to the morgue, where they were gently led to Susan. "Identification was most easy," wrote Hoggan to Susan's mother, "a sweet, peaceful smile sat upon her countenance, as if she felt pleased that the anchor had been cast in the haven of eternity, and that the tempest-tossed voyager was now at rest...."

Dr. Hoggan's observations were typically Victorian, both romanticizing and idealizing the death and demeanor of such a pure, young soul.

"The remains had been carefully swathed by women's hands," Hoggan explained in his letter, "and the rough, navy men had strewed flowers over her body. These men had all of them something to tell me about Miss Dimock, and of the special mourning that had been held over her by the whole community. The peaceful beauty of her dead face left a deep impression on all of them who saw her brought ashore; and, when rumor told them of her great talents, noble character, and useful life, they all affirmed that her loss was a calamity which towered far above the rest of the disaster. One officer (Mr. Ferris), who stood by me while we gazed at the face of the dead, said: 'Look there! that woman died like a hero. I warrant ye she neither showed nor felt any fear of death. I would willingly meet death to-morrow, if I could wear the same expression on my face afterwards.'"[36]

In Boston, the Rev. James Freeman Clarke summarized it thus: "You, who knew her, all know this; but it is remarkable to find that the same power remained with her after death."[37]

A night of despair and a week of recoveries ended in a month of funerals.

The first funeral was held on St. Mary's, the largest of the Isles of Scilly at two-and-a-half by one-and-a-half miles in size. After successions of lifeless bodies were brought into the island's Hugh Town harbor by gigs, pilot boats, and fishing vessels, Scillonians gently moved the shipwreck victims from the pier to stone storehouses on the shore. In these makeshift morgues, bodies were cleaned, wrapped in calico winding sheets by two elderly widows, identified as best as possible, and tagged accordingly. Dozens of cheap wooden coffins were swiftly built—both on St. Mary's and in Penzance—then painted black and readied for the corpses.

On late Monday afternoon, May 10, just two days after the disaster, the first of several funeral processions began. Horses and ponies were hitched to a cortège of two-wheeled farm carts, each carrying a pair of black coffins topped with sprays of fresh-cut flowers. The funeral carts snaked down the Hugh Town pier, passed by crowds lining the main thoroughfare, then edged up the hillside toward Old Town Cemetery. A sea of grieving islanders, survivors, relatives, and journalists followed close behind, eventually arriving at the ancient terraced burying ground overlooking the bay. While many were forced to stand outside, others squeezed into the small stone cemetery chapel—a rustic, bell-less structure that still

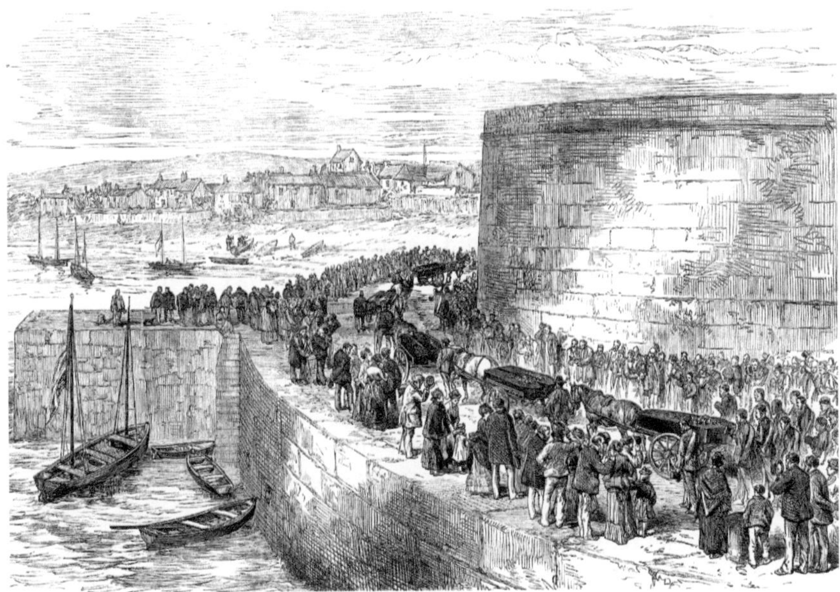

Just two days after the shipwreck, the first of several funeral processions began from the Hugh Town pier transporting victims to Old Town Cemetery. Horses and ponies were hitched to a cortège of two-wheeled farm carts, each carrying a pair of black coffins topped with sprays of fresh-cut flowers (The Wreck of the *Schiller*: Funeral Procession at the Burial of the Drowned, St. Mary's, Scilly Isles; *Illustrated London News*, May 22, 1875, 481; courtesy the Morrab Library, Penzance, Cornwall, UK).

included segments of its ancient Norman origins—for what turned out to be multiple services.

At the moment, there was silence interspersed with hushed prayers and tears. But both before and after the funeral services, the noise was literally earthshaking, as gravediggers blasted and excavated the cemetery's rocky terraces to create three temporary group graves. As coffin after coffin arrived on the carts, most were stacked one upon another and side-by-side in long trenches marked with identifying tags. As it turned out, some of the *Schiller* victims were to remain there for eternity, while others were more fleeting residents. Wealthy families were advised to collect their loved one's remains. A few had already retrieved their deceased kin directly from the harborside morgues, while others arrived at the graveyard just before their beloved's coffin was lowered into the trenches. Though most of these victims were escorted to their homelands for reburial and commemoration, a few stayed in Old Town Cemetery, separated from the others and marked with individual headstones.[38]

The thirty-seven survivors, many too traumatized to speak, gathered in Hugh Town's two inns. Given new clothing by John Banfield, who was the agent for Lloyd's as well as the German Consul, they rested briefly, then were encouraged to move on. From St. Mary's they ferried to Penzance, where most stayed at the Queens Hotel on the Esplanade before boarding trains to Plymouth, London, or beyond. Of those thirty-seven, only fifteen were passengers: three from first cabin, three from second, and nine from steerage. The majority of those who survived the *Schiller* wreck were crewmembers, ranging from officers, sailors, and stewards to stokers, boilermakers, boatswains, and sailmakers. It was common for ships' crews to survive wrecks more often than the passengers; they were more skilled at sea, were better swimmers, and were alerted to impending dangers before the guests. Yet the man in charge of it all, the valiant Captain George Thomas, had gone down with his vessel.[39]

Susan Dimock, we know, was not one of the fortunate thirty-seven. Neither were the other New Englanders on the trip—including the extended Ridgway family, the Caverly family, Captain Daniel Percival, and Susan's friends Bessie and Carrie. Though Susan's body was among the first located and pulled from the waters near the battered *Schiller*, Bessie Greene's was never found. Still, those who knew of Bessie and Susan's intimate relationship were consoled that at least the two had perished together. "In death they were not divided," wrote Susan's mother, "and we must think that they are enjoying Heaven more for having entered it together."[40]

Carrie Crane's grieving aunt and uncle, waiting anxiously for news at the American Embassy in Italy, were dealt a different, but equally painful, blow. Carrie's body was located almost a week after the shipwreck, floating fifteen miles south of the island of St. Agnes. John Dunn, the master of the fishing lugger *Victory*, based in Porthleven on the Cornwall mainland, wrote about her discovery: "On the 13th day of May 1875 ... at about 11 o'clock in the morning.... I saw the Body of a Female floating with a Life belt or Jacket around her, and with the assistance of my Crew I got her into the Boat. I then found it was the Body of a Young Lady with long hair, light blue Eyes,—dressed in Silk plaid Dress with long Waterproof Cloak over same...."[41]

Among the items Dunn found on the lovely young woman was a gold ring, inscribed "E.M. to C.M.C." and dated April 26, 1875—one day before the *Schiller*'s departure from New York. Dunn and his small crew, however, were more interested in finishing their scheduled day of chasing mackerel than collecting the fees paid to vessels that returned with shipwreck victims' remains. He and his six crewmen pulled the ring and other identifying items off Carrie's body, wrapped her in a canvas shroud, weighted her with rocks, and buried her at sea.[42]

Carrie Crane's ring was not the only piece of gold that was salvaged or sought in the wake of the *Schiller* shipwreck. While the initial mission of many of the boatmen was to retrieve survivors or corpses—duties for which they were duly reimbursed—others were eager to salvage the wreck's material treasures: the 250-odd mailbags that had been stored below decks, for example, as well as luggage, trunks, sea chests, boxed farm machinery, mower parts, and other sundries that were rapidly scattering across the waters. The ultimate prizes, however, turned out to be thirty precious barrels of twenty-dollar gold coins, most of which were retrieved intact within three months of the disaster. One keg, split open by accident or by overzealous divers, dumped three hundred or more coins into the wreckage and onto the ocean bed below. To this day, professional divers still scour the area near these treacherous underwater ledges hoping to find the last of those gold coins.[43]

With Bessie's body lost and Carrie's re-interred at sea, Susan Dimock's were the only remains from the trio brought back to the island of St. Mary's. Curiously, various documents alternately assigned May 7 and May 8, 1875, as her official date of death. Though *Schiller* survivor Leo Weste claimed he saw Susan and Bessie swept off the deck together at 11:00 p.m., no one knew how long the two survived in the water. Susan's mother assumed both women succumbed to the turbulent seas within the hour. "What a comfort to know, that with those precious Souls, but one hour intervened between the joys of earth and the impending great joys of Heaven," she wrote to Lilian Freeman Clarke.[44] Others guessed that Susan's time of death was 3:53 the following morning, based on the time frozen on her gold watch. "Her watch (if not run down) marks the moment of her death," observed Dr. George Hoggan, "—seven minutes to four, on the morning of Saturday, 8th of May." Linking death to the time shown on the hands of a clock was common in the Victorian era. It was deemed appropriate, for example, to stop clocks at the moment of a loved one's death, then draw curtains over the windows and cover the mirrors. In the absence of hard evidence, Susan's official death certificate from the New York City Health Department read May 7, 1875, while the records at her final resting place, Forest Hills Cemetery in Jamaica Plain, Boston, read May 8. Her tombstone was likewise engraved May 8, 1875.[45]

When Dr. Hoggan and Anna Dahms arrived from London to identify Susan's body, they already knew she was scheduled to return to Boston. Bessie's grieving father, Colonel William Batchelder Greene, had pledged to pay all expenses incurred in Susan's homecoming. Dr. Hoggan personally embalmed Dr. Dimock in the makeshift morgue near the Hugh Town pier, to prepare the twenty-eight-year-old for her final journey—on the boat to Penzance, the train to Plymouth and London, and the steamer from Bristol to New York. Meanwhile, Lilian Freeman Clarke, Susan and Bessie's close friend and colleague from Boston, arrived to accompany Susan's coffin home. "When we left the island, with the case containing her body in our care," remembered Clarke, "those who followed it insisted on putting it on board with their own hands; and one remarked to me. 'There! we have placed her on board as gently as ever her mother laid her to her breast as a baby.'"[46]

On May 18, 1875, Susan's coffin in tow, Lilian Freeman Clarke boarded the steamer *Arragon* and departed Bristol, England, for New York. Meanwhile, the New England Hospital had appointed George W. Bond of Jamaica Plain to chair the committee that ensured Susan's return to Boston and arranged for her funeral and burial. Since Bond needed permission to receive the remains in Manhattan, Colonel Greene wrote to Susan's mother on May 21, requesting she declare Bond her approved agent. "I suppose it will be a week or ten days before the body arrives," explained Greene in his letter, "but it will be well to make such arrangements as we may ... because we will have many new things to attend to...."[47]

Upon arrival in New York City on June 2, Susan's casket was held overnight at the W.D. Morgan shipping agency on 70 South Street. The next morning, George Bond settled Lilian and the coffin on the train to Boston. Benjamin F. Smith Undertakers of 251 Tremont Street met the women at the station later that afternoon. The next day, the Rev. James Freeman Clarke—who was both Susan's friend and Lilian's father—would host the funeral service for Susan, Bessie, and Carrie at his Church of the Disciples in Boston's South End.

Friday, June 4, 1875, should have been just another lovely late spring day in Boston. For many, it was a time to shop the "black and fancy silks" sales at Jordan Marsh, buy lawn mowers at Hovey & Co. near Faneuil Hall, or row a rental boat across the Public Garden's lagoon. Others were eager to catch a show at the Boston Museum or the Music Hall, or exchange gossip about the successful "sound transmission experiment" Alexander Graham Bell had made two days earlier, from his fifth-floor workshop on Court Street.

But for the friends, family, and admirers of Susan Dimock, the destination of necessity for the fourth of June was the Reverend Clarke's Church of the Disciples. Dominating the corner of West Brookline and Warren streets, the church was an imposing presence. Seven arched Gothic windows set under rows of ornate dentils lined each side of the geometric brick building, while the steeply sloped roof ascended to a broad hexagonal cupola topped by a stone chalice and cross. As guests entered the church through a trio of impressive Gothic arches, they were struck by the high Victorian motifs inside.

Reflecting the bereavement of those in attendance with typical Victorian excess, the church's altar, arches, fresco windows, and tables fairly overflowed with the most splendid classical symbols of death and mourning. Mounds of lilies, magnificent wreaths, weeping willow, floral crosses, and flowing fabrics were hung, strung, and draped throughout the spacious chamber, befitting a personage as significant as the New England Hospital's resident physician. Instead of the traditional black popularized by Queen Victoria through decades of mourning her late husband, many of the fabrics and flowers were in hues of violet, purple, and white—colors that symbolized youth and the unmarried.[48]

The arch behind Dr. Clarke's pulpit was festooned with "passion-vine and larch, surmounted with rich purple wisteria," which, in the eyes of Ednah Dow Cheney, "drooped as if in sympathy."[49] Since Susan's was the only body recovered, there was but one casket present, covered by a violet drape. On the table near her head was a vase of ascension lilies, which friends recognized as Susan's favorite flowers. At the foot of her coffin, a second table held three floral bouquets of white and violet—one each for Susan, Bessie, and Carrie.

As a woman of purpose and simplicity, it's likely that Susan Dimock would have been chagrined by the grandeur and ceremony that followed, despite her love for her old friend, Dr. Clarke.

Major local newspapermen attended and chronicled the event, as well as a reporter from *The New York Times*.[50] Once the church was filled with mourners and the organ music resounded throughout the stone chamber, Dr. James Freeman Clarke began his scripture reading, followed by

Alice Parker singing "Come Unto Me" from Handel's *Messiah*. It was Dr. Clarke's subsequent remarks, however, that most moved both the newspapers and assembled mourners. "We have the sad satisfaction to-day of coming together for one last united expression of love and reverence toward our dear friends …," he began. "Having loved such souls as these, we shall always love them. Having known them once, we shall never cease to know them."[51]

Though the loss of Boston's beloved young woman doctor was arguably the central theme of the service—in part because of her standing, and in part because hers was the only body present—the Reverend Clarke was deliberately inclusive, especially with Bessie Greene. "When we heard of this great disaster," he continued, "it seemed almost too much to lose with Susan Dimock her intimate friend, another soul, also so rare and radiant; … These two dear friends, each so noble, so needed, went away together, and a part of our own life seems to have gone with them. … [Bessie], too, was so young and yet so wise; so full of enjoyment, always happy, bright as a sunbeam, and also taking the most serious and most noble tasks of life into her young hands, becoming an arm of aid to the weak, and a hand of help to … the most helpless of her human sisters."[52]

More extensive and eloquent remarks by Dr. Clarke were followed by additional organ music, "an impressive prayer" by Clarke, and the full congregation singing the popular hymn, "Nearer, my God, to Thee." That same hymn became associated with the sinking of RMS *Titanic* in 1912, since some survivors claimed it was played by the ship's string ensemble as the vessel sank.

After the benediction, the tearful assemblage inside the Church of the Disciples arose and remained standing as eight pallbearers bore Susan's coffin from the church. Every reporter present specifically mentioned the names of those eight men: Henry Ingersoll Bowditch, Samuel Cabot, Edward Hammond Clarke, Benjamin Joy Jeffries, Charles Pickering Putnam, Reginald Heber Fitz, Francis Minot, and J.P. Oliver. The eight men's names were worth listing since they were all prestigious Boston physicians from socially prominent families, were largely Harvard-educated, and had all, in different ways and at different times, actively supported Susan and the New England Hospital. It was particularly notable that Edward Hammond Clarke, the author of the anti-feminist *Sex in Education*, was among them. All eight doctors were influential members of the Massachusetts Medical Society, which had refused Dimock membership, as it had done with every woman applicant. Perhaps ironically, and certainly symbolically, the eight male pallbearers were viewed that day as Dr. Susan Dimock's peers.[53]

Undertaker Benjamin F. Smith parked a horse-drawn hearse just outside the church entrance. Once Susan's casket was placed on the wagon, a long train of mourners followed along the four-mile journey to Forest Hills in Jamaica Plain, Boston's most beautiful and largest rural garden cemetery. Such long treks were typical by the mid–nineteenth century, since all the downtown burying grounds had been filled to capacity. After passing through the cemetery's majestic Gothic-gated entrance, they wound past well-manicured, tree-shaded knolls *en route* to one of the most desirable sections of the memorial park. There, on the hill called Mount Dearborn, Susan's coffin was gently lowered into a freshly dug hollow at 3056 Sweet Briar Path. That her grave site was near several prestigious old Bostonians—including members of the Weld and Agassiz families, famed clockmaker Simon Willard, and General Henry A.S. Dearborn, the cemetery's founder and co-designer—was a clear statement of esteem for the young doctor.

"When we had reached the spot where our dear friend's body was to be laid to rest," remembered a friend, "we stood around her open grave, and the minister repeated from the Gospel of John the passage beginning, 'Let not your heart be troubled.' Then Dr. Bowditch said: 'I know no one for whom I have a more sincere love and respect than I had for Dr. Dimock; and I now propose that, instead of allowing the last services to be performed by strangers, we, who knew her and loved her in life, should with our own hands lay the earth in her grave.'"

Hearing their cue, the undertaker's men handed their spades to the physicians present, who lifted earth into the grave, then passed the shovels on to the many friends who came forward. One onlooker described those final moments: "Very gently, with reverent hands, the earth was placed upon the coffin, the birds singing, and the trees waving, and the blue June sky looking down as if with a blessing all the time. And when the last spadeful had been tenderly laid down, we covered the grave with flowers, and came away; leaving, indeed, the precious body in the earth, but with a memory and a hope that will never die out of our hearts, making each day of our lives more beautiful and blessed with the thought of one whose own life was a perpetual benediction."[54]

Susan Dimock would certainly have been happier working at the hospital, teaching her young nurses, performing complex surgeries, and calming her patients.

But instead, she and her remarkable journey had come to an end.

For months after her death, Susan Dimock was mourned, analyzed, and eulogized through words—in obituaries, articles, and letters written from Boston, North Carolina, Zurich, London, Paris, Vienna, and other regions where the young surgeon had touched people's hearts and captivated their imaginations. In her hometown of Washington, North Carolina, the news "fell with crushing weight upon the hearts of her family and friends, [and] shrouded our community in gloom and sadness." In her chosen city of Boston, Susan's death "brought to our own community … grief and pain as great possibly as the death of any private persons could possibly produce." Internationally acclaimed artist Anne Whitney, writing from Florence, Italy, summarized it well when she observed, "Miss Dimick's [sic] death will pierce a great many hearts."[55]

The words, not surprisingly, invited comparisons of Susan to another strong and independent Boston woman who had been similarly lost at sea, twenty-five years earlier. "Among all the bright lives that have been engulfed in this dreadful shipwreck, none is more valuable than [Susan Dimock's]," wrote Mary Putnam Jacobi, MD. "Perhaps no woman's life of equal social value has met this tragic fate since the body of Margaret Fuller was washed ashore on the western coast of the Atlantic."[56] Like Dimock, Fuller had successfully forged through a world and a profession dominated by men, challenging stereotypes of "woman's work" along the way.[57]

Words were also shared mourning the loss of Susan's close companion, Bessie Greene. Poet John Greenleaf Whittier, a relative of the Greene family, exclaimed, "How strange that we shall never see her more! That that young, bright, beautiful life is gone out of the world!"[58] Another literary light, Maine-based writer Sarah Orne Jewett, lamented to her friend Annie Fields in Boston about Bessie and Susan's simultaneous demise: "I am full of sadness and of sympathy over this terrible disaster. Hardly can I think of anything else, and those two dear people haunt my little room, the sunny piazza, the little garden; I see and hear them everywhere. How gentle they were, how sweet and good and noble. How can we spare them, and fools and knaves are cumbering the earth! I have such a letter of sorrow from S. C., who grew so attached to them here: 'That dear, splendid little doctor! To think of the cruelty of her tender body being beaten on the rocks!'"[59]

Many fondly remembered the close bond between Susan and Bessie. "Beside her in that dreadful hour was the beloved friend who had been with her in so many scenes of joy and sorrow, herself as fair and beloved and full of life," recalled Ednah Dow Cheney. "A friendship on so high a plane between such gifted souls was as beautiful as that of David and Jonathan. Truly, they were 'lovely and pleasant in their lives, and in their death they were not divided.'"[60]

It was the same Ednah Dow Cheney who collected many of these letters, obituaries, and tributes, then arranged them alongside some original text, augmented by correspondence to and from Susan during her European sojourn. The result was a 103-page volume, the cloth-bound *Memoir of Susan Dimock, Resident Physician of the New England Hospital for Women and Children*. Released in Boston six months after the *Schiller* shipwreck, the book was printed by Roberts Brothers, a publisher with offices across from the Old South Meetinghouse on Washington Street.[61]

Roberts Brothers had skyrocketed to fame seven years earlier with the release of Louisa May Alcott's *Little Women*. Curiously, the 1875 Dimock *Memoir* foreshadowed the future direction of Roberts, both in author attribution and subject matter. Though Cheney wrote Dimock's *Memoir*, her name appears nowhere on the book. Beginning in 1876, Roberts Brothers inaugurated a "No Name" series, which deliberately left out authors' names

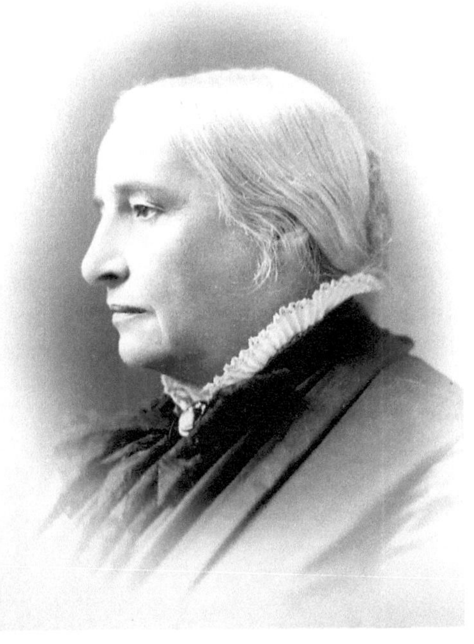

Ednah Dow Littlehale Cheney (1824–1904) was an American philanthropist, writer, and reformer who supported the New England Hospital for Women and Children as volunteer secretary, president, friend, and donor. Following the death of Susan Dimock in 1875, Cheney assembled letters, obituaries, and reminiscences about the young doctor into a *Memoir* (used by permission of the Dimock Center, Roxbury, Massachusetts).

in the hopes that the contents of the books would sell themselves. Cheney wrote the Dimock *Memoir* as a brief biography and anthology in 1875. In the 1880s and '90s, Roberts Brothers ran its "Famous Women Series," featuring women authors writing women's biographies, including heroes like Margaret Fuller, Mary Wollstonecraft, and Jane Austen.[62]

As limited as Cheney's sympathetic *Memoir of Susan Dimock* was in historical content—it was, after all, assembled in a mere five months—it served an admirable purpose. "I would be glad if every woman in the land could read a record of [Dr. Dimock's] life," wrote Mary E. Little, a friend and former student of Susan's. "It would inspire them to loftier views, to purity of life. It would make them better wives, better mothers, better citizens."[63]

It would also, of course, have made them better doctors.

After the words of reverence and remembrance came countless requests for keepsake images. Though the camera had been invented in 1839, professional portrait sittings were still a relative rarity in the 1870s, and Kodak snapshot cameras would not be available to the public-at-large until 1888. As a result, Susan sat for only two known photo sessions: the first, following her graduation from medical school while studying in Vienna, and the second after she returned home to Boston. While two different poses from the Vienna sitting show a younger woman than her Boston patients, pupils, and friends remembered, most agreed that these albumen photographs captured her essence, "with a clear, fresh complexion, a full but not very high forehead, … dark hair, and a mouth expressing as much gentleness as firmness."[64] The later Boston sitting resulted in

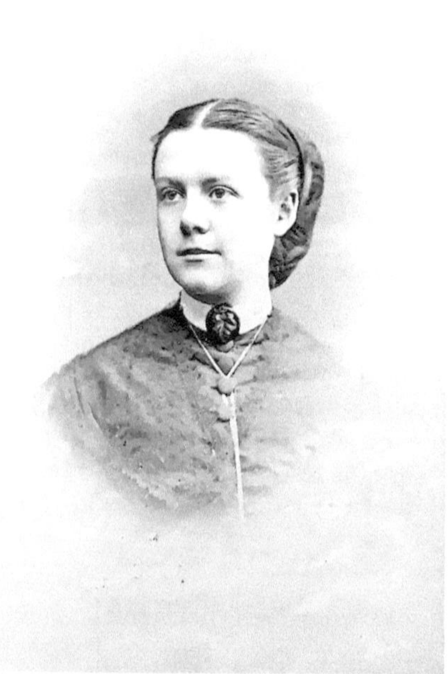
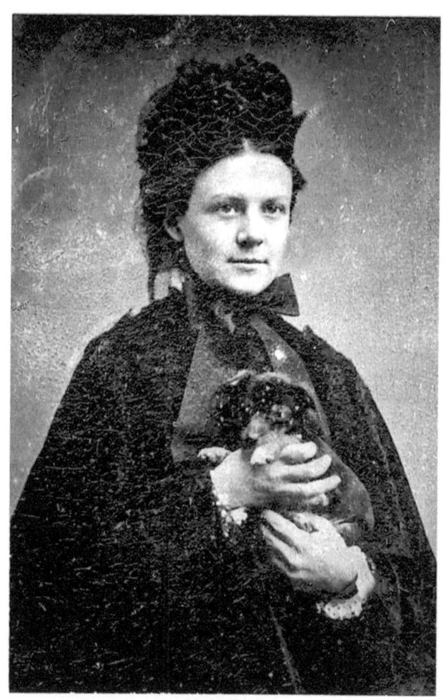

Though the camera had been invented in 1839, professional portrait sittings were still a relative rarity in the 1870s. Susan Dimock sat for two known photograph sessions: the first (left) following her graduation from medical school while studying in Vienna, and the second (right) cradling her pet spaniel Dotty after returning home to Boston (New England Hospital for Women and Children Records, Sophia Smith Collection, Smith College, Northampton, Massachusetts; used by permission of the Dimock Center, Roxbury, Massachusetts; the private collection of Susan Wilson, courtesy Kay Hicks, Lynchburg, Virginia).

a small ambrotype depicting a more mature Dr. Dimock cradling her pet spaniel, Dotty. The latter photograph was taken specifically for her mother, Mary Malvina Dimock, and was not published until more than a century after her death.[65]

Ednah Dow Cheney lamented of the photos that "[n]one of them are entirely satisfactory to her friends, since it was impossible, in mere mechanical light and shadow, to reproduce the brightness of her countenance and the bloom of her color." Still, she admitted, "they all have value as records." The issue of "light and shadow" also caused considerable delay in acquiring several dozen copies of the first photo from Vienna. In an era before electricity and mechanical enlargers in darkrooms, many photographic images were still made using "sun-printing," where negative plates were laid on treated paper, then exposed to the sun for ten to twenty minutes. Anna H. Clarke, the wife of the Rev. James Freeman Clarke, explained that the holdup in delivery was "said to be caused by the fact that there is so little sun in Vienna at this season." Still, she argued, "This Vienna photograph is the most satisfactory likeness which we have I think—but oh how we long to hear the sweet, gentle voice, which is never absent from our memory of that dear face."[66]

When the stack of albumen sun-prints finally arrived in Boston, they were published, duplicated, mailed, and shared with friends, family, colleagues, and the press. Copies of the photo were also given to the Swiss-born Boston painter, Edward L. Custer, whose Boston studio was located at 128 Tremont Street. Though best known for his artistic studies of cattle, Custer also painted landscapes, still lifes, and portraits, and exhibited his work for over two decades at the Boston Athenaeum (the latter served as Boston's *de facto* art museum before the Museum of Fine Arts opened in 1876). According to the *Boston Transcript*, despite his penchant for bovine subjects, Custer's portraits "were uniformly good likenesses, for no man was more accurate in the observation of traits or more faithful in their reproduction. He had the genius of patience and attention, and his power of concentration kept him from the sentimental and the over-emphatic style of treatment."[67]

Custer's oil portrait of Susan Dimock was given to her mother, then returned to the New England Hospital following Mary Malvina Dimock's death.[68] In the painting, Susan is shown in her typical and classically simple black dress, albeit with an unusually frilly collar. She gazes slightly away from the viewer, as if thoughtfully planning her next surgery or nursing lecture. Her mouth is closed in a pleasant, yet determined, manner. Her face looks more rounded and cherubic, and her lips fuller, than the photographic prints on which it was based. Set on a dark Rembrandt-esque background, the portrait exudes youth, poise, and professionalism. It was, one could argue, a fitting testament to the esteem in which the young, exceptionally skilled, and clearly driven doctor was held.

On June 4, 1875, when the twenty-eight-year-old doctor was permanently laid to rest at Forest Hills Cemetery, mounds of fresh flowers were left covering her grave on Mount Dearborn's Sweet Briar Path. For months thereafter, plans for her "simple stone" monument were discussed, debated, disagreed-upon, and, as a result, delayed. More than eight months after the burial, Anna H. Clarke wrote to Susan's mother that she had just seen a new sketch for the stone, adding, "No action has yet been taken on this design, but we all like it better than the first one."[69] A few months later, a finished carved memorial was finally set in place. The gleaming marble stone—fashionable at the time for its "pure white clarity without mineral inclusions"[70]—was topped by a carved floral variation on the classic Celtic cross. Just below the cross, set in a sunken frame, a brief inscription read simply:

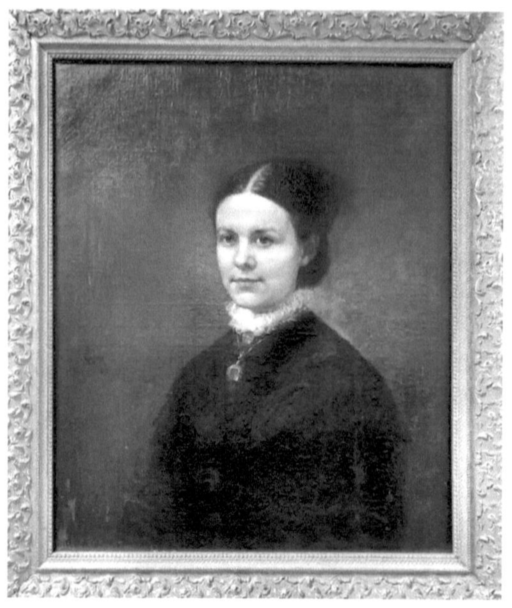

Set on a dark Rembrandt-esque background, the posthumously painted oil portrait of Dr. Dimock by Swiss-born Boston painter Edward L. Custer exudes youth, poise, and professionalism (used by permission of the Dimock Center, Roxbury, Massachusetts; photograph © the author).

SUSAN DIMOCK, M.D.
28 YEARS
BEING MADE PHYSICIAN IN A
SHORT TIME, SHE IS REMB'D
A LONG TIME.

Further details on Susan's life and death graced the back of the monument:

SUSAN DIMOCK
SURGEON AND PHYSICIAN
TO THE NEW ENGLAND HOSPITAL

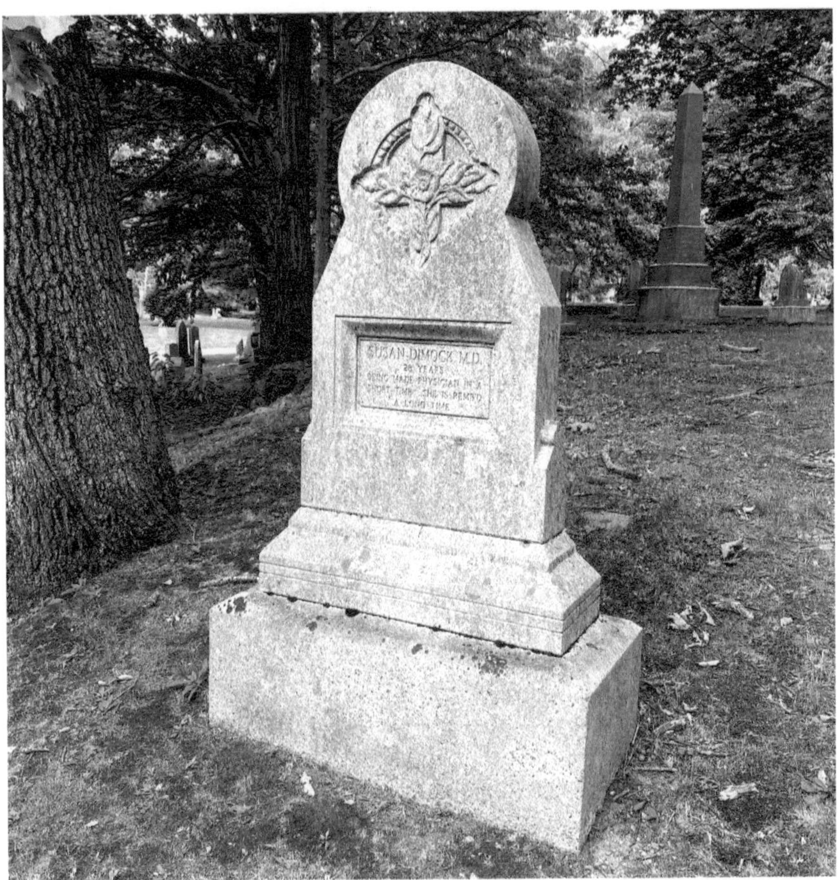

Susan Dimock's marble gravestone at Forest Hills Cemetery in Jamaica Plain was decorated with a carved floral variation on the classic Celtic cross (photograph © the author).

FOR WOMEN AND CHILDREN
LOST IN THE STEAMER SCHILLER
ON THE SCILLY ROCKS
MAY 8, 1875

Still, those who knew Susan well realized that none of these commemorations—words, images, or stone monuments—would have mattered to the young doctor. Hence, her closest colleagues and friends arranged to have something more substantial celebrate her legacy, something that would continue "the work she loved and served."[71] The result was a campaign to establish the Susan Dimock Free Bed at the New England Hospital for Women and Children. Knowing that $5,000 would endow such a free bed in perpetuity for needy patients, the fundraising committee began collecting donations through public subscription. Local papers, including the *Boston Daily Globe* in its "City and Suburbs" column, regularly published updates of the fund's progress. According to the *Globe*, an impressive $2,523 was accumulated by July 29, 1875. In addition, the paper reported, an additional $805 had been donated "for funeral expenses, portrait and other memorials of Dr. Susan Dimock."[72] Two months later, the New England Hospital's Annual Report announced that the $5,000 had "already nearly been collected." Ednah Dow Cheney explained that the money had come "from various classes of patients, pupils, and friends; and even those who knew her only in Europe have rejoiced at the opportunity to unite themselves with this testimony to her worth."[73]

That same New England Hospital Annual Report ended with a poignant philosophical note: "Hawthorne said that the Pilgrims never really loved their New-England home until they had laid one of the dearest of their little band under its soil. Perhaps we have never known how this Hospital of ours is entwined with our heart's affections until it has become sacred with the memory of those on whom death has set its sanctifying seal."[74]

An editorial in the *Philadelphia Medical Times* published two months after Susan's death acknowledged that the young doctor was a standard-bearer for women entering the field of medicine. "A chronicler of the passing events of the day cannot fail to note the continued growth of the 'woman movement' in medicine," the article began. "Abroad, Mrs. Garrett Anderson appears to be received freely in the best medical circles of London ... and in Boston the *Medical Journal* lavishes praise on Miss Susan Dimock, who was lost in the *Schiller*."

The seemingly enlightened analysis, however, finished with a backhanded compliment about the advances of women and African Americans. "As we said some time since, the day for discussion is over; and, although the brain of the average woman does weigh less than that of the average man, and although some may believe the profession is being deteriorated, going to ruin, or what not, yet it is becoming more and more apparent that, like the negro at the South, woman in medicine is a fact which it is wiser to adapt ourselves to than to knock out our brains against."[75]

More than just a standard-bearer for women entering the field of medicine, Susan Dimock had also set a precedent of excellence for women pursuing a specialty in surgery. Initially, Dr. Marie Zakrzewska worried that "Many years will probably elapse before Dr. Susan Dimock's place can be filled." Dr. Mary Putnam Jacobi quite agreed that "both the surgical talents and surgical training of Dr. Dimock are certainly, at the present date, exceptional among women. It is on this account that her loss is literally irreparable, for at this moment there seems to be no one to take her place."[76]

Yet Susan had forged a path—one that many other well-trained women physicians followed in the decades after her death. "In the beginning of our work it was received as an axiom that women might become skilful [sic] physicians and midwives, but could never be equal to the demands of surgery," read a hospital report at the turn of the twentieth century. "Dr. Susan Dimock was the first in our own city to prove the fallacy of this opinion. Her season of active work was too soon fatally closed, but she had already demonstrated the special fitness of women for surgical work; and her example was not lost, for many a bright young woman has since chosen this branch...."[77]

Susan Dimock was a leader not only in the surgical profession, but also in the fight for women's inclusion in previously all-male medical associations. In June of 1872, she was accepted as the first female member of the North Carolina Medical Society. It was an honorary position, however, since she was no longer a state resident. Three months after accepting this honor—and only a few weeks after taking the helm at the New England Hospital—the young doctor sought a more elusive goal: full membership in the adamantly and exclusively male Massachusetts Medical Society.

The Mass. Medical Society was a prestigious organization Susan had dreamed about since her days as a student in Zurich. In October of 1868, she wrote to her friend and mentor, Dr. Samuel Cabot, "I hope to get my Degree here in three and a half years, and then to spend a year in Paris, pass my examinations there also, and get that Degree too to take home to the Mass. Med. Society."[78] Four years later, it appeared that her dream might become a reality. On October 2, 1872, the council of the Mass. Medical Society accepted a letter requesting that Susan be examined for admission. Despite agreement among council members that the request be considered early in 1873, and despite the fact that the idea was argued and fought for, a small but vocal group of dissenting male doctors caused the request to ultimately be shelved. And there it sat, shelved and unacted upon, for more than two years.

Then in 1875, Susan died in the dreadful *Schiller* shipwreck. Newspapers and journals around the world featured remembrances and accolades for this exceptional woman doctor. Seizing the moment, Dr. Henry Bowditch took immediate action. On June 8, 1875, just four days after Susan Dimock's funeral, Bowditch formally proposed that a committee be appointed to create a plan for admitting qualified female physicians into the Mass. Medical Society. Still, nothing was decided. Over the following years, "animated discussions" and heated debates about female inclusion often included references to the remarkable Dr. Dimock. But each time the decision was stalled by minority protests. Finally, on June 13, 1882—ten years after Susan's initial request and seven years after her death—the subject of admitting women to the Society came to a vote and was accepted by a clear majority of the members.

Forty years later, a chronicler of the Mass. Medical Society's history observed, "Since that time the subject has not been revived, women have become fellows of the society in ordinary course, and we marvel that there could be so much and so long sustained opposition to what today we regard as the obvious."[79]

On September 25, 1884, Dr. Emma Louise Call of Cambridge, Massachusetts, a former student and current physician at the New England Hospital, was admitted to the Massachusetts Medical Society—the first woman to be granted membership.[80] Less than a month later, on October 20, Codman Street, the small road leading into and through the New England Hospital's hillside campus, was officially renamed Dimock Street.

Susan Dimock, it seemed evident, would always remain in memory. "All that we could do for her has been done," reflected Dr. Elizabeth Garrett Anderson, "but what she has done for *us*, for service, for women, for humanity—that remains a vital and permanent good which cannot perish."[81]

When Susan Dimock died, she left a grieving mother, 53-year-old Mary Malvina Owens Dimock. Mary Malvina's final letter to her daughter had been written on May 2, 1875, five days before the fateful shipwreck. The intent, of course, was to ensure that Susan had a letter in hand shortly after arriving in Europe. In her sweet, rambling, four-page missive to "Susie dear," Mrs. Dimock wrote about Susan's pet dog and cat, Dotty and Dainty, chronicling in abundant detail their daily escapades in and about the doctor's private chambers at the New England Hospital. "Give my best love to Bessie," she entreated her daughter, "and tell her I am sure her Mother's letters won't be near so long and interesting as mine, for she has no Dot and Dainty to write of." Meanwhile, Mrs. Dimock admitted that "I have done little since you left but 'putter' around, picking up your things and arranging them with my own for the summer."

When not puttering and picking up, Mary Malvina found a surrogate daughter in Dr. Mary E. Little, a former New England Hospital student who agreed to serve as resident physician during Dr. Dimock's five-month sabbatical. Shortly after putting her daughter on the train to New York *en route* to the Hoboken piers, Mrs. Dimock had even led Dr. Little on the first of several downtown Boston shopping sprees that ultimately yielded a new Neapolitan bonnet (a woman's head-covering with a small crown and wide, rounded, front brim), decorative trimmings, and two long combs. After personally coiffing Dr. Little's hair, Mrs. Dimock proudly announced that the final package was "a very great improvement…. I say she looks quite *Doctor Dimocky*."[82]

Following the shocking news of *Schiller*'s wreck, the days of hope and despair, and finally, the funeral, Mary Malvina Dimock left Boston and settled back in North Carolina, where relatives and friends tried to offer comfort. "I have placed in divers [*sic*] places in my room and on the wall the many little treasures, on which the eyes of my dear departed once delighted to rest," Mrs. Dimock wrote to a friend, "so as to have my surroundings speak as much as possible of her precious presence." It was perhaps a fruitless effort, since "the vacant chair by my side, spoke of the great sorrow that I have been called to pass through."[83]

Susan Dimock's heartbroken mother eventually relocated to Greensboro, in Guilford County, North Carolina, where she lived with the extended Murray family—relatives by both blood and marriage. When Mary Malvina Owens Dimock died in 1910 at the age of 88, she had outlived her husband by forty-eight years, and her only child by thirty-five. Her husband's headstone stood in the cemetery of St. Peter's Episcopal Church, only a block from the Dimocks' old home in Washington, North Carolina. Since that graveyard had long since been filled to capacity, Mrs. Dimock was buried in Oakdale Cemetery, more than a mile away from her husband—and 700 miles from the Boston gravesite of her daughter.[84]

Mary Malvina Dimock was a survivor. In contrast to the long life of Mrs. Dimock, many of those who knew, loved, and worked with her daughter had passed on long before the nineteenth century even came to a close. Colonel William Batchelder Greene, clouded with grief over the death of his own daughter Bessie, died at age 58, only three years after the *Schiller* shipwreck. Susan Dimock's most significant male medical mentors—Dr. Solomon Satchwell in North Carolina (d. 1892), Dr. Jefferson Pratt in Hopkinton (d. 1883), and Drs. Samuel Cabot (d. 1885) and Henry Ingersoll Bowditch (d. 1892) in Boston—didn't live to see the twentieth century. Neither did Dimock's friend and New England Hospital colleague, Dr. Lucy Sewall, who was just 52 when she passed away in 1890. Both the perennially supportive James Freeman Clarke of Boston, and Susan's aunt, Maria Dimock Mann of Sterling, died respectively in 1888 and 1892.

In 1912, when the New England Hospital for Women and Children held a festive gala celebrating its fiftieth anniversary, it was immediately apparent that those of Susan Dimock's peers and promoters who lived to

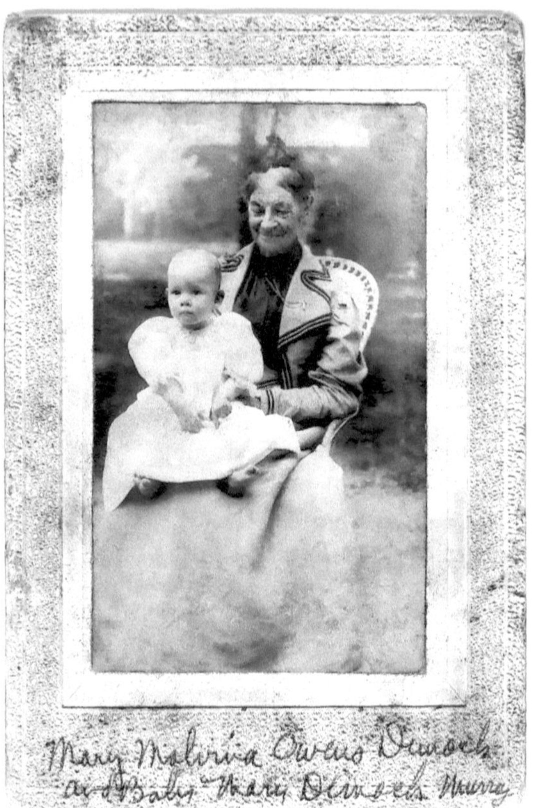

Susan Dimock's heartbroken mother eventually relocated to Greensboro, North Carolina, where she lived with the extended Murray family—relatives by both blood and marriage. When Mary Malvina Owens Dimock died in 1910 at the age of 88, she had outlived her husband by forty-eight years and her only child by thirty-five (photograph of Mary Malvina Dimock with baby Mary Dimock Murray, 1898; courtesy Kay Hicks, Lynchburg Virginia).

greet the new century had not lasted much past the first decade. Among those fondly remembered in a variety of anniversary speeches were Dr. Marie Zakrzewska, the founder, face, and guiding spirit of the hospital, who retired in 1890 and died in 1902 at the age of 72. Recalled also was Ednah Dow Cheney, the hospital's benefactor, secretary, and second president, who died at age 80, two years after Dr. Zak.[85] Meanwhile, Mary Putnam Jacobi, the pioneering American medical physician, teacher, scientist, writer, and suffragist passed in 1906. And fellow medical pioneer Sophia Jex-Blake—the English physician, teacher and feminist who had battled beside Susan Dimock to gain entry into Harvard Medical College in the late 1860s—died early in 1912.

The medical-feminist "old guard" had, with a few exceptions, departed.

With family and so many familiar faces gone, the legacy, the accomplishments, and the remarkable life story of Susan Dimock remained in collective memory as the twentieth century progressed—but to a diminishing degree.

In Susan's native town of Washington, North Carolina, remembrance of the young doctor and her family continued, despite the passing of old friends and fading of personal memories. In April of 1937, historian Pauline Marion Worthy wrote a glowingly detailed full-length feature about Dr. Dimock's life, family, and work in the *Raleigh News & Observer*. It was by far the most extensive piece written about the young doctor since the years immediately following her death in 1875.[86] In 1939, on the eve of the Second World War, the North Carolina Department of Conservation and Development commissioned four historic markers to be erected in the town. Three commemorated events from the Civil War—*The Capture of Washington*, *The Burning of Washington*, and *Fort Hill*, the last being an earthwork battery where Confederate forces set up camp to reclaim the town from Union troops. Only one of the markers honored an individual, and that was the town's illustrious young doctor, Susan Dimock.

On January 19, 1940, presentation exercises were held for all four markers at the Washington High School Auditorium. After the Washington School Band's renditions of "America" and the "Star Spangled Banner," and the High School Glee Club's performances of "Dixie" and "Carolina," distinguished guests were introduced, presentations made, and the four markers were accepted and explained. The memorial plaque for Susan Dimock was formally recognized by Betsy Blount, while Sally Bogart relayed the historical significance of all four.[87]

Happily, those commemorative markers remain in place to this day. Marker B14, perched atop a pole on East Main Street, between Market and Bonner streets, is inscribed to "Dr. Susan Dimock: Native of Washington, Zurich graduate, head of a Boston hospital, 1st woman member N.C. Medical Society, 1872. Her girlhood home was here." Though the sentiment was endearing, the historical facts were not entirely accurate. Dimock was not the "head of a Boston hospital," but the hard-working and under-paid resident physician and chief surgeon. She was a member of the North Carolina Medical Society, but only an honorary one. And the building that once stood on that site was not just Susan's home, but also the Lafayette Hotel, a landmark establishment operated by her mother and aunt.

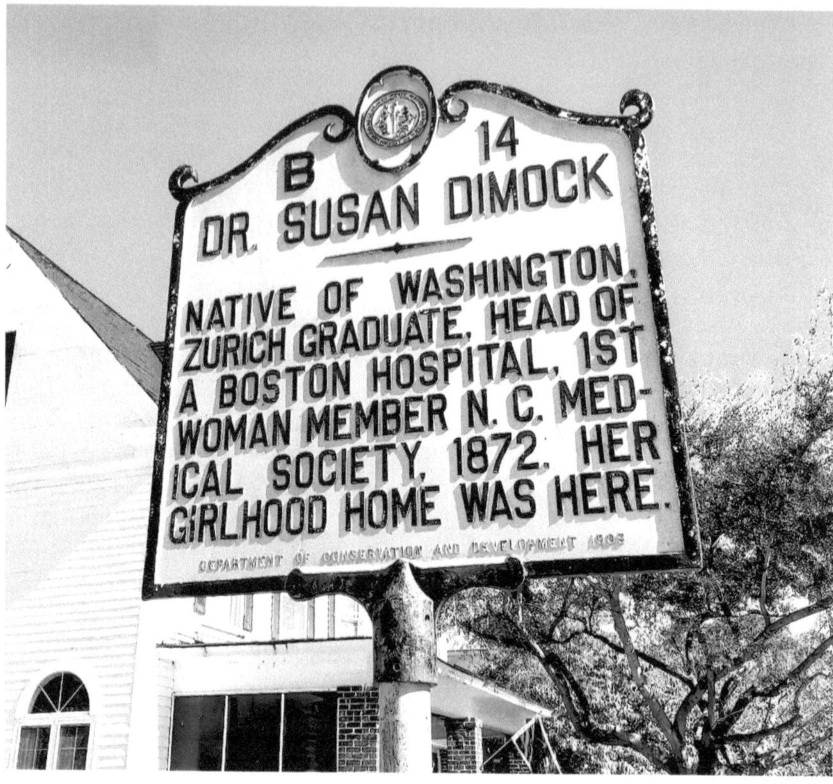

In 1939, the North Carolina Department of Conservation and Development commissioned historic marker B14 to be created and erected on East Main Street, between Market and Bonner streets, in Washington, North Carolina. The lot was the former site of the Lafayette Hotel, Susan Dimock's family home and business (photograph © the author).

Up north in Boston, Susan's pioneering work as a skilled surgeon at the New England Hospital was periodically recalled as younger women began gaining credibility and success in the world of American medicine. In the book produced for the hospital's fiftieth anniversary in 1912, Dr. Augusta Pope acknowledged that "Dr. Dimock's mantle fell on worthy successors."[88] As noted earlier, nine years after Susan's death, in 1884, obstetrician Dr. Emma Call of the New England Hospital was the first woman to receive membership in the Massachusetts Medical Society. Over the next decade, other women doctors who worked at the hospital, including Fanny Berlin and sisters Augusta and Emily Pope, were voted in as well. Still, none of the hospital's founding physicians—like doctors Zak, Sewall, and Dimock—were ever similarly accepted, even posthumously.[89] Nevertheless, an important precedent had been set. When the American

College of Surgeons was established in 1913, two generations after Susan *et al* began their journey, the first five females admitted were all doctors affiliated with the New England Hospital for Women and Children.[90] Clearly, some kind of legacy had been left, both by the hospital and by Susan Dimock herself.

Despite those gains, in the Greater Boston area, the memory of Susan Dimock faded as the twentieth century progressed. Many of the founding or sustaining mothers and fathers of the New England Hospital for Women and Children were memorialized over the years in buildings spread across the campus. The original High Victorian hospital structure (1872) was officially renamed the Dr. Marie E. Zakrzewska Medical Building, later shortened to "The Z Building." The Georgian-Revival style Sewall Maternity House (1892) was inaugurated in honor of Dr. Lucy Sewall and her father, Samuel E. Sewall. The Cheney Surgical Pavilion (1899) was named for Ednah Dow Cheney, while the Goddard Nursing Home (1909) celebrated the Goddard family, whose various members had served as hospital president, director, and treasurer. Colonel Albert Augustus Pope, the much-heralded "founder of American bicycle industries," donated the downtown Pope Dispensary in the name of his twin physician sisters, Emily and Augusta Pope. The last building added to the Roxbury campus while the hospital was still run exclusively by women was the Classical-Revival Richard's Children's Building. Constructed in 1930, it commemorated Linda Richards, America's first professionally trained nurse, who passed away that same year.

But no building was ever named for Dr. Susan Dimock.

In 1969, the New England Hospital finally closed its doors after 107 years of existence and several decades of decline.[91] That century of existence, of course, was heralded for many successes. It was the first hospital in New England to be staffed entirely by women physicians, the first in New England to admit women as interns, and the first in New England to offer obstetrics, gynecology and pediatrics under one roof. It created the first professional school of nursing in the U.S., was the first institution in America to graduate a trained nurse, the first to graduate an African American nurse, and the first to have Visiting Nurses.[92] As mentioned earlier, the New England Hospital also sponsored the first women accepted into the Massachusetts Medical Society and the first accepted into the American College of Surgeons.

Ultimately, however, the New England Hospital for Women and Children proved a victim of its own success. In the nineteenth century, faced with discrimination against professional women, Marie Zakrzewska and her colleagues had created and nourished their hospital by maintaining a policy of separatism—hiring and teaching women to provide healthcare for other women. In the twentieth century, such gender segregation steadily weakened as formerly all-male medical colleges and medical careers increasingly opened up to women.[93] As a result, the refuge once offered to aspiring female physicians by NEHWC seemed less necessary—and to many women, less desirable. In line with national trends, the New England Hospital eventually dropped "for Women and Children" from its name and began hiring male doctors and accepting adult male patients. Perhaps even more significant to its eventual demise was the fact that that beginning in the 1930s, the aging hospital found that it could no longer compete with the wealth of excellent, innovative, well-funded medical institutions booming throughout Greater Boston.

Finally, after years of controversy—and downsizing both bed capacity and services—the decision was made to close the facility as a hospital and reopen it as a more realistic entity: an outpatient clinic serving people in nearby neighborhoods. Hence, in July of 1969, the Dimock Community Health Center was born. When Dr. Zak launched the New England Hospital for Women and Children in Roxbury in 1872, the area was largely populated by wealthy white Bostonians. After a century of demographic shifts, however, much of the local population was neither wealthy nor white. Early brochures promoting the new Dimock Center proudly acknowledged that fact, noting that "what was begun more than 100 years ago as a reaction to discrimination against women" continued now as "a reaction to discrimination against the nation's poor and near poor who do not receive adequate health care."[94]

Given her history of inclusiveness and care for people of all races and socio-economic circumstances, it's likely that Dr. Susan Dimock would have been pleased that, almost a century after her passing, her old women's hospital had become a community-based organization providing health and human services to some of Boston's most underserved, largely African American, neighborhoods.

Naming the new institution the Dimock Community Health Center suggests that in 1969, Boston and the medical community were finally giving Susan Dimock her due recognition and remembrance. But apparently that wasn't so. "We decided to call it Dimock because that was the name of the street it was on," explained hospital board member and director emeritus Richard M. Karoff in a 1994 interview with the author. It was true that community health centers were frequently named for the streets on which they were located. But what many had apparently forgotten by 1969 was the backstory: when NEWHC opened on this site in 1872, the road was called Codman Street; but on October 20, 1884, it had been renamed to honor the late Susan Dimock.

That Susan Dimock had largely passed from collective memory

in Boston was attested to in the late spring of 1964, when Rosa Heinzen Roewer was visiting Forest Hills Cemetery, three miles from what was then still known as the New England Hospital. The eighty-year-old Heinzen Roewer, a former suffragist and longtime progressive activist, was the granddaughter of both radical German journalist Karl Heinzen and famed lithographer and "Father of the American Christmas Card," Louis Prang. When Heinzen Roewer walked up the cemetery's Sweet Brier Path, on the outer slope of the historic area known as Mount Dearborn, she encountered several grave markers ascending the hillside in a neat row: first was Karl Heinzen and family, followed by a cenotaph for Louis Prang[95]; next came Dr. Marie Zakrzewska and her younger sister Minna, and, finally, Dr. Susan Dimock. Though Heinzen Roewer had presumably come to visit the Heinzen family gravesite—a site where her own ashes would be interred fourteen years later—she noticed that Susan Dimock's once-pristine marble memorial was badly decaying. In response to Heinzen Roewer's request, Forest Hills Cemetery officials sent a service order to the New England Hospital, asking if they had a fund "which might take care of replacing of stone or deepening inscription so it may be readable."[96]

There was, apparently, no such fund. And, amidst all the turmoil the hospital was experiencing in its final decade, the matter was quickly forgotten.

In 1994, thirty years after Rosa Heinzen Roewer's visit to Forest Hills Cemetery, I discovered Susan Dimock's near-illegible gravestone while working on an article for the *Boston Globe*. I was in my eighth year of writing history columns for the *Globe*, where I was encouraged by my editors to uncover stories of people, landmarks, and events from the city's remarkably rich past. While pursuing many of these long-forgotten tales, I often embedded myself in the microfilm room of the Boston Public Library, where I spent hours scrolling though pages of eighteenth and nineteenth-century newspapers in search of fascinating nuggets.

One particular series of news stories that fired my imagination was the ongoing front-page coverage about the shocking wreck of S.S. *Schiller* and the loss of Boston's beloved young surgeon, Susan Dimock. Piqued with curiosity, I reached out to the Dimock Community Health Center in Roxbury and Forest Hills Cemetery in Jamaica Plain. As it turned out, President Erling ("Bud") Hanson, Jr., and his staff at Forest Hills Cemetery had no idea of Dr. Dimock's story or significance. She was not yet in the cemetery's collective consciousness nor in their visitors' guide to famous gravesites. As for the Dimock Community Health Center, CEO Jackie Jenkins-Scott and her colleagues were unaware that they owned a lot at the cemetery where both their founder, Marie Zakrzewska, and

Susan Dimock were interred. Together we began to dig into and unearth all the facts we could find. Aided by materials held in the Sophia Smith Collection of Women's History, at Smith College in Northampton, Massachusetts, I was able to finish my article. The story ran on May 8, 1994, exactly 169 years after Dimock's death on S.S. *Schiller*.[97]

In some ways, however, a new chapter to the story had just begun. There was, after all, that decaying headstone. In order to honor Dr. Dimock's memory, our group agreed that it was high time to finally get it fixed.

My friends at the Dimock Center and Forest Hills Cemetery were joined by the Jamaica Plain Historical Society, the Boston Women's Heritage Trail, local nursing associations, a distant cousin of Dr. Dimock's in Virginia, and a battery of friends from the historic community and beyond in establishing what became known as the Dimock Heritage Fund.[98] After analyzing Susan Dimock's marble memorial with stone carver Carol Driscoll, we began to understand the underlying problem. "The Dimock memorial was made from marble (calcium carbonate)," explained Driscoll, whose previous work included archeological digs on Easter Island and preservation projects for the city of Boston's Historic Burying Grounds initiative. "It must have been a conscious choice to use this stone for the original monument due to its pure white clarity without mineral inclusions. Today, marble cannot stand up to acid rain …," Driscoll continued. "Marble deteriorates quicker in northeastern cities because of manufacturing and car exhaust settling on the stone surface. The deteriorated inscription was caused by acid precipitation—a chemical reaction of sulfur dioxide gas and water breaking down the crystal structure and washing away the surface."[99]

Realizing that repairing the stone was physically impossible, we decided to create a more durable replica in granite—a decision approved by Dimock's distant cousin in Virginia. While the rest of us in the Heritage Fund began holding regular meetings to develop fundraising initiatives and public events promoting the project, Carol Driscoll faced the initial task of deciphering illegible elements on the Dimock stone. Though much of the text could be read with some effort, one section was so badly worn that it required special treatment. Working with a fellow sculptor, Driscoll applied a water-soluble material (alginate)[100] to the marble surface to produce a mold. From the mold, they cast a plaster form that helped reveal the subtle markings from the original letters. Particularly vexing was the word "remembered," which was carved simply as "REMB'D." "It was a challenge and adventure to interpret the missing text," recalled Driscoll. "We used raking light to create the shadows on the cast plaster form and reveal more information about the letters. It was easier to eliminate certain letters and through this process discover the inscription. It was like solving a mystery from the past."[101]

Meanwhile, Jackie Jenkins-Scott of the Dimock Center confirmed that we had collected adequate monies to purchase the granite and begin processing the new stone. Granite Importers in Barre, Vermont, prepared the granite profile and honed the surface to be carved. The piece was then trucked to Driscoll's studio at the Settimelli Granite Company in Quincy, Massachusetts, where a chain hoist was used for lifting and a forklift for moving the dense rock. Once the stone was placed in the sandblasting booth, Driscoll began sketching the layout of the letters and floral design.

After close to a year of preparation, members of the Dimock Heritage Fund Steering Committee were ready to host a gala community event, which was held on September 10, 1995. "Monumental Women: 19th Century Heroes in Health and Harmony" featured a walking and trolley tour of famous women interred at Forest Hills Cemetery that included several of Susan Dimock's contemporaries, like hospital founder Dr. Marie Zakrzewska, nursing pioneer Linda Richards, and feminist journalist Lucy Stone. Among the other Forest Hills residents remembered, both on the tour and in an afternoon concert by internationally acclaimed pianist Virginia Eskin, was Amy Beach, the first American woman to write a symphony.[102] The tour's centerpiece was the ceremonial unveiling and dedication of Susan Dimock's replica stone, accompanied by stories about the doctor and her gravestone as well as selections read from the original sermon given by the Rev. James Freeman Clarke in 1875. More than one hundred people of diverse ages, ethnicities, and backgrounds attended the event. Several of us mused that Susan Dimock would have been proud of the inclusive assemblage—though dismissive of such attention focused on herself.

Over the next year, I gave multiple talks and tours about Susan Dimock's life and work. History professor Virginia Drachman—author of *Hospital with a Heart*, the definitive history of the New England Hospital[103]—expanded her previous service on the Dimock Heritage Fund Steering Committee by involving her students at Tufts University in Medford, Massachusetts, in the Dimock Center's on-site archives. During the 1995 fall semester, these Tufts undergraduates sorted through, organized, and filed the center's historic papers, letters, pamphlets, and artifacts, then wrote term papers on select topics from the New England Hospital's history.

It seemed that our mission had been more than accomplished, albeit with one caveat. Susan Dimock's original marble headstone, which was legally owned by the Dimock Community Health Center, remained in storage near the greenhouses at Forest Hills Cemetery. Since there was no

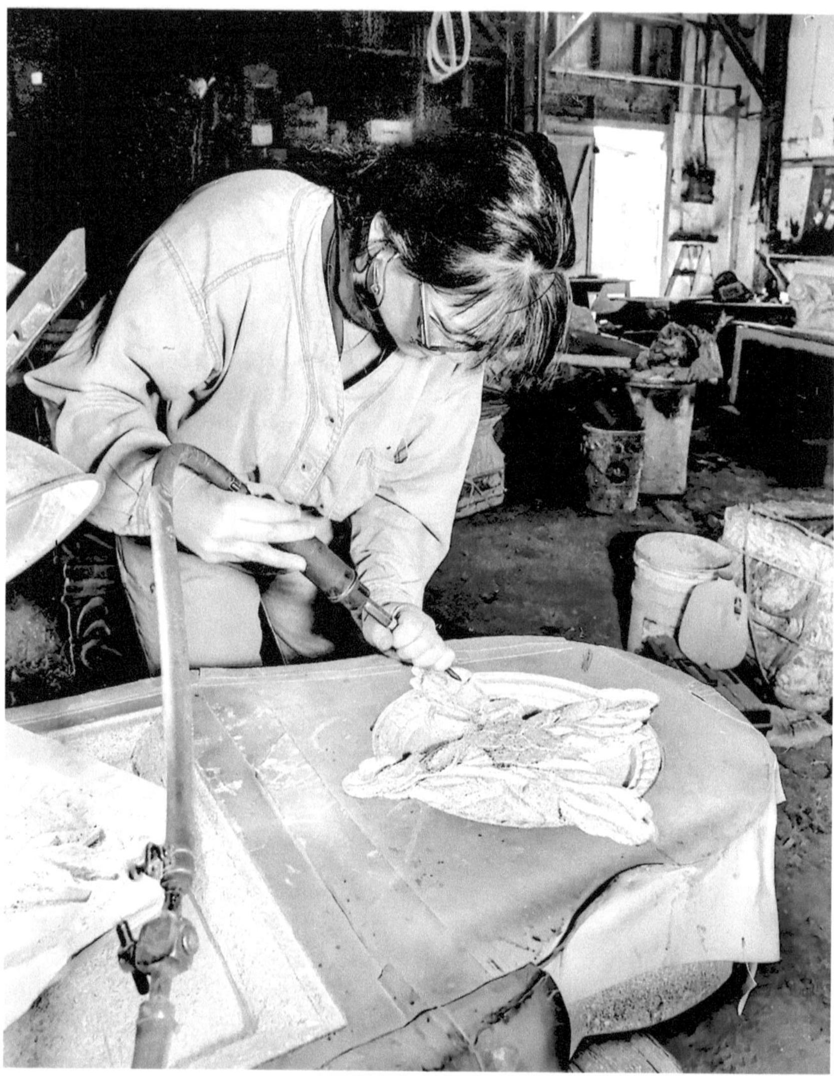

After deciphering illegible elements on Susan Dimock's badly eroded marble headstone with the aid of a mold and a plaster cast, sculptor Carol Driscoll began the process of sketching and carving the original letters and floral design into a dense granite replica (photograph © the author)

practical reason to keep it at the cemetery or the health center, we wondered what might be an appropriate adoptive home for this piece of women's medical history.

After an exchange of phone calls and letters between Bud Hanson from Forest Hills Cemetery and Carolyn Stroud, Director of Public Affairs for the city of Washington, North Carolina—and many more phone calls and meetings within Washington itself—it was agreed that Susan Dimock's weathered headstone would be welcomed in her old hometown.[104] Though we originally thought it might be placed in some indoor museum, the decision was made to set it in the same cemetery where Susan's father had been laid to rest—a block from Susan's historic marker on the site of the Dimocks' former home. The churchyard cemetery at St. Peter's Episcopal Church did not have space for another coffin, but it did have room for a vertical headstone commemorating one of the town's nineteenth-century heroes.

The question of how to move an 800-pound, nineteenth-century marble headstone from Boston to Washington was solved by Johanna and Leonard Huber, relative newcomers to Washington who were members of the Washington Area Historic Foundation. The Hubers had already planned a fall driving vacation to visit relatives in Concord, New Hampshire, an hour north of Boston. After conferring with their friend Carolyn Stroud, the couple agreed to pick up the Dimock monument on their return trip to North Carolina. Both Leonard and Johanna had some prior experience with burying grounds: Leonard had spent time working in a cemetery owned by his grandfather in New Orleans, while Johanna and her sister often accompanied their father, a college professor and amateur photographer, on his sojourns into Louisiana and Mississippi, where they studied tombstones, iron work, and curious old homes.[105]

On October 15, 2006, the Hubers arrived at Forest Hills in their white Ford pickup truck. With the aid of industrial dollies and sturdy cemetery staff members, the stone was boosted into the rear of the wagon. Once the papers were signed and thank-yous exchanged, the couple began their seven-hundred-mile trip to Little Washington, replete with the most unusual baggage—a tombstone in their trunk. "I think we brought it directly to St. Peter's Church cemetery, to its final resting place," Johanna Huber recalled more than two decades later. "Although we got a lot of

Susan Dimock signature (letter from Susan Dimock to Dr. Cabot, October 25, 1868; New England Hospital for Women and Children Records, Sophia Smith Collection, Smith College, Northampton, Massachusetts; used by permission of the Dimock Center, Roxbury, Massachusetts).

teasing from our friends in Washington, most were interested in history and were delighted we had brought the headstone to Washington."[106]

With two headstones in place—and a flurry of new interest in one of the nineteenth century's most compelling female physicians—it seemed that now, at last, the final chapter of Susan Dimock's remarkable journey was complete.

Chapter Notes

Chapter 1

1. The term "Yankee" was popularized as a disparaging term for New Englanders in the nineteenth century. In the years leading up to, during, and after the Civil War, it was used by many Southerners to refer to all Northerners and Union loyalists. The term "Damn Yankees" was so common during this era that it inspired an oft-repeated joke: "It wasn't until I was 18 that I realized 'damnyankees' was two words." Even in 1860, the reference was not a new one. "Yankee" had been used by both the Dutch residents of New York and the British as a contemptuous reference to American colonists as early as 1740. The British ditty "Yankee Doodle" was meant to mock those colonists, though American rebels later turned it around and proudly sang the song, adopted it as their own, and briefly used it as America's national anthem.

2. Descriptive quotes about the fire are from a letter from M.M. [Martha Matilda] Fowle to "My dear sisters," May 3, 1864, Brown Library Archives, Washington, North Carolina, and "Statement of Mrs. M.M. Wiswall [Martha M. Wiswall] in regard to the Fire that occurred in Washington North Carolina 30th April 1864," notarized by L.A. Squires, Beaufort County Notary Public, Brown Library Archives, Washington, North Carolina.

3. The DeMilles (alternately spelled DeMill) were the family of famed Hollywood film director, producer, and showman Cecil B. DeMille (1881–1959). Although his father was born in Washington, North Carolina, in 1853, Cecil was born in 1881 in Ashfield, Massachusetts, where his family was on summer vacation. Several DeMille family members are buried in Washington cemeteries.

4. Ed Hodges (local history educator), interview with author, St. Peter's Episcopal Church, Washington, North Carolina, October 17, 2016.

5. Betty Cochran with C.A. Mann, *On This Rock: A History of St. Peter's Church* (Washington, North Carolina, 1997), 10–11. Another version of this saving-the-bell story suggests that a parishioner removed the church bell before the flames engulfed the steeple. No reliable sources appear to exist corroborating one tale or the other.

6. Lucy Wheelock Warren Myers, "By-Gone Days," in Ursula Loy and Pauline Worthy, *Washington and the Pamlico* (Washington-Beaufort County Bicentennial Commission, 1976), 33–36. *Washington and the Pamlico* remains the single best source for stories from the history of Washington, North Carolina.

7. Porte Crayon [David Hunter Strother], *The Old South Illustrated*, edited by Cecil D. Eby, Jr. (Chapel Hill: University of North Carolina Press, 1959).

8. Myers, "By-Gone Days," 35.

9. *Ibid.*

10. The Dimock family traced its American ancestry to Englishman Thomas Dimick [sic] and his wife Anne, who arrived in Massachusetts Bay on the ship Hopewell in 1635. Genealogy chart from Edward C. Dimock Jr., included in a letter addressed to Mary Smoyer, January 23, 1995. William Dimock (1817–83) established a store in Limington Village in 1864. His son Charles (1854–1917) joined him in 1877, and created a clothing "salework" shop, with 15–20 employees,

in the building that became Grange Hall. Charles Dimock also ran the Post office there. See Robert L. Taylor, *Early Families of Limington, Maine* (Bowie, Maryland: Heritage Books, 1991).

11. "Dimock Headmaster of 'Lower Jamaica,'" *The Boston Globe*, February 18, 1955, 16.

12. Congressman Lindsay C. Warren, "Beaufort County's Contribution to a Notable Era of North Carolina History," printed in the Congressional Record, April 29, 1930, in Loy and Worthy, *Washington and the Pamlico*, 17–18.

13. Loy and Worthy, *Washington and the Pamlico*, 13–14; Kay Hicks (Dimock distant cousin), phone interview with author, from Lynchburg, Virginia, February 2, 2021.

14. The Whig Party dissolved in 1854; that same year, Dimock's *North State Whig* ceased publication.

15. Craven County Marriage Bonds, North Carolina, U.S., Marriage Records, 1741–2011. https://www.ancestry.com/discoveryui-content/view/64671:60548?_phsrc=uCX130&_phstart=successSource&gsfn=Henry&gsln=Dimock&ml_rpos=1&queryId=b726f11895ee767de4b2c91ee0dc3831

16. According to Beaufort County Sheriff records, Stephen Owens served from 1801–1806, 1821–1822, 1823–1826, 1827–1828, and 1831–1832. The sheriff's office was in Washington, N.C. http://www.beaufortcountysheriff.org/2015/10/14/sheriff/

17. Pauline Marion Worthy, "Susan Dimock, Pioneer in Medicine," *Raleigh News & Observer*, April 25, 1937. Memories of Mrs. Dimock were still fresh in the 1930s, since she lived in North Carolina until her death in 1910.

18. Rena Harding Davenport, "Early Customs of Washington," undated typed manuscript of recollections from her father, Edmund H. Harding, Brown Library Archives, Washington, North Carolina, 11.

19. *Ibid.*, 1.

20. Ednah Dow Cheney (anon.), *Memoir of Susan Dimock* (Boston: Press of J. Wilson, 1875), 6; and Pauline Worthy, "Susan Dimock, M.D.," in Loy and Worthy, *Washington and the Pamlico*, 450–451.

21. As late as 1880, the illiteracy rate in North Carolina was 48.3%; in contrast, that of Massachusetts was 6.5%. From Charles L. Coon, *Facts About Southern Education Progress* (Durham, North Carolina: The Campaign Committee of the Southern Education Board, 1905), 41.

22. "Female School," recurring advertisement in the *North State Whig*, beginning August 16, 1853.

23. "Schools—Private & Public (up to 1974)," paper donated by Mrs. Joe Kornegay, Brown Library Archives, Washington, North Carolina, 1–5. After the Civil War, many individuals took up private teaching again, including Mrs. William DeMill, who ran an excellent school in the DeMill house at the corner of Bridge and Second streets. She was the grandmother of Cecil B. DeMill, who grew up in Washington, North Carolina, added an "e" to his surname, and became a founding father of the American cinema, producing some seventy feature films, both silent and sound. Also, Lucy Wheelock Warren Myers, "By-Gone Days," in Loy and Worthy, *Washington and the Pamlico*, 36.

24. "Schools—Private & Public," 3; "School Books," recurring advertisement in the *North State Whig*, beginning December 5, 1849.

25. From the *Washington Echo*, N.C., quoted in Cheney, *Memoir*, 92.

26. The author is probably referring to a yaupon bush, a hardy evergreen holly shrub native to the southeastern U.S. and once used by Native Americans to make a caffeine-rich tea.

27. Luola, "Jennie's Tooth-ache," originally published in the *North Carolina Presbyterian* (Fayetteville, North Carolina: Geo. McNeill & Bart'w Fuller), 1858; from a clipping found in Caroline Fowle's family Bible, Brown Library Archives, Washington, North Carolina.

28. Washington Public Schools, "One Hundred and Sixty Years of Culture in Washington, North Carolina: A Pageant of Local Education in collaboration with the State-wide plans for the Celebration of the Hundredth Anniversary of the Beginning of Public Education in North Carolina," December 1936 (Washington City Schools, recopied from the original in December 1956), Brown Library Archives, Washington, North Carolina, 1–2.

29. *Cyclopedia of eminent and representative men of the Carolinas of the nineteenth century* (Madison, Wisconsin: Brant & Fuller, 1892), II, 223.

30. Luola, "Jennie's Tooth-ache." "Pillentary" was a local nickname for Zanthoxylum clava-herculis, a spiny tree or shrub native to the southeastern United States and known as "the toothache tree" or "tingle tongue," since chewing on the bark, twigs, or leaves was shown to cause numbness in the mouth, gums, or teeth.

31. Cheney, *Memoir*, 7.

32. *Ibid.*, 8.

33. *Ibid.*

34. E.D. Sloan Jr., to Mrs. Vonnie Marsh, July 26, 1987, in "Memories of Elizabeth Satchwell" (Satchwell genealogy), Brown Library Archives, Washington, North Carolina.

35. Lilian Freeman Clarke, "The Story of an Invisible Institution," *Outlook*, December 15, 1906, 932.

36. Sloan, "Memories of Elizabeth Satchwell."

37. E.D. Sloan Jr., "SOLOMON SAMPSON SATCHWELL, M.D. 1821–1892 HIS LIFE FROM 1841 TO 1865," draft document, April 4, 1999 (Satchwell genealogy), Brown Library Archives, Washington, North Carolina. After war's end, Dr. Satchwell continued his successful medical practice and was made President of the North Carolina Medical Society.

38. Slave advertisements, June 1829 and March 1839, courtesy the Washington Waterfront Underground Railroad Museum, Washington, North Carolina. See Anya Jabour, *Topsy-Turvy: How the Civil War Turned the World Upside Down for Southern Children* (Lanham, Maryland: Rowman & Littlefield, 2010).

39. Author's italics. Congressman Lindsay C. Warren, "Beaufort County's Contribution to a Notable Era of North Carolina History," printed in the *Congressional Record*, April 29, 1930, in Loy and Worthy, *Washington and the Pamlico*, 16.

40. Martha Wiswall, undated typed manuscript read by her daughter, Mrs. Sarah Wiswall, at the Addisco Book Club meeting, Brown Library Archives, Washington, North Carolina.

41. U.S. Census Bureau, Seventh Census of the United States, 1850, and Eighth Census of the United States, 1860, Slave Schedule, Beaufort County, North Carolina.

Federal Slave Schedules were used in only two U.S. censuses, those of 1850 and 1860. See also Samantha Winer, "A Brief History of slavery in North Carolina," Walter Clinton Jackson Library, The University of North Carolina at Greensboro (UNCG) http://libcdm1. uncg.edu/cdm/history/collection/RAS Accessed April 19, 2021.

42. David S. Cecelski, *The Waterman's Song: Slavery and Freedom in Maritime North Carolina* (Chapel Hill: University of North Carolina Press, 2001), xii.

43. The term "peculiar institution" is often misconstrued in the modern day as meaning that slavery was odd or strange. The reference, which came into general use in the 1830s, originally meant that the institution was "peculiar to" the South in the U.S.; the intended implication was that Southern slavery was not as harsh as in other countries and that it had no impact on the residents of the American North. See also W.E.B. (William Edward Burghardt) Du Bois, 1868–1963. The war to preserve slavery, February 1960. W.E.B. Du Bois Papers (MS 312). Special Collections and University Archives, University of Massachusetts Amherst Libraries. http://credo.library.umass.edu/ view/full/mums312-b217-i035 Accessed April 21, 2021.

44. U.S. Census Bureau, Fourth Census of the United States, 1820; Records of the Bureau of the Census, Record Group 29, National Archives, Washington, D.C. 1830 United States Federal Census; Census Place: Washington, Beaufort, North Carolina; Series: M19; Roll: 119; Page: 9; Family History Library Film: 0018085; "$15 REWARD," *American Recorder*, January 10, 1823, North Carolina Runaway Slave Advertisements, Digital Collection, The University of North Carolina at Greensboro. http://libcdm1. uncg.edu/cdm/search/collection/RAS/ searchterm/Beaufort%20County/field/ county/mode/exact/conn/and/order/date/ ad/asc/cosuppress/0

45. Worthy, "Pioneer in Medicine;" Cheney *Memoir*, 5; Beaufort County Register of Deeds, Washington, North

Carolina, Book 29, 159. The phenomenon of Southern women slaveholders is explored in Stephanie E. Jones-Rogers, *They Were Her Property: White Women as Slave Owners in the American South* (New Haven: Yale University Press, 2019).

46. U.S. Census Bureau, Seventh Census of the United States, 1850, Slave Schedule, Beaufort County, North Carolina; Eighth Census of the United States, 1860, Slave Schedule, Beaufort County, North Carolina; Beaufort County Register of Deeds, Beaufort County Courthouse, Washington, North Carolina, Book 29, 159.

By the time of the 1860 slave census, the Dimocks reportedly owned a 60-year-old female and a 60-year-old male. This may have meant that an older slave couple was living together with the family by then.

47. The definitive study on this topic is found in David S. Cecelski, *The Waterman's Song: Slavery and Freedom in Maritime North Carolina* (Chapel Hill: University of North Carolina Press, 2001).

48. "Ranaway," *Newbernian and North Carolina Advocate*, New Bern, North Carolina, July 31, 1849, North Carolina Runaway Slave Advertisements, Digital Collection, The University of North Carolina at Greensboro http://libcdm1. uncg.edu/cdm/search/field/source/searchterm/North%20Carolina%20Runaway%20Slave%20Advertisements%20Digital%20Collection/mode/exact

49. Wanda Hunt McLean, "Washington North Carolina Waterfront Network to Freedom Application," National Park Service National Underground Railroad Network to Freedom, July 3, 2014, 4-10. Since 2014, the Washington North Carolina Waterfront has been an official site in the National Underground Railroad Network to Freedom, a program of the National Park Service that honors, preserves, and promotes the history of resistance to enslavement through escape and flight. There are currently more than 700 Network to Freedom locations in 39 states, plus Washington, D.C., and the U.S. Virgin Islands.

50. The burning of Charleston, South Carolina, occurred on Dec. 11, 1861, and of Alexandria, Virginia, on May 13, 1864. Leesa Jones (local historian and educator), interview with author, Washington Waterfront Underground Railroad Museum, Washington, North Carolina, October 15, 2016. In 2016, Leesa Jones founded the Washington Waterfront Underground Railroad Museum in a refurbished, bright orange railroad car packed with images, articles, and artifacts. In her animated talks and tours, Jones shares facts as well as twentieth century folklore about the Underground Railroad. https://whda.org/underground-railroad-museum/.

51. Cheney, *Memoir*, 7.

52. Clarke, "The Story of an Invisible Institution," 932.

Chapter 2

1. Martha M. Fowle Wiswall, undated typed manuscript. Wiswall Papers #41, Brown Library Archives, Washington, North Carolina, 1.

2. *Ibid.*, 2.

3. There remains disagreement as to whether or not it was local citizens who hoisted the pro–Union banner that day, and, if it was, what their reasons were for doing so. Lindsay Warren, a U.S. Congressman from North Carolina (served 1925–40), wrote, "It is baseless calumny lodged both during and after the war that there was disloyalty on the part of the citizens of Washington to the Confederate government. ... The hoisting of the banner across Main Street welcoming the invading Federals can be dismissed as an act of a very few cowed and whipped citizens who felt that their government (Confederate) had deserted them. The fact that the banner was even raised by local people is not admitted, for immediately afterwards no one would take responsibility for it."

Congressman Lindsay Warren, "Beaufort County's Contribution to a Notable Era of North Carolina History," *The Congressional Record*, April 29, 1930, in Ursula Loy and Pauline Worthy, *Washington and the Pamlico* (Washington-Beaufort County Bicentennial Commission, 1976), 25.

Alfred S. Roe, *The Twenty-Fourth Regiment Massachusetts Volunteers, 1861–1866, "New England Guard Regiment"*

(Worcester, Massachusetts: Twenty-Fourth Veteran Association, 1907), 103.

4. *Ibid.*

5. John G. Barrett, *The Civil War in North Carolina* (Chapel Hill: University of North Carolina Press, 1963), 122–123. Barrett's *The Civil War in North Carolina* is an intricately detailed and indispensable source for wartime stories in the state of North Carolina.

6. Though the Dimock's Lafayette Hotel was destroyed in the second fire of 1864, the homes mentioned here all survived into the twenty-first century: the Myers (built circa 1780) and Marsh houses (1795) on Water Street, the Hollyday House (1840) on West Second Street, the Fowle House on West Main (1816), and the Havens House on West Main (1820).

7. Susan had already lost regular contact with Dr. Satchwell in 1860, when he visited Paris for several months for additional medical schooling. Satchwell returned to Washington, North Carolina, then moved to Wilson for active military medical service. E.D Sloan Jr., to Mrs. Vonnie Marsh, July 26, 1987, in "Memories of Elizabeth Satchwell" (Satchwell genealogy), 2, Brown Library Archives, Washington, North Carolina.

8. According to a spokesperson for the county, their Register of Deeds only extends back to 1913. St. Peter's interments are listed in their volume of Burial Records, which show that activities during the tumultuous war years went largely unrecorded. The church itself was lost in the same 1864 fire that incinerated the Dimock's hotel. Unlike the Lafayette Hotel, St. Peter's Episcopal Church was rebuilt after the war.

9. U.S. Census Bureau, Seventh Census of the United States, 1850, Slave Schedule, Beaufort County, North Carolina, and Eighth Census of the United States, 1860, Slave Schedule, Beaufort County, North Carolina; Henry Dimock rolling account, 1856–59, Ledger from Dave Fowle's General Store, Brown Library Archives, Washington, North Carolina.

10. Robert Krulwich, "Successful Children Who Lost a Parent—Why Are There So Many of Them?," Krulwich Wonders: Robert Krulwich on Science, October 16, 2013, NPR https://www.npr.org/sections/krulwich/2014/09/24/35088

8287/this-blog-is-ending-soon Accessed January 16, 2022.

11. "Excerpts from Recollections of the Civil War by Annie Blackwell Sparrow," in Joy W. Sparrow, ed., *Sparrows' Nest of Letters* (Wake Forest, N.C.: The Scuppernong Press, 2011), 244–45.

12. *Ibid.*, 245.

13. *Ibid.*, 248.

14. Barrett, *The Civil War in North Carolina*, 133–134. Additional information from Charles F. Warren, "The September Attack," from article in *The Confederate Reveille*, 1898, reprinted in Loy and Worthy, *Washington and the Pamlico*, 38–41, and http://www.pamlico.com/washington-history.html.

15. Sparrow, *Sparrows' Nest*, 247–48; Warren, "The September Attack," 40.

16. Adrienne Dunn, "Contraband Camps," The North Carolina History Project, Encyclopedia, http://north carolinahistory.org/encyclopedia/contraband-camps/ Accessed June 4, 2020.

17. Barrett, *The Civil War in North Carolina*, 133.

18. Sparrow, *Sparrows' Nest*, 252.

19. Charles F. Warren, "The Civil War Era," in Loy and Worthy, *Washington and the Pamlico*, 41; Barrett, *The Civil War in North Carolina*, 156–157.

20. Barrett, *The Civil War in North Carolina*, 158–159.

21. Dr. H.G. Jones, Associated Press, "In Light of History: Washington Woman Left NC to Practice Medicine," ND, Brown Library Archives, Washington, North Carolina.

22. Massachusetts, U.S., State Census, 1865, Middlesex, Hopkinton https://www.ancestry.com/imageviewer/collections/9203/images/41265_316179-00163?ssrc=&backlabel=Return.

National Archives, Milestone Documents, Emancipation Proclamation. https://www.archives.gov/milestone-documents/emancipation-proclamation.

Beaufort County Register of Deeds, Beaufort County Courthouse, Washington, North Carolina, Book 29, 159.

President Lincoln's Emancipation Proclamation, issued on January 1, 1863, announced "that all persons held as slaves" within the rebellious areas "are, and henceforward shall be free." However, it wasn't until December 4, 1865, that North

Carolina's legislature agreed to abolish slavery when the state ratified the 13th Amendment to the U.S. Constitution. Tracking the lives of Lewis and Ellen after their arrival in Massachusetts proved almost futile because of the dearth of available records. There is no thread for Ellen and only minimal information on Lewis. In 1875, Susan Dimock's medical student, M.E. Little, noted that despite the care Susan tried to give him, Lewis "became tired of the quiet life, and went to a city where, unused to the world, he fell into bad company, was led into crime by men older than himself, and was finally sentenced to five years in State Prison." Prison records indicate that Lewis was twice convicted of "breaking, entering, stealing" in Worcester, Massachusetts. Two months after his release in 1880, Lewis married Alice M. Williams and held a job as a waiter. No further information could be found. M.E. Little, "Letter from a Pupil of Dr. Dimock," in Cheney, *Memoir*, 47; Warden's memorandum of prisoners, 1858–1902 (bulk 1880–1886), Massachusetts State Prison, Commonwealth of Massachusetts State Archives. https://www.familysearch.org/ark:/61903/3:1:3Q9M-CSFH-4SDX-S?cat=730034. Accessed October 25, 2022; Massachusetts, U.S., Town and Vital Records, 1620–1988.

https://www.ancestry.com/search/collections/2495/?name=Lewis+J_Dimmock&birth=1852_washington-north+carolina-usa_3067&birth_x=1-0-0&gender=m&keyword=negro&marriage=1880_worcester-worcester-massachusetts-usa_4771. Accessed October 25, 2022.

23. "For a brief period mother and daughter refuged in Wilson. Then, in some way, they managed to obtain transportation to New England, eventually reaching the Dimock relatives in Sterling, Massachusetts"; quoted in Pauline Marion Worthy, "Susan Dimock, Pioneer in Medicine," *Raleigh News & Observer*, April 25, 1937.

24. Though the town of Wilson, North Carolina, became an Amtrak stop in the late twentieth century, the Wilson depot predated Amtrak and a unified rail system by more than 130 years. That depot had been an established rail stop since 1839, when the area was still known as Toisnot Junction and Hickory Grove.

25. Based on research by Boston historian Charlie Bahne, the patchwork of trains the Dimocks might have taken would have been daunting: "First, it helps to understand that rail travel in the Civil War era was not as we understand it in the 20th century, not even as it was in the early 20th century circa 1900. ... Individual railroad companies tended to cover rather short distances and when you got to the end of one company's lines, you'd have to transfer to another company. That might mean transferring to another depot in some intermediate city along your route. Information on schedules was not widely available beyond the area that a given company served. The first edition of the Official Railway Guide—a monthly publication of timetables from railroads across the nation—wasn't published until 1868. So you really couldn't plan a trip of this nature in advance. You'd take the train to one major city along your route, have to change trains and quite probably depots, and when you got to that intermediate point, then you'd have to ask locally about the schedule to the next major city along the way...In the south, development of rail lines was slower than in the north, and disruptions caused by war of course made it even harder to plan a trip in advance. Many large rivers, especially in tidewater areas, had not yet been bridged by railroads. In some rural areas—such as the Thames and Connecticut Rivers in CT—the entire train would be put on a ferry to cross the river. Dickens describes this in *American Notes*." Charlie Bahne (historian), email message to author, August 14, 2016.

26. The Sterling Historical Society, Sterling, Massachusetts, *A Pictorial History Commemorating the 200th Anniversary of Incorporation, 1781–1981* (Sterling MA, 1981).

27. There is a longstanding controversy about whether famed nineteenth century editor Sarah Josepha Hale wrote her version of "Mary's Lamb" after seeing Jon Roulstone's version or as an independent literary act. See Sandra Sonnichsen, "Who wrote Mary Had a Little Lamb?" (Richards Free Library, Newport, New Hampshire, August, 2016) https://newport.lib.

nh.us/sarah-josepha-hale/who-wrote-mary-had-a-little-lamb/

28. "Further History of This Place," typed, undated notes from the Mann family files; and "Valuation and Description of Estates Taxed, Town of Sterling, 1855," Sterling Historical Society, Sterling, Massachusetts.

29. Boston directories listed the following years and addresses for Mann's dental and surgical practice: 1839, 175 Tremont Street;1840, 16 Summer Street; 1854, 13 Avery Street (formerly "Mann and Melbourne"); 1858, 11 Suffolk Place; 1863, 146 Harrison Ave.

30. Walter M. Merrill, ed., *The Letters of William Lloyd Garrison*, Volume 5, 1861–1867 (Cambridge, Massachusetts: Belknap Press of Harvard University Press, 1979), 283.

31. Harriet Hyman Alonso, *Growing Up Abolitionist: The Story of the Garrison Children* (Amherst and Boston: University of Massachusetts Press, 2002), 129. By the time Susan Dimock arrived at the Manns' in 1864, Aunt Maria and cousin Birney were present, but Daniel Mann was probably no longer there. Initially, he had left his wife, son, farm, and dental practice to join the Union army in the Civil War. After completing his service— which included working as a surgeon for the Massachusetts 35th Regiment U.S. Colored Infantry—Daniel seems to have abandoned his Sterling family. Four years later, in 1868, he married one "Rocksy Ann" Bailey in Rockville, Massachusetts, which may explain the reason for his continued absence. Yet another of Susan relatives, Uncle Alonso Dimock, also lived in Sterling, though records of his life, work, and connections to other family members appear to be lost.

32. David W. Gibbs (local historian), email message to author, June 21, 2016.

33. David W. Gibbs (local historian) and Kathy Bogosian (resident), interview with author, Sterling, Massachusetts, July 19, 2016.

34. Ednah Dow Cheney (anon.), *Memoir of Susan Dimock* (Boston: Press of J. Wilson, 1875), 8.

35. Lilian Freeman Clarke, "The Story of an Invisible Institution," *Outlook*, December 15, 1906, 932.

36. Dean Grodzins, *American Heretic: Theodore Parker and Transcendentalism* (Univ of North Carolina Press, 2002), 177.

37. "William Batchelder Greene," https://spartacus-educational.com// USAgreeneW.htm. Accessed June 20, 2020.

38. Sumner quote from Edward L. Pierce, ed., *Memoir and Letters of Charles Sumner* (Boston: Roberts Brothers, 1893), III, 179. Two of the old Boston families who profited profusely from the slave trade or slave labor were the Cabots and the Lowells. Given the vast number of intermarriages between the Brahmin elite, few families could completely distance themselves from some historic connection to slavery. In the mid–nineteenth century, Russell Sturgis (1805–87) was a Boston merchant who became a partner and eventual head of Barings Bank, a London firm whose eighteenth-century roots included financing the lucrative slave trade; Russell was the older brother of Sarah Blake Sturgis (1815–82), the sister-in-law of Anna Blake Shaw. The Sturgis family was also related to a variety of other old Boston families, including the Parkmans, Perkins, and Paines. William Batchelder Greene was part of the vast and complex Greene family tree, which included Gardiner Greene (1753–1832), a merchant who made his initial fortune in the Demerara sugar plantations on the northern coast of South America, worked by enslaved laborers. Familial connection from Louise Brownell Clarke, *The Greenes of Rhode Island, with Historical Records of English Ancestry, 1534–1902. Compiled from the Mss. of the Late Major-General George Sears Greene, U.S.V.* (New York: The Knickerbocker Press 1903).

39. James S. Pula, "A Passion for Humanity: Founding the New England Hospital for Women and Children," *The Polish Review*, Vol. 57, No. 3, 67–82. (University of Illinois Press on behalf of the Polish Institute of Arts & Sciences of America, 2012.), 77.

40. Cheney, *Memoir*, 8–9.

41. Mrs. Frances A. Safford, *A Brief History of Hopkinton, Prepared for the Town's Bicentennial Celebration in 1915* (Hopkinton Public Library, 1915), 4.

42. Massachusetts, U.S., State Census, 1865, Middlesex, Hopkinton. https://www. ancestry.com/imageviewer/collections/

9203/images/41265_316179-00163?ssrc=&
backlabel=Return.

43. *Ibid.*

44. Massachusetts Historical Commission, Form B-Building, Community: Hopkinton; No: G-407; Property name: 112 Main Street, recorded by A. Forbes for the Hopkinton Historical Commission, 6/89. Mrs. Dimock's hotel went through several other owners and names over the decades. The decrepit building endured through most of the twentieth century. In December of 1994, it was razed and replaced by the current Respite Center.

45. The original schools for training teachers were meant to create a standard, model, or "norm" for their students, so were called "Normal Schools." The Commonwealth of Massachusetts opened its first Normal School in 1839; that institution evolved into Framingham State University.

46. James F. Ward, *The Common Uncommon: Stories of the Past, Hopkinton, Massachusetts* (Damianos Publishing, 2014), 14–15, 69.

47. Berkshire Medical College was founded in Pittsfield, Massachusetts in 1823; its graduates included the second African American in the nation ever awarded a medical degree, James Skivring Smith, who later became the president of Liberia; the college closed in 1867. In the early 1860s, the Pratts' ever-changing household included their daughter Sarah, their daughter and son-in-law Mary J. and Gary H. Bowen, a seemingly unrelated family, Eliza A. Cutter and three Cutter children in their teens and twenties, as well as the two Irish servants. Massachusetts Historical Commission, Form B-Building, for 25 Main Street, Hopkinton, Form HPK.192, recorded by Jennifer B. Doherty, Hopkinton Historical Commission, April 2018; Harold S. Wood, "Hopkinton, Massachusetts, Physicians and Surgeons, 1750 to 1800," (Hopkinton Historical Society, 1959), unpublished document in the Hopkinton Public Library, Hopkinton, Massachusetts; Cheney, *Memoir*, 9.

48. Alfred Lord Tennyson, "The Princess," Part V, lines 427–431. The Project Gutenberg EBook of The Princess, by Alfred Lord Tennyson. https://www.gutenberg.org/files/791/791-h/791-h.htm, Accessed August 20, 2020.

49. Modern scholarship has questioned the two-spheres theory, wondering how many women paid heed to, or were constrained by, those concepts, and suggesting that rather than actually penetrating the men's public sphere, nineteenth-century women created an alternate public sphere for themselves (a "female public sphere") or simply expanded the boundaries of their domestic sphere ("increased publicness of the women's sphere"). Moreover, the spheres theory did not explain, but merely constrained, women of lower socio-economic classes and women of color, who were long used to taking care of home and hearth while simultaneously contributing to the family's economic survival through labor. See Eyal Rabinovitch, "Gender and the Public Sphere: Alternative Forms of Integration in Nineteenth-Century America," *Sociological Theory* 19, no. 3 (American Sociological Association, Nov. 2001), 344–370. During this era in Boston, Mary Baker Eddy founded the Church of Christ, Scientist; Isabella Stewart Gardner created her namesake museum; and Marie Zakrzewska opened the New England Hospital for Women and Children. Susan Wilson and the Boston Women's Heritage Trail, "Enterprising Women, 1862–1914," *The Atlas of Boston History*, Nancy S. Seasholes, ed. (Chicago: University of Chicago Press, 2019), plate 36, 102–103.

50. Mrs. Ednah D. Cheney, "The Women of Boston," in Justin Winsor, ed. *The Memorial History of Boston: Including Suffolk County, Massachusetts, 1630–1880* (Boston: Ticknor and Company, 1881), IV, 331.

51. *The Bostonians* features an intensely romantic friendship between two of its ardent feminist characters, Olive Chancellor and Verena Tarrant. Henry James explored the notion in part because his sister, diarist Alice James, was in a life-long companionship with educator Katherine Peabody Loring.

52. The groundbreaking study on the history of lesbian relationships was Lilian Faderman's *Surpassing the Love of Men: Romantic Friendship and Love Between Women from the Renaissance to the Present* (New York: William Morrow and Company, 1981).

53. Arleen Marcia Tuchman, *Science Has No Sex: The Life of Marie Zakrzewska, M.D.* (Chapel Hill: University of North Carolina Press, 2006), 114–115.

54. In an 1874 letter to a friend in Zurich, Susan wrote that she would be traveling to Europe with Bessie the following year and was looking for accommodations. "As it is my dearest friend," she wrote, "one room will do for us both." Susan Dimock to Sophie Heims, May 31, 1874, in the private collection of Kay Hicks, Lynchburg, Virginia; accessed 1995. Among the multiple sources that classify Susan and Bessie's relationship as a "Boston Marriage" are Arleen Marcia Tuchman, *Science Has No Sex: The Life of Marie Zakrzewska, M.D.* (Chapel Hill: University of North Carolina Press, 2006); The History Project, *Improper Bostonians: Lesbian and Gay History from the Puritans to Playland* (Boston: Beacon Press, 1998); and Olivia Campbell, "The Queer Victorian Doctors Who Paved the Way for Women in Medicine," History Stories (The History Channel, A+E Networks, Jun 1, 2021).https://www.history.com/news/queer-victorian-doctors-women-medicine.

Though Susan Dimock expressed no apparent interest in having a boyfriend, that feeling was not necessarily mutual. Gustav Adolf Tobler (1850–1923), for example, a male student at the University of Zurich who later became one of the richest men in Zurich, was extremely attracted to Susan when she attended the medical school there in 1870. Though Susan was three years his senior, Tobler wrote about her in his diaries and hoped his feelings would be reciprocated. See Verena E. Müller, *Marie Heim-Vögtlin—die erste Schweizer Ärztin (1845–1916): Ein Leben zwischen Tradition und Aufbruch* (Baden 2007, vierte Auflage 2016), Kindle, chapter 15, paragraphs 20–21. Bessie Greene was apparently idealized and appreciated by many. In 1871, Transcendentalist poet (William) Ellery Channing (1817–1901)—the nephew of famed Unitarian minister William Ellery Channing—based his character Miranda on Bessie Greene in an epic poem published as *The Wanderer: A Colloquial Poem*. In the poem, Miranda/Bessie is described as a "Goddess of an isle that sleeps in Grecian seas," who explains, "I crave a real passion …May I meet human sympathies not less /Demanding lovely truth of me than I/Of them!" and wonders, "May be that saints and lovers stupefy/Themselves and others with a threadbare dream." William Ellery Channing, *The Wanderer: A Colloquial Poem* (Boston: James R. Osgood and Company, 1871), 72.

55. Cheney, *Memoir,* 77; Worthy, "Pioneer in Medicine."

56. 1 Samuel 18:1–5, 1 Samuel: 20:41, 2 Samuel 1:23–27.

57. Examples of the contradictory arguments about David and Jonathan's relationship are found in Robert A.J. Gagnon, *The Bible and Homosexual Practice: Texts and Hermeneutics* (Nashville: Abingdon Press, 2001); Susan Ackerman, *When Heroes Love: The Ambiguity of Eros in the Stories of Gilgamesh and David* (New York: Columbia University Press, 2005); Martti Nissinen, *Homoeroticism in the Biblical World: A Historical Perspective* (Minneapolis: Augsburg Fortress, 2004); Jennie Rothenberg Gritz, "But Were They Gay? The Mystery of Same-Sex Love in the 19th Century," *The Atlantic,* September 7, 2012; Franklyn Salzman, "Gay or Nay, Modern Readings of the David and Jonathan Narrative," Winner 2015 Henry A. Bern Memorial Essay Competition (Bloomington: Indiana University).

58. Professor Douglas O. Linder, "Famous Trials: The Three Trials of Oscar Wilde (1895)," University of Missouri-Kansas City School of Law. https://famous-trials.com/wilde Accessed August 18, 2020.

59. During a four-month period in 1873, when Susan Dimock was resident physician at the New England Hospital for Women and Children and Bessie Greene was a live-in patient at the same hospital, the two women did technically live in the same building. But Dr. Dimock resided at the hospital full-time, as required by her job. Bessie's legal residence was the Clarendon House Hotel in Boston's South End.

60. Cheney, *Memoir,* 50.

61. Marie E. Zakrzewska, "In Memoriam," in Cheney, *Memoir,* 83.

62. Cheney, *Memoir,* 9.

63. *Ibid.*

64. Marie E. Zakrzewska, "In Memoriam," in Cheney, *Memoir*, 83–84.

65. Agnes C. Vietor, ed., *A Woman's Quest: The Life of Marie Zakrzewska, M.D.* (New York: Arno Press, 1972), 67. Among the most valuable books on Marie Zakrzewska's life are Vietor's *A Woman's Quest* and Arleen Marcia Tuchman's *Science Has No Sex*. The only comprehensive study of the New England Hospital for Women and Children is Virginia G. Drachman's *Hospital with a Heart: Women Doctors and the Paradox of Separatism at the New England Hospital, 1862–1969* (Ithaca NY: Cornell University Press, 1984).

66. Vietor, *A Woman's Quest,* 140; Drachman, *Hospital with a Heart*, 34. For an excellent biography of the Blackwell sisters, see Janice P. Nimura, *The Doctors Blackwell: How Two Pioneering Sisters Brought Medicine to Women—and Women to Medicine* (New York: W.W. Norton & Company, 2021).

67. James S. Pula, "A Passion for Humanity: Founding the New England Hospital for Women and Children," *The Polish Review*, Vol. 57, No. 3 (University of Illinois Press on behalf of the Polish Institute of Arts & Sciences of America, 2012), 73.

68. Shirley Phillips Ingebritsen, "Lucy Ellen Sewall," in *Notable American Women, 1607–1950; A Biographical Dictionary*, James, Edward T., ed. (Cambridge, Massachusetts: Belknap Press of Harvard University Press, 1971), III, 268.

69. Ednah Dow Cheney, *Reminiscences of Ednah Dow Cheney* (Boston: Lee & Shepard, 1902), 60.

70. Pula, "A Passion for Humanity," 76.

71. Cheney, *Reminiscences*, 60.

72. K. Codell Carter, PhD., "Leechcraft in nineteenth century British Medicine," *Journal of the Royal Society of Medicine* 94 (January 2001): 38–42. For centuries, barbers in western civilization were known to cut hair, trim beards, bloodlet, extract teeth, and perform other types of surgery, including amputation.

73. Alice B. (Mrs. William O.) Crosby, *The Story of the New England Hospital for Women and Children Through Seventy-Five Years, 1862–1937* (Boston, Massachusetts: New England Hospital for Women and Children, 1937), 4; Mary Roth Walsh, *Doctors Wanted: No Women Need Apply* (New Haven and London: Yale University Press, 1977), 86.

74. Tuchman, *Science Has No Sex*, 168.

75. *Fair at the Hotel Vendome for the Benefit of the New England Hospital for Women and Children, December 4th to 9th, 1899* (Boston, 1899), 8.

76. Mary Putnam Jacobi, MD, "An Obituary of the Author [Susan Dimock, M.D.]." *The Medical Record: A Weekly Journal of Medicine and Surgery* 10 (January 2–December 25, 1875): 358.

77. *History of the New England Hospital for Women and Children, 1859–1899*, 10.

78. "Circular," handwritten appeal in Box 1, Series I. History, Publications, Circulars, 1859, 1860s, New England Hospital for Women and Children Records, 1792–1994: MS 339, Sophia Smith Collection, Smith College, Northampton, Massachusetts; statistics from the Massachusetts Civil War Research Center, http://www.massachusettscivilwar.com/statistics.asp, Accessed October 12, 2020.

79. *Annual Report of the New-England Hospital for Women and Children, No. 14, Warren Street, For the Year Ending November 1, 1866* (Boston: Prentiss & Deland, 1866), 12. The reference is to a classic quote from Charles Dickens' *Oliver Twist* (1838). While a resident in the parish workhouse, young Oliver is hungry, barely subsisting on three meager meals of gruel per day. So he begs of Mr. Bumble, "Please, sir, I want some more." Many mid–nineteenth-century Americans knew those lines well.

Chapter 3

1. Although the American Medical Association, founded in 1847, attempted to set standards for medical education, their early successes were erratic and licensing remained state-mandated. In the nineteenth century, many so-called physicians attended, but never graduated from, medical schools, while others simply apprenticed with practicing doctors. Individuals also called themselves "doctors" who were outside of "orthodox," mainstream (allopathic) medicine in fields such as homeopathy,

phrenology, and mesmerism. Shauna Devine, "Health Care and the American Medical Profession, 1830–1880," *The Journal of the Civil War Era*, July 6, 2017. https://www.journalofthecivilwarera.org/2017/07/health-care-american-medical-profession-1830-1880/; Robert G Slawson, MD, FACR, "Medical Training in the United States Prior to the Civil War," *Journal of Evidence-Based Complementary & Alternative Medicine* 17(1) (Accepted for publication September 28, 2011):11–27. https://journals.sagepub.com/doi/full/10.1177/2156587211427404 Accessed Dec. 2, 2020.

2. Agnes C. Vietor, ed., *A Woman's Quest: The Life of Marie Zakrzewska, M.D.* (New York: Arno Press, 1972), 156.

3. Margaret Todd, M.D., *The Life of Sophia Jex-Blake* (London: MacMillan and Co., 1918), 174.

4. *Ibid.*, 162.

5. *Annual Report of the New-England Hospital for Women and Children, No. 14, Warren Street, For the Year Ending November 1, 1867* (Boston: Prentiss & Deland, 1867), 12.

6. *Ibid.*, 11–12, 19.

7. Dr. Lindsey Fitzharris, "An appointment at the house of death: the horror of the early Victorian hospital," *History Extra: The official website for BBC History Magazine*, BBC History Revealed and BBC World Histories https://www.historyextra.com/period/victorian/an-appointment-at-the-house-of-death-the-horrors-of-the-early-victorian-hospital/ Accessed Dec. 16, 2020.

8. *Annual Report of the New-England Hospital for Women and Children, No. 14, Warren Street, For the Year Ending November 1, 1866* (Boston: Prentiss & Deland, 1866), 15. $100 in 1866 would be worth about $1,665 today.

9. *1867 Annual Report*, 15.

10. *Ibid.*, 6, 17.

11. *Ibid.*, 17.

12. New England Hospital for Women and Children, Records of Medical Wards [B MS 19.2, vol. 1], Boston Medical Library in the Francis A. Countway Library of Medicine, Harvard University, Boston, Massachusetts.

13. *Annual Report of the New-England Hospital for Women and Children, No. 14 Warrenton Street, For the Year Ending November 1, 1868* (Boston: Prentiss & Deland, 1868), 20.

14. *Ibid.*

15. Mary Dobson, *Disease: The Extraordinary Stories Behind History's Deadliest Killers* (London, England: Quercus Books, 2008), 74.

16. Hilary J. Lane, MLS; Nava Blum, PhD; Elizabeth Fee, PhD., "Oliver Wendell Holmes (1809–1894) and Ignaz Philipp Semmelweis (1818–1865): Preventing the Transmission of Puerperal Fever," *American Journal of Public Health* 100, Issue 6 (Washiungton: June 2010): 1008–1009. https://search.proquest.com/docview/347504583?accountid=9703&pq-origsite=primo Oliver Wendell Holmes' colleagues decided to largely ignore his warnings and herald him as a poet more than as a physician. Ignace Semmelweis' work was fiercely disputed by European obstetricians; when he began to denounce them as murderers, the backlash led him to depression and drink, and finally forced him into an insane asylum.

17. Sophia Jex-Blake, *Puerperal Fever: An Enquiry into its Nature and Treatment, with an historical retrospect of some of the chief epidemics recorded under that name, and of the principal theories successively entertained respecting it. With notes of personal observations* (Graduation Thesis presented to the Medical Faculty of the University of Bern, 1877), 22–24.

18. *1867 Annual Report*, 17.

19. Emma L Call, M.D., "Evolution of Modern Maternity Technique. Illustrated by Records of the New England Hospital for Women and Children, Boston, from 1862 to 1907," *The American Journal of Obstetrics and Diseases of Women and Children* 59, no. 1, Brooks H. Wells, M.D., ed. (July–December, 1908): 393.

20. Susan J. Dimock, *Ueber die verschiedenen Formen des Puerperalfiebers. Nach Beobachtungen in der Züricher Gebaranstalt.* (inaugural-Dissertation, Zürich: Druck von Zürcher und Furrer, 1871); Sophia Jex-Blake, *Puerperal Fever.*

21. Ednah Dow Cheney (anon.), *Memoir of Susan Dimock* (Boston: Press of J. Wilson, 1875), 10–11.

22. *Ibid.*

23. "Students Term of 1866–7," *Nineteenth Annual Catalogue and Report of*

the New England Female Medical College (Boston: Published by the Trustees, Wright & Potter Printers, 1867).

24. Cheney, *Memoir*, 50.

25. Dimock family genealogy from Robert L. Taylor, *Early Families of Limington, Maine* (Bowie, Maryland: Heritage Books, 1991).

26. Vietor, *A Woman's Quest*, 496.

27. Kenneth M. Ludmerer, "Reform at Harvard Medical School, 1869–1909," *Bulletin of the History of Medicine* 55, no. 3 (The Johns Hopkins University Press, 1981), 345. http://www.jstor.org/stable/44441382

28. Charles Snyder, "Massachusetts Eye and Ear Infirmary: Studies on Its History" (Boston: Massachusetts Eye and Ear Infirmary, 1984), 129. https://archive.org/stream/massachusettseye00snyd/massachusettseye00snyd_djvu.txt

29. Thomas Neville Bonner, *To the Ends of the Earth: Women's Search for Education in Medicine* (Cambridge: Harvard University Press, 1992), 7; Snyder, "Massachusetts Eye and Ear Infirmary," 129. After years of well-received practice and her brief inclusion and expulsion from Harvard, Harriot Hunt (1805–75) was granted an honorary medical degree from the Female Medical College of Pennsylvania as a tribute to her pioneering work.

30. Founded as the Boston Female Medical College in 1848, then renamed the New England Female Medical College in 1850, the NEFMC merged with Boston University in 1874 to become the first accredited coeducational medical school in the nation. The Female Medical College of Pennsylvania was founded in 1850 and became the Woman's Medical College of Pennsylvania in 1867. In 1970, the school began accepting men as the newly renamed Medical College of Pennsylvania. Since 2003, it has been part of the Drexel University College of Medicine.

31. George Cheyne Shattuck (1813–93) was the Dean of the Harvard Faculty of Medicine from 1864–69. A professor of clinical medicine at Harvard Medical School (1855–74), he—along with John Collins Warren and others—founded the medical library for physicians in Boston.

32. Todd, *The Life of Sophia Jex-Blake*, 190. Jex-Blake's biographer Margaret Todd was in a Boston Marriage with Sophia Jex-Blake. Twenty years younger than her life partner, Todd was a novelist and a former medical student of Jex-Blake.

33. *Ibid.*, 190–91. Thomas Hill (1818–91) was the president of Harvard from 1862–68. During his tenure, admissions standards were raised, the Peabody Museum of Archaeology and Ethnography was begun, and the dental school (the first university dental school in the nation) was founded. Among Harvard College undergraduates at the time was Robert Todd Lincoln, the son of the U.S. president.

34. "The Beginning of the End," *The Advocate* 3, no. 4 (Cambridge MA: The Students of Harvard College), April 27, 1867): 61.

35. Todd, *The Life of Sophia Jex-Blake*, 191; Carolyn Ticknor, ed., *Dr. Holmes's Boston* (Boston: Houghton Mifflin Company, 1915), 31.

36. Snyder, "Massachusetts Eye and Ear Infirmary,"126–127; Todd, *The Life of Sophia Jex-Blake*, 192.

37. Todd, *The Life of Sophia Jex-Blake*, 196, 199.

38. Marie E. Zakrzewska, "In Memoriam," in Cheney, *Memoir*, 84.

39. Susan Dimock to the Dean of the Medical College of Zurich, March 17, 1868, in New England Hospital for Women and Children Records, 1792–1994, Sophia Smith Collection, Smith College, Northampton, Massachusetts.

40. *1868 Annual Report*, 20–21; Cheney, *Memoir*, 13–14.

41. Todd, *The Life of Sophia Jex-Blake*, 165–66.

42. Tuchman, *Science Has No Sex*, 213; Sophia Jex-Blake to her mother, August 18, 1865, in Todd, *The Life of Sophia Jex-Blake*, 164–66. In the Muggins card game, players watch the others to see if anyone breaks the rules with a wrong play or card. Should someone make a mistake, the player who sees it yells "Muggins!"

43. "Holmes Coins the Term 'Anaesthesia,'" Center for the History of Medicine at Countway Library, https://collections.countway.harvard.edu/onview/exhibits/show/introduction/holmes-anesthesia Accessed 01.14.21; "The surprising (and Long) story of the first use of anesthesia in surgery," The

Conversation https://theconversation. com/the-surprising-and-long-story-of-the-first-use-of-ether-in-surgery-113340 Accessed 01.14.21 Oliver Wendell Holmes (1809–94) was also the gentleman who first wrote "Boston State-House is the Hub of the Solar System," which was later distorted by others into the popular phrase, "Boston is the Hub of the Universe."

44. *The Fiftieth Anniversary of the New England Hospital for Women and Children, Dimock Street, Boston, Mass., October Twenty-Nine, Nineteen Hundred Twelve* (Boston: Press of Geo. H. Ellis Co., 1913), 48; Cheney, *Memoir*, 51–52; Tuchman, *Science Has No Sex*, 118–119.

45. Well into the twentieth century, professional women—whether in Boston Marriages or not—often believed that "a wedding-ring led to the graveyard of a medical woman's ambitions." Wendy Moore, *No Man's Land: The Trailblazing Women Who Ran Britain's Most Extraordinary Military Hospital During World War I* (New York: Basic Books, 2020), 26.

46. Mary Putnam Jacobi, MD, "An Obituary of the Author [Susan Dimock, M.D.]." *The Medical Record: A Weekly Journal of Medicine and Surgery* 10 (January 2-December 25, 1875): 358.

47. Verena E. Müller, *Marie Heim-Vögtlin—die erste Schweizer Ärztin (1845–1916): Ein Leben zwischen Tradition und Aufbruch* (Baden 2007, vierte Auflage 2016), Kindle, chapter 14, paragraph 2.

48. *Ibid.*

49. The Massachusetts Institute of Technology (M.I.T.) was founded in Boston in 1861 but did not begin classes until 1865 due to the intervening Civil War. M.I.T. relocated from Boston to Cambridge in 1916. Zurich's Polytechnikum, now known as ETH Zurich and often referred to as "Zurich's counterpart to M.I.T.," was founded even earlier, in 1855. ETH Zurich was given its present name, Swiss Federal Institute of Technology (Eidgenössische Technische Hochschule), in 1911.

50. Thomas Neville Bonner, *To the Ends of the Earth: Women's Search for Education in Medicine* (Cambridge: Harvard University Press, 1992), 33.

51. The venerable University of Basel, founded in 1460, did not admit a woman into its medical college until 1890. The University of Zurich, a far newer and more liberal institution, was founded in 1833. Switzerland itself, long a grouping of cantons, was not united into a nation state until 1848.

52. "Frauenstudium im deutschen Sprachraum," https://de.wikipedia.org/ wiki/Frauenstudium_im_deutschen_ Sprachraum

53. Bahnhofstrasse emerged in 1864 when Zurich's old city fortifications were demolished and the ditch in front of those walls was filled. The former name of that area was Fröschengraben ("Ditch of the Frogs"), then changed to Bahnhofstrasse for its new incarnation.

54. Susan Dimock to her mother, October 18th, 1868, in Cheney, *Memoir*, 16.

55. *Ibid.*, 17.

56. Susan Dimock to her mother, October 25th, 1868, in Cheney, *Memoir*, 17–18.

57. *Ibid.*, 18. The "lake" Susan refers to is the Lake of Zurich, at the east end of the River Limmat.

58. *Ibid.*, 17.

59. Susan Dimock to Dr. Marie Zakrzewska, January 9, 1870, in Cheney, *Memoir*, 21.

60. Müller, *Marie Heim-Vögtlin*, Kindle, chapter 14, paragraph 1.

61. *Ibid.*, chapter 16, paragraph 14.

62. Cheney, *Memoir*, 17–18.

63. In the nineteenth century, medical students were expected to know their plants and value natural history. A discipline then called "natural philosophy" consisted of botany, zoology, geology, and physics. Scott A. Norton, "Whither medical botany?," in *CMAJ* (Canadian Medical Association Journal), June 20, 2006.

64. Müller, *Marie Heim-Vögtlin*, Kindle, chapter 16, paragraph 6.

65. *Ibid.*, chapter 16, paragraph 7.

66. Susan Dimock to her mother, November 15th, 1868, in Cheney, *Memoir*, 19.

67. Müller, *Marie Heim-Vögtlin*, Kindle, chapter 11, paragraph 6.

68. *Ibid.*, chapter 14, paragraph 8.

69. Susan Dimock to Dr. Marie Zakrzewska, January 9, 1870, in Cheney, *Memoir*, 20. Susan Dimock's years in

Zurich are well chronicled in her own words thanks to letters she wrote to friends, colleagues, and family, later collected by Ednah Dow Cheney and published as the *Memoir of Susan Dimock* following Dimock's death.

70. Susan Dimock to Dr. Cabot, Feb. 8, 1869, in New England Hospital for Women and Children Records, 1792–1994: MS 339, Sophia Smith Collection, Smith College, Northampton, Massachusetts.

71. The Dennison Manufacturing Company and the Avery Dennison company of Pasadena, California, were descendants of the paper box manufacturing company created by Aaron Dennison and his younger brother, Eliphalet Whorf Dennison.

72. Dimock to Zakrzewska, January 9, 1870, in Cheney, *Memoir*, 20.

73. Müller, *Marie Heim-Vögtlin*, Kindle, chapter 20, paragraph 13.

74. Verena E. Müller (author), email message to author, January 20, 2018.

75. Cheney, *Memoir*, 27.

76. Advertisements from issues of the Swiss-German daily newspaper, *Tagblatt*, 1870–71, city archives of Zurich (Stadtarchiv Zürich).

77. Verena E. Müller (author), email message to author, February 19, 2018.

78. Dimock to Marie Zakrzewska, December 10, 1870, in Cheney, *Memoir*, 23.

79. Susan Dimock to Marie Zakrzewska, January 9, 1870, *Ibid.*, 21.

80. Müller, *Marie Heim-Vögtlin*, Kindle, chapter 13, paragraph 4.

81. *Ibid.* version chapter 11, paragraph 7.

82. Dimock to Zakrzewska, January 9, 1870, in Cheney, Memoir, p. 20.

83. Müller, *Marie Heim-Vögtlin* Kindle, chapter 16, paragraph 4.

84. *Ibid.*, chapter 22, paragraph 13.

85. Karl Victor Böhmert, "from a Berlin Newspaper," quoted in Cheney, *Memoir*, 25–26.

86. Müller, *Marie Heim-Vögtlin*, Kindle, chapter 16, paragraphs 10–11. According to legend, an oath of the Old Swiss Confederacy was taken on the Rütli, a meadow above Lake Uri. The oath is featured in the play *Wilhelm Tell* by Friedrich Schiller. Schiller was a German poet, philosopher, playwright, physician, and historian—and a favorite of Susan Dimock.

87. *Ibid.*

88. Böhmert, in Cheney, *Memoir*, 26–27.

89. Susan Dimock to Marie Zakrzewska, January 9, 1870, in Cheney, *Memoir*, 20–21.

90. There is a long-standing, unresolved controversy over whether or not the symbol of the Red Cross was created by simply reversing the colors of the Swiss flag; the first is a red cross on a white background, the second a white cross on red. When the war between the Second French Empire of Napoleon III and the German states of the North German Confederation broke out in July of 1870, the International Committee of the Red Cross created an International Agency for Aid to Wounded Military Personnel in Basel, Switzerland, a city close to both the French and German borders. Among the agency's activities was bringing aid to the battlefield and to conflict victims, compiling lists of prisoners of war, and repatriating the wounded. https://www.icrc.org/eng/resources/documents/misc/57jnvw.htm, Accessed February 14, 2018.

91. August Forel, *Out of My Life and Work* (New York: Norton, 1937), 68–73.

92. Edmund Rose, *Der Zürcher Hülfszug zum Schlactfeld bei Belfort* (Zurich: Cäsar Schmidlt, 1871) 17, cited in Bonner, *To the Ends of the Earth*, 40.

93. Susan Dimock to her mother, November 1, 1868, in Cheney, *Memoir*, 18.

94. Marie Vögtln to Marie Ritter, January 17, 1869, in Johanna Siebel, *Das Leben von Frau Dr. Heim-Vögtlin 1845–1916* (Zurich: Rascher, 1928), 75.

95. Scott A. Norton, "Whither medical botany?," in *CMAJ* (Canadian Medical Association Journal), June 20, 2006.

96. Dimock to Zakrzewska, January 9, 1870, in Cheney, *Memoir*, 20–21.

97. *Ibid.*, 19–20.

98. *Ibid.*, 23.

99. Edmund Rose was the successor in Zurich to the eminent surgeon, Theodor Billroth, who had moved to the University of Vienna. Rose was quoted in "Vögtlin, Marie (1845–1916)," Women in World History: A Biographical Encyclopedia, Encyclopedia.com, Gale Research Inc.

https://www.encyclopedia.com/women/encyclopedias-almanacs-transcripts-and-maps/vogtlin-marie-1845-1916 Accessed May 13, 2021.

100. Müller, *Marie Heim-Vögtlin*, 139–140. The debate over Russian female students in Zurich became moot in 1873 when Tsar Alexander II banned all Russians from studying there starting January 1, 1874, due to what he perceived as the Swiss city's anarchist, revolutionary influences. Seven years later, the Tsar was assassinated by a radical nihilist group.

101. Susan Dimock to Dr. Samuel Cabot, Oct. 9, 1873, in New England Hospital for Women and Children Records, 1792–1994: MS 339, Sophia Smith Collection, Smith College, Northampton, Massachusetts.

102. Forel, *Out of My Life and Work*, 56.

103. *Ibid.*

104. Bonner, *To the Ends of the Earth*, 2.

105. Cheney, *Memoir*, 27; Susan J. Dimock, *Ueber die verschiedenen Formen des Puerperalfiebers. Nach Beobachtungen in der Züricher Gebaranstalt* (inaugural-Disseration, Zürich: Druck von Zürcher und Furrer, 1871). Puerperal fever was a major cause of death for new mothers and newborns throughout much of the nineteenth century. Among the first doctors to write extensively on the subject was Oliver Wendell Holmes, Sr., of Boston, often remembered more today for his literary accomplishments than for his contributions to medicine.

106. Müller, *Marie Heim-Vögtlin*, Kindle, chapter 14, paragraph 1; and Bonner, *To the Ends of the Earth*, 2.

107. Thomas Neville Bonner, "Rendezvous in Zurich: Seven Who Made a Revolution in Women's Medical Education, 1864–1874," *Journal of the History of Medicine and Allied Sciences*, Vol. 44. No. 1 (Oxford University Press, 1989), 17.

108. August Forel to his mother, June 19, 1869, Medizinhistorisches Institut, University of Zurich, cited in Bonner, *To the Ends of the Earth*, 37.

109. The definitive biography of Marie Vögtlin is Verena E. Müller's *MarieHeim-Vögtlin—die erste Schweizer Ärztin (1845–1916): Ein Leben zwischen Tradition und Aufbruch* (Baden 2007, vierte Auflage 2016.)

110. Bonner, "Rendezvous in Zurich," 26.

111. Cited in Vögtlin, Marie (1845–1916), *Women in World History: A Biographical Encyclopedia* http://www.encyclopedia.com/women/encyclopedias-almanacs-transcripts-and-maps/vogtlin-marie-1845-1916 Accessed May 13, 2021.

112. Vietor, *A Woman's Quest*, 359.

113. Boston University began as the Newbury Biblical Institute in Newbury, Vermont, in 1839. The school moved to Boston in 1867 and was granted a charter with the name "Boston University" by the Massachusetts Legislature in 1869. For the history of John Hopkins and women medical students, see "Women Gaining Access to Medical Education," Johns Hopkins Medicine, History https://www.hopkinsmedicine.org/about/history/women-med-ed.html Accessed May 14, 2021.

114. There were non–Ivy League schools with even worse records than Harvard. It wasn't until 1948, for example, that the medical colleges at St. Louis University and Georgetown University admitted women. And not until 1960 did Jefferson Medical College in Philadelphia become co-educational.

115. See Karel B. Absolon, *The Surgeon's Surgeon: Theodor Billroth 1829–1894*, Volume II (Lawrence, Kansas: Coronado Press, 1981). The Austro-Hungarian Empire, also called Austria-Hungary or the Dual Monarchy, was created in 1867 with Emperor Franz Joseph I at its helm. Although it was one of the greatest powers in central Europe, the empire was dissolved on November 12, 1918, following its defeat in the First World War.

116. August Forel, *Briefe Correspondance 1864–1927*, Hans H. Walser, ed. (Bern: Verlag Hans Huber, 1968), 83 (translated from French and German by Megan Catalano).

117. Return address noted in a letter from Susan Dimock to Marie Zakrzewska, Nov. 22, 1871, in Cheney, *Memoir*, 24–25.

118. "Billroth always felt uncomfortable about women in medicine and he never gets over this feeling he acquired in early life. He was positive that women are unsuitable for certain professions." Quoted in Absolon, *The Surgeon's Surgeon*, 140.

119. Absolon, *The Surgeon's Surgeon*, 81, 103; Erna Lesky, *The Vienna Medical*

School of the 19th Century (Baltimore: Johns Hopkins University Press, 1976), 262. The medical school at the University of Vienna traced its origins back to the fourteenth century. The Vienna General Hospital opened in 1784. In 1842, what became known as the "Second Viennese Medical School" emerged as a companion surgical clinic within the General Hospital itself. Having two surgical clinics allowed separate surgical procedures to co-exist in different work areas.

120. Absolon, *The Surgeon's Surgeon*, 20. For a detailed study of the medical school in this era, see Erna Lesky, *The Vienna Medical School of the 19th Century*.

121. Absolon, *The Surgeon's Surgeon*, 8, 12, 19, 103. For details and a modern analysis on Dr. Dimock's neck tumor surgery, see two journal articles: Jane Petro, MD, FACS, Susan Wilson, and Megan Catalano, "Susan Dimock, pioneering American physician," *Bulletin of the American College of Surgeons* (March 2021). https://www.facsbulletin.com/acs bulletin/march2021/MobilePagedReplica. action?pm=2&folio=26#pg28; Jane Petro, MD, FACS, Susan Wilson BA, MA History, and Megan Catalano BS, MS Health Policy, "Susan Dimock, Pioneering 19th Century American Surgeon/Physician," *Annals of Surgery Open* 3, no. 4 (December 2022): e208. https://journals.lww.com/aosopen/ Fulltext/2022/12000/Susan_Dimock,_ Pioneering_19th_Century_American.5.a spx?context=LatestArticles

122. Lilian Freeman Clarke, "The Story of an Invisible Institution," *Outlook*, December 15, 1906, 932; Cheney, *Memoir*, 28–29.

123. Susan Dimock to Marie Zakrzew-ska, Nov. 22, 1871, in Cheney, *Memoir*, 24–25.

124. Absolon, *The Surgeon's Surgeon*, 37. "An der schönen, blauen Donau," known as "By the Beautiful Blue Danube" in English, was composed by Johann Strauss II (1825–1899) in 1866. It was first performed in Vienna in a choral version in 1867, followed by a purely orchestral version that same year at the Paris World's Fair.

125. August Forel, *Briefe Corre-spondance 1864–1927* (Bern Und Stuttgart: Verlag Hans Huber, 1968), 85.

126. *Ibid.*, 84.

127. Absolon, *The Surgeon's Surgeon*, 119.

128. "L'homme tatouage de Birmanie," *Wiener Medizinische Wochenschrift*, No. 2, 1872. https://www.whonamedit. com/doctor.cfm/621.html Accessed June 6, 2021. The man whose real name was George Constantine Alexandrinos became one of the most recognized Greeks in the United States. See Steve Frangos, "Captain Costentenus: The Tattooed Greek of New York City," *The National Herald*, Feature 7, June 3, 2006. http://hellenicgenealogygeek. blogspot.com/2017/09/captain-costen tenus-tattooed-greek-of.html Accessed June 8, 2021.

129. Frangos, "Captain Costentenus."

130. Susan Dimock to Marie Zakrew-ska, December 10, 1870, in Cheney, *Memoir*, 22–23.

131. David McCullough, *The Greater Journey: Americans in Paris* (New York: Simon and Schuster, 2011), 193.

132. Marilyn Brouwer, "The Paris Morgue: A Gruesome Tourist Attrac-tion in the 19th Century," *Bonjour Paris: The Insider's Guide*, Oct 7, 2019. https://bon jourparis.com/history/the-paris-morgue-a-gruesome-tourist-attraction-in-19th-century/?utm_source=Bonjour+Paris &utm_campaign=0ba6be207a-EMAIL_ CAMPAIGN_2019_03_07_02_50_ COPY_01&utm_medium=email&utm_ term=0_306bdf7563-0ba6be207a-294026465&mc_cid=0ba6be207a&mc_ eid=b555450a09

The site of the old Paris Morgue is now occupied by the Mémorial des Martyrs de la Deportation, an underground commemoration of the more than 200,000 people deported from Vichy France to Nazi concentration camps during World War II. The memorial was dedicated in 1962.

133. Müller, *Marie Heim-Vögtlin*, 111–112.

134. Pauline Marion Worthy, "Susan Dimock, Pioneer in Medicine," *Raleigh News & Observer*, April 25, 1937.

135. *Transactions of the Nineteenth Annual Meeting of the Medical Society of the State of North Carolina, Held at Newbern, N.C., May 1872* (Raleigh: Edwards & Broughton, 1872).

136. From the *Washington Echo*, N.C., quoted in Cheney, *Memoir*, 93–94.

Chapter 4

1. Ednah Dow Cheney (anon.), *Memoir of Susan Dimock* (Boston: Press of J. Wilson, 1875), 49–50; Lilian Freeman, Clarke, "The Story of an Invisible Institution," *Outlook,* December 15, 1906, 932–933.

2. *Annual Report of the New-England Hospital for Women and Children, Codman Avenue, Boston Highlands, For the Year Ending September 30, 1872* (Boston: Press of W.L. Deland, 1873), 11.

3. Oliver Wendell Holmes, Sr., dubbed the Boston State House the "Hub of the Solar System" in his *Autocrat of the Breakfast Table* in 1858. The quote was later misremembered as Boston being the "Hub of the Universe." During Susan's first years at the New England Hospital for Women and Children, Boston continued absorbing neighborhood towns: Brighton and Roslindale were annexed in 1873; Jamaica Plain, Allston, Charlestown, and West Roxbury were independent towns that became Boston neighborhoods in 1874. Immigration statistics from Frederick A. Bushee, "The Growth of the Population of Boston," *Publications of the American Statistical Association* 6, no. 46 (1899), 260–261.

4. After less than a decade, Howe's "Mother's Day for Peace" disappeared. In 1914 it was replaced by the Mother's Day we now celebrate as a national holiday, initiated by Anna Jarvis of Philadelphia and West Virginia in honor of her late mother. Both Howe and Jarvis would have been disappointed by the maudlin, non-political, highly commercialized celebration Mother's Day later became.

5. Cheney, *Memoir*, 31.

6. Nabby Joy (1791–1869), the sole heir of Joseph G. Joy, was a wealthy Boston heiress who lived at 32 Mount Vernon Street. The executors of her will gave substantial funds to 53 charitable societies and institutions in May of 1872, including $5,000 to NEHWC. "A Joy Forever: Bequests Amounting to $280,560 Paid to Massachusetts Charitable Institutions," *New York Times*, May 24, 1872. Among Nabby Joy's other bequests were the "Joy Scholarships" at M.I.T, intended to "benefit of one or more women studying natural science at the institute," and the donation of sculptor Richard Saltonstall Greenough's "Carthaginian Girl" to the Boston Athenaeum.

7. Alice B. (Mrs. William O.) Crosby, *The Story of the New England Hospital for Women and Children through Seventy-Five Years, 1862–1937* (Boston, Massachusetts: New England Hospital for Women and Children, 1937), 7.

8. Emma L Call, M.D., "Evolution of Modern Maternity Technique. Illustrated by Records of the New England Hospital for Women and Children, Boston, from 1862 to 1907," *The American Journal of Obstetrics and Diseases of Women and Children* 59, no. 1, Brooks H. Wells, M.D., ed. (July-December, 1908): 395.

9. In the course of the second half of the nineteenth century, germ theory—buoyed by the studies of Louis Pasteur in the 1860s—eventually replaced miasmic theory. In the 1870s, the work of Joseph Lister helped establish the practical application of sanitation to medical procedures.

10. Charles Amos Cummings and Willard T. Sears had established their architectural office in Boston in 1864. Among their works following the New England Hospital for Women and Children (1872) were the New Old South Church in Boston (1873), the chapel at Phillips Academy in Andover (1876), and the Cyclorama building in Boston (1884). Willard T. Sears' greatest renown was for his work on Isabella Stewart Gardner's "Venetian palace" in Boston (1901).

11. Crosby, *The Story of the New England Hospital*, 7.

12. *Ibid.*; *1872 Annual Report*, 6; Virginia G. Drachman, *Hospital with a Heart: Women Doctors and the Paradox of Separatism at the New England Hospital, 1862–1969* (Ithaca NY: Cornell University Press, 1984), 74.

13. Drachman, *Hospital with a Heart*, 73–74.

14. *The Woman's Journal*, July 13, 1872, 221.

15. Crosby, *The Story of the New England Hospital*, 7.

16. *1872 Annual Report*, 6.

17. "Childbed Fever and Lying in Hospitals," in https://duallovedoula. wordpress.com/history-of-childbirth Accessed November 14, 2019.

18. Call, "Evolution of Modern Maternity Technique," 393.

19. Drachman, *Hospital with a Heart*, 75.

20. *1872 Annual Report*, 14–15.

21. *New England Hospital for Women and Children: Fair at Tremont Temple, December 1–6, 1896* (souvenir booklet), 35.

22. "Hospital for Women and Children," *The Woman's Journal*, June 15, 1872, 192. The Providence Railroad boarded at Boylston Station in downtown Boston, quite close to the New England Hospital's Dispensary.

23. Crosby, *The Story of the New England Hospital*, 9. In 1880, the New England Hospital purchased a building on Fayette Street, where the Dispensary would be located for the next decade and a half. A small dispensary was also included in the basement of the new Roxbury hospital.

24. When Susan began work in 1872, her three fellow dispensary physicians were Dr. Lucy Sewall, Dr. C. Annette Buckel, and Dr. Helen Morton. *1872 Annual Report*, 2.

25. *Annual Report of the School Committee of the City of Boston* (Boston: Geo. C. Rand & Avery, 1874), 29–33.

26. *The Washington Echo*, N.C., in Cheney, *Memoir*, 93–94.

27. Dr. Augusta Pope, quoted in *The Fiftieth Anniversary of the New England Hospital for Women and Children* (Boston: Press of Geo. H. Ellis Co., 1913), 46.

28. *1872 Annual Report*, 11; Crosby, *The Story of the New England Hospital*, 7.

29. William Randall King, *Ghost Dance: The Legacy of Susan Dimock, Nineteenth Century Surgeon* (Yale University School of Medicine, 1997), 56. In 1836, a German Lutheran minister named Theodore Fliedner created the Kaiserwerther Diakonie as a hospital and deaconess training center where young women could learn both theology and nursing skills. In 1850, thirty-year-old Florence Nightingale received her first nurses' training there; Nightingale went on to become the "founder of modern nursing."

30. Alfred Worcester, A.M., M.D., *Nurses for Our Neighbors* (Boston: Houghton Mifflin Company, 1914), 58–59.

31. *Ibid.*

32. *The New England Hospital, One Hundred Years, 1862–1962* (1962), 22; Linda Richards, "Early Days in the First American Training School for Nurses," *The American Journal of Nursing* 16, no. 3 (Lippincott Williams & Wilkins: December, 1915), 174. When Dr. Dimock opened her formal nurses' training program at the NEHWC on September 1, 1872, it was a year before the much-heralded "Nightingale schools" of nursing began. The first three were at Bellevue Hospital, New York, NY; the New Haven Hospital (originally called the Connecticut Training School at the State Hospital); and the training school at Massachusetts General Hospital (MGH), Boston.

33. Richards, "Early Days," 174–176.

34. *1872 Annual Report*, 8; *The New England Hospital, One Hundred Years*, 16.

35. Linda Richards, *Reminiscences of America's First Trained Nurse* (Boston: Whitcomb & Barrows, 1911), 11; *The New England Hospital, One Hundred Years*, 22; *1872 Annual Report*, 8; Drachman, *Hospital with a Heart*, 80–81.

36. Richards, *Reminiscences*, 10–11.

37. Cheney, *Memoir*, 50–51.

38. *The New England Hospital, One Hundred Years*, 16.

39. Richards, *Reminiscences*, 11; Richards, "Early Days," 177; *The New England Hospital, One Hundred Years*, 22.

40. *The New England Hospital, One Hundred Years*, 16.

41. *1872 Annual Report*, 8.

42. Cheney, *Memoir*, 34.

43. Call, "Evolution of Modern Maternity Technique," 401.

44. Crosby, *The Story of the New England*, 8; *Fiftieth Anniversary*, 47.

45. Clarke, "The Story of an Invisible Institution," 933.

46. *The New England Hospital, One Hundred Years*, 23.

47. "The Horse Epidemic," *Boston Transcript*, October 31, 1872, 2. Horses pulled all of Boston's trolleys, since the first electrified streetcars didn't arrive in the city until 1888. Over the next dozen years, horsecars were gradually phased out.

48. *Annual Report of the New-England Hospital for Women and Children, Codman Avenue, Boston Highlands, for the*

Year Ending September 30, 1873 (Boston: Press of W.L. Deland, 1874), 5.

49. Susan Wilson, "History Notebook: The Great Fire of 1872," City Weekly, *The Boston Sunday Globe*, November 7, 1993, 1. How badly the loss of horsepower affected the speed and efficacy of the firefighting process during the Great Fire of 1872 can only be conjectured.

50. Harriet Hyman Alonso, *Growing Up Abolitionist: The Story of the Garrison Children* (Amherst and Boston: University of Massachusetts Press, 2002), 244.

51. Oliver Wendell Holmes, "After the Fire," 1872, http://www.ibiblio.org/eldritch/owh/fire.html. Accessed September 19, 2020.

52. Wilson, "The Great Fire of 1872." Though no precise numbers will ever be available, the death toll for the Great Fire of 1872 is estimated to be around 30–40 individuals, more than a quarter of whom were firefighters.

53. *1872 Annual Report*, 4.

54. *1873 Annual Report*, 6.

55. *Fiftieth Anniversary*, 46–47.

56. Harriet Hyman Alonso, *Growing Up Abolitionist: The Story of the Garrison Children* (Amherst and Boston: University of Massachusetts Press, 2002). 244; L.S. (Lucy Stone), "The Great Fire," *The Woman's Journal*, November 16, 1872, 364.

57. *1872 Annual Report*, 6–9; *History of the New England Hospital for Women and Children, 1859–1899*; and *Fair at the Hotel Vendome for the Benefit of the New England Hospital for Women and Children, December 4th to 9th, 1899* (Boston, 1899), 15.

58. *Fiftieth Anniversary*, 47.

59. Mary Roth Walsh, *Doctors Wanted: No Women Need Apply* (New Haven and London: Yale University Press, 1977), 112–113.

60. Quoted by Dr. Zakrzewska in Agnes C. Vietor, M.D., F.A.C.S., *A Woman's Quest: The Life of Marie E. Zakrzewska, M.D.* (New York: D. Appleton and Company, 1924), 343.

61. Walsh, *Doctors Wanted*, 119.

62. Nina Renata Aron, "The father of American gynecology fought to criminalize abortion in the 1850s: Horatio Storer's legacy remains even after Roe v. Wade," *Timeline*, March 27, 2017.

63. Elaine Showalter, *The Civil Wars of Julia Ward Howe* (New York: Simon & Schuster, 2016), 197–198.

64. Edward H. Clarke, M.D., *Sex in Education; or, A Fair Chance for Girls* (Boston: Houghton, Mifflin and Company, 1884), 39.

65. Drachman, *Hospital with a Heart*, 55.

66. Susan Speaker, "The Question of Rest for Women," *Circulating Now: From the Historical Collections of the National Library of Medicine*, July 29, 2014. Jacobi's work was so impressive that she was encouraged to enter the Harvard Medical Faculty's Boylston competition, since the topic was the effect of menstruation on women. Her well-written, well-researched, and expertly documented piece, "The Question of Rest for Women During Menstruation," won the Boylston Prize Essay of Harvard University for 1876.

67. Cheney, *Memoir*, 13.

68. *1873 Annual Report*, p. 5. Calling the New England Hospital a "Beacon on a hill" harkens back to a 1630 sermon by John Winthrop of the Massachusetts Bay Colony, who founded the town of Boston. Winthrop predicted that their settlement would be a beacon of hope for the world: "We shall be as a city upon a hill, the eyes of all people are upon us." The center of Boston, where the Massachusetts State House was later erected, came to be called Beacon Hill.

69. Boston City Hospital, opened in 1864, didn't offer gynecological treatment until 1873; they had no gynecology department until 1892. Children's Hospital, opened in 1869, offered only pediatric services. Mass. General Hospital, opened in 1821, didn't offer obstetric services until the twentieth century; in the nineteenth century, they had only medical and surgical care for women. The only other hospital in the city that specialized in obstetrics, Boston Lying-In, closed in 1856; though it reopened in 1873, it closed three more times over the next thirteen years due to epidemics in its wards.

70. Cheney, *Memoir*, 38; James Freeman Clarke, *Memorial and Biographical Sketches* (Boston: Houghton, Osgood and Company, 1878), 217.

71. Cheney, *Memoir*, 50.

72. Clarke, "The Story of an Invisible Institution," 933.

73. Cheney, *Memoir*, 40.

74. *Ibid.*, 24.

75. Call, "Evolution of Modern Maternity Technique," 177.

76. *Ibid.*, 395, 401.

77. *1873 Annual Report*, 11.

78. Ignaz Philipp Semmelweis (1818–1865), known as the "Savior of Mothers," was a Hungarian-born scientist and physician and an early pioneer of antiseptic procedures. Though he discovered that the incidence of puerperal fever in obstetrical clinics could be cut drastically when doctors washed and disinfected their hands, he could not scientifically prove his findings and was largely rejected by the medical community. His findings were not widely accepted until many years after his death, when Louis Pasteur confirmed the germ theory of disease. An infamous chapter in the lack of antiseptic intervention occurred in 1881, when U.S. President James Garfield suffered two gunshot wounds on July 2 of that year. The president survived for 80 days, finally succumbing to complications from sepsis, a result of his surgeon probing the wound with unwashed hands. Garfield's assassin noted, "Yes, I shot the president, but his physicians killed him." Ehrhardt, J.D., Jr., O'Leary, J.P., & Nakayama, D.K., "Yes, I Shot the President, but His Physicians Killed Him." The Assassination of President James A. Garfield. *The American surgeon*, vol. 84,11 (2018): 1711–1716.

79. Cheney, *Memoir*, 40.

80. *Ibid.*

81. *1873 Annual report*, 9.

82. *Ibid.*, 14.

83. *1872 Annual Report*, 7.

84. Call, "Evolution of Modern Maternity Technique," 395.

85. Drachman, *Hospital with a Heart*, 14.

86. Susan Dimock, "Report of Resident Physician," *1873 Annual Report*, 11–12.

87. Cheney, *Memoir*, p. 39; Drachman, *Hospital with a Heart*, 61–63.

88. Cheney, *Memoir*, 38–39.

89. While Susan's mother was a slave-holding Southerner, her father was a Northerner who agreed to keep a few enslaved workers for the family, but only with reluctance. When Susan and her mother fled North near the end of the Civil War, after Susan's father died and their home and hometown were consumed by fire, they had few possessions left; that Susan's childhood doll was still with her several years later was extraordinary.

90. Susan Dimock, "Report of Resident Physician," *1873 Annual Report*, 12.

91. Clarke, "The Story of an Invisible Institution," 932.

92. S. Dimock, Resident Physician, "Surgical Wards record #5," February 9, 1873," New England Hospital 1873 Cases, Boston Medical Library in the Francis A. Countway Library of Medicine, Harvard University, Boston, Massachusetts, New England Hospital for Women and Children, Records of Surgical Wards [B MS b19.1 vol. 1B and 2].

93. Untitled article, *The Independent … Devoted to the Consideration of Politics, Social and Economic Tendencies*, February 19, 1891, 13.

94. Call, "Evolution of Modern Maternity Technique," 394–396; Arleen Marcia Tuchman, *Science Has No Sex: The Life of Marie Zakrzewska, M.D.* (Chapel Hill: University of North Carolina Press, 2006), 13.

95. The relationship between David and Jonathan is primarily recounted in the Hebrew Bible's Book of Samuel. David was slayer of Goliath and the King of Israel; Jonathan was the son of Saul and the presumed heir to the crown of Israel. The two shared what has been called an intense "romantic friendship," though some scholars believe they were lovers (see a more detailed discussion in Chapter 2: Transitions).

96. Clarke, "The Story of an Invisible Institution," 933.

97. *Ibid.*

98. Alice B. (Mrs. William O.) Crosby, *The Story of the New England Hospital for Women and Children through Seventy-Five Years, 1862-1937*, 8; *The New England Hospital, One Hundred Years, 1862-1962* (Boston: 1962), 16.

99. Marie E. Zakrzewska, "In Memoriam," in Cheney, *Memoir*, 86; David Lowenthal, *George Perkins Marsh: Prophet of Conservation* (Seattle: University of Washington Press, 2000), 360–361.

100. M.E. [Dr. Mary E.] Little, "Letter from a Pupil of Dr. Dimock," in Cheney, *Memoir*, 45–46.

101. Cheney, *Memoir*, 43–44.

102. *Ibid.*, 35.

103. *Ibid.*, 36.

104. Susan Dimock, "Report of Resident Physician," *Annual Report of the New-England Hospital for Women and Children, Codman Avenue, Boston Highlands, for the Year Ending September 30, 1874* (Boston: Press of W.L. Deland, 1875), 12–13.

105. The first public demonstration of diethyl ether as a general anesthetic was in 1846, at the place now known as the Ether Dome of Massachusetts General Hospital. Though the United States phased ether out in the 1970s, largely due to its flammability, some developing countries still use it today due to its low cost and minimal respiratory and cardiac depression.

106. Tuchman, *Science Has No Sex,* 13; Call, "Evolution of Modern Maternity Technique," 396–398.

107. William Randall King, "Ghost Dance: The Legacy of Susan Dimock, Nineteenth Century Surgeon" (Thesis submitted to the Yale University School of Medicine, 1997), 64–6; James M. Edmonson, Ph.D., *Nineteenth Century Surgical Instruments: A Catalogue of the Gustav Weber Collection at the Howard Dittrick Museum of Historical Medicine* (Cleveland, Ohio: Historical Division, The Cleveland Health Sciences Library, 1986).

108. King, "Ghost Dance," 66.

109. Dr. Samuel Cabot, quoted by James Freeman Clarke, in "Susan Dimock," *Boston Daily Advertiser,* May 15, 1875.

110. Boston Medical Library in the Francis A. Countway Library of Medicine, Harvard University, Boston, Massachusetts, New England Hospital for Women and Children, Records of Medical Wards [B MS b19.2 vol. 1] and Surgical Wards [B MS b19.1 vol. 1B and 2]. Two of the author's lengthy articles about this surgery, along with 21st century analysis, were printed in American medical journals in 2021 and 2022. See Jane Petro, MD, FACS, Susan Wilson, and Megan Catalano, "Susan Dimock, pioneering American physician," *Bulletin of the American College of Surgeons* (March 2021). https://www.facsbulletin.com/acsbulletin/march2021/MobilePagedReplica.action?pm=2&folio=26#pg 28; Jane Petro, MD, FACS, Susan Wilson BA, MA History, and Megan Catalano BS, MS Health Policy, "Susan Dimock, Pioneering 19th Century American Surgeon/Physician," *Annals of Surgery Open* 3, no. 4 (December 2022): e208. https://journals.lww.com/aosopen/Fulltext/2022/12000/Susan_Dimock,_Pioneering_19th_Century_American.5.aspx?context=LatestArticles

111. Records of Medical Wards and Surgical Wards. Nineteenth century apothecaries used the "drachm" or "dram," a unit of weight which was the equivalent of an eighth of a fluid ounce or sixty grains. Long before vitamins and proteins were discovered or understood, British doctors had tried to understand why beef had nutritional value; they came up with a kind of beef broth, called "beef tea," which seemed to soothe and comfort patients. Sadly, almost two years after that successful neck tumor operation, young patient Sarah died of "dropsy," an old term for edema.

112. Mary Putnam Jacobi, MD, "An Obituary of the Author [Susan Dimock, M.D.]," *The Medical Record: A Weekly Journal of Medicine and Surgery* 10 (January 2–December 25, 1875): 358. Born Mary Corinna Putnam in London, England, Putnam Jacobi (1842–1906) was the daughter of the founder of the G.P. Putnam's Sons publishing firm. A writer, educator, physician, and suffragist, she became one of the most preeminent female doctors of her era.

113. Records of Medical Wards and Surgical Wards.

114. Susan Dimock, M.D., "A Case of Successful Operation for Recto-Vaginal Fistula," *The Medical Record* 9 George F. Shrady, ed. (New York: William Wood & Company, 1874), 458; Susan Dimock, M.D., "A Case of Congenital Anal Occlusion of an Unusual Kind," *The Medical Record* 10, George F. Shrady, ed. (New York: William Wood & Company, 1875), 357–358; Records of Medical Wards and Surgical Wards.

115. "The medical ethics of Dr J Marion Sims: a fresh look at the historical record," *Journal of Medical Ethics,* June 2006, Volume 32, Number 6, 346–50. James Marion Sims (1813–1884) was one of nineteenth century America's most famous physicians. Among other

accomplishments, he developed the first effective operation to cure vesicovaginal fistula, a dreadful childbirth complication wherein a hole develops between a woman's vagina and bladder, resulting in uncontrollable urinary incontinence and social ostracism. Inspired in part by the outcry that accompanied Harriet Washington's 2007 book, *Medical Apartheid: The Dark History of Medical Experimentation on Black Americans from Colonial Times to the Present*, a statue of Sims was removed from Central Park in New York City in April 2018 by unanimous vote of the New York City Public Design Commission.

116. Drachman, *Hospital with a Heart*, 86–88.

117. Call, "Evolution of Modern Maternity Technique," 400.

118. Street ledger, Ward 9, 1874, part 2, 197, City of Boston Archives, West Roxbury, Massachusetts.

119. Cheney, *Memoir*, 80–81.

120. Bessie Greene to Lilian Freeman Clarke (n.d.), Perry-Clarke Collection: Lilian Freeman Clarke correspondence, Ms. N-109, Massachusetts Historical Society. For all of the nineteenth and the first half of the twentieth century, it was common for individuals and families to live in hotels. The Clarendon, at 521–523 (sometimes listed as 517–529) Tremont Street, boasted in an August 20, 1872 advertisement that it was an "excellent family hotel" with "handsome airy rooms" that could be rented by the day, week, month, or year. It also proudly stated that it was "on one of the broadest avenues in the city" and that "horse cars pass the door day and evening."

121. Susan Dimock to Sophie Heim, May 31, 1874, in the private collection of Kay Hicks, Lynchburg, Virginia; accessed 1995.

122. Cheney, *Memoir*, 52. Osgood & Company was the successor firm to the innovative Ticknor & Fields and the nucleus of what became Houghton Mifflin and Company. Oliver Ditson ran one of America's greatest nineteenth century music publishing companies, which was also a manufacturer and retailer of musical instruments.

123. Dimock to Heim, May 31, 1874.

124. *Ibid.*

125. *Ibid.*

126. Cheney, *Memoir*, 43.

Chapter 5

1. Susan Dimock to Dr. Elizabeth Garrett Anderson, April 14, 1875, in Ednah Dow Cheney (anon.), *Memoir of Susan Dimock* (Boston: Press of J. Wilson, 1875), 57. Fearing that he was too successful and might therefore suffer a reversal of fortune, the ancient Greek tyrant Polycrates took the suggestion of Egypt's Pharoah and threw his most treasured item, a jewel-encrusted ring, into the sea. A few days later, while Polycrates' cooks were preparing a freshly caught fish for his meal, they found the ring inside. Polycrates told Pharaoh, who immediately broke their alliance, fearing that such a lucky man would come to a sad end.

2. Cheney, *Memoir*, 16.

3. *Ibid.*, 52. A beautifully illustrated history of Susan Dimock's ship is Keith Austin, *The Victorian Titanic: The Loss of the S.S Schiller in 1875* (Tiverton, Devon, Great Britain: Halsgrove House, 2001). It's possible that Dimock's love of Friedrich Schiller (1759–1805) grew during her years in Zurich, since the German poet, philosopher, physician, historian, and playwright was enjoying renewed popularity in that city for more than a decade leading up to Susan's arrival. "Der Ring des Polykrates" was written by Friedrich Schiller in June 1797 and first published in his 1798 *Musen-Almanach* annual. In 1914, Erich Wolfgang Korngold wrote the one-act opera, *Der Ring des Polykrates*, Op. 7, which made its debut in Munich. Germany's Nationaltheater in 1916.

4. Keith Austin, *The Victorian Titanic: The loss of the S.S Schiller in 1875* (Tiverton, Devon, Great Britain: Halsgrove House, 2001), 55–57.

5. "Miss Bessie Greene, obituary signed "W.," *The Boston Evening Transcript*, in Cheney, *Memoir*, 82.

6. Marie Zakrzewska, "In Memoriam," Cheney, *Memoir*, 86.

7. Crane Family Papers, 1819–1944, New York Public Library, Manuscripts and Archives Division; Nick Greene, email

message to author, Jan 16, 2019; Miss Jenn Winslow Coltrane, *Lineage Book—National Society of the Daughters of the American Revolution* (Washington, D.C.: Judd & Detweiler, 1922), Vol. 62, item 61079.

The Marshes were a prominent Vermont family. George Perkins Marsh (1801–1882) served as United States Ambassador to Italy from 1861–1882. In 1839 he married his second wife, Caroline Crane (1816–1901). While Ambassador Marsh himself has been heralded as America's first conservationist, his wife Caroline was equally impressive: a poet, author, translator, and women's rights advocate, she was apparently as strong and smart as her husband, as well as the impetus behind some of his major accomplishments. Vermont Senator George Franklin Edmunds (1822–1919) married Susan Marsh Lyman (1831–1916), a niece of George Perkins Marsh, in 1852 (Susan was the daughter of Marsh's sister and Wyllys Lyman, a lawyer and friend of Marsh's from Burlington, Vermont). A constitutional lawyer by profession, Senator Edmunds had a long and prestigious tenure in the U.S. Senate, playing a role in some of the most significant developments of his era, including the move to impeach President Andrew Johnson, the Edmunds Acts against polygamy in Utah, and the Sherman Antitrust Act to limit monopolies.

8. By the time of its opening in 1883, the East River Bridge was already known by its permanent name, "The Brookyln Bridge." Castle Garden, later known as Castle Clinton or Fort Clinton, is in Manhattan's Battery Park today. New York's most heralded entrance point for immigrants, Ellis Island, opened in 1892. The welcoming Statue of Liberty made its debut six years earlier, in 1886.

9. Austin, *The Victorian Titanic*, 21–24, 48.

10. *Ibid.*, 49–50, 58–59, 76. Mad Jack's father, John Percival (1740–1802), was the cousin of Thomas Percival (1759–1816), the great-grandfather of *Schiller* passenger Daniel Webster Percival (1841–1875).

11. S.S. *Schiller* exhibit at the Isles of Scilly Museum, Church Street, Hugh Town, St. Mary's, Isles of Scilly, Cornwall, accessed June 15, 2018; and Austin, *The Victorian Titanic*, 79.

12. S.S. *Schiller* exhibit at the Isles of Scilly Museum; and Austin, *The Victorian Titanic*, 53–56. The estimated value of those gold coins today would be almost seven million dollars. The kegs of gold were addressed to E.S. Ballin & Company, Paris. Eugene S. Ballin was on the Finance Committee of the New York Gold Exchange; his company offices were on Boulevard Haussmann in Paris and Exchange Place in New York City.

13. "The Ocean Steamer," *Harper's New Monthly Magazine*, August 1870, 185–198.

14. *Newburyport Daily Herald*, May 11, 1875.

15. Various sources in family history list the name as "Ridgeway" or "Ridgway," sometimes using both spellings in the same document. Joseph Ridgway is erroneously referred to as George Joseph Ridgway in some texts. Back in 1858, Mary Ridgway, her husband Joseph, and their daughters Elizabeth ("Lizzie") and Clara, had happily relocated to Cambridge, Massachusetts, where they intersected with "all the right people." They leased a home that had been the residence of celebrated sculptor Horatio Greenough, sent Lizzie and Clara to a school founded by the equally celebrated Harvard College scientist, Professor Louis Agassiz, and delighted when Lizzie later married New York merchant Charles W. Walter. A decade later, the family fortunes began to spiral downward: daughter Clara, now a mother of two, died while on a "health cure" in Southern France; Mary and Joseph brought her body home to the States, only to discover that their other daughter, Lizzie, had gone to South Carolina due to her own ill-health. The sorrowing parents rushed south, where father Joseph died "of a broken heart." After Lizzie's health improved, she travelled to the Tyrolean Alps, where she too passed away. *Newburyport Daily Herald*, May 11, 1875; *Springfield Republican*, May 12, 1875; *Newburyport Daily Herald*, cited from St. Louis Paper, June 7, 1875.

16. Amanda Martin (museum curator), interview with author, Isles of Scilly Museum, St. Mary's, Isles of Scilly, June 17, 2018; Austin, *The Victorian Titanic*, 72.

17. Assessor of wrecks note, London, May 15, 1875, chronicling items returned with Susan Dimock's body; Brown Library Archives, Washington, North Carolina.

18. Austin, *The Victorian Titanic*, 66.

19. S.S. *Schiller* exhibit at the Isles of Scilly Museum; "How the Schiller Was Lost," *The Saturday Review*, July 3, 1874, 17; and Austin, *The Victorian Titanic*, 82–87.

20. Oliver Hawker (photographer), interview with author, Penzance, Cornwall, June 19, 2018. As ships approached the English Channel from the Atlantic Ocean, they also had to contend with the Rennell Current from the Bay of Biscay, which could push vessels northward. James Rennell, Esq. F.R.S., *Observations on a Current That Often Prevails to the Westward of Scilly; Endangering the Safety of Ships That Approach the British Channel* 83(London: Philosophical Transactions of the Royal Society of London, 1793): 182–200.

21. The precise number of islands in the Isles of Scilly varies with the tides and the times; various sources have listed 140 to 200 islands total. An 1847 precursor to the 1858 lighthouse washed away before it was completed.

22. S.S. *Schiller* exhibit at the Isles of Scilly Museum.

23. "How the Schiller Was Lost," 17; Austin, *The Victorian Titanic*, 95; and S.S. *Schiller* exhibit at the Isles of Scilly Museum.

24. Austin, *The Victorian Titanic*, 93.

25. *Ibid.*, 91–99; and S.S. *Schiller* exhibit at the Isles of Scilly Museum.

26. Austin, *The Victorian Titanic*, 108; Mikael Elinder and Oscar Erixson, "Gender, Social Norms, and Survival in Maritime Disasters," *Proceedings of the National Academy of Sciences* 9, no.33 (August 14, 2012): 13220–13221.

27. Mary Malvina Dimock to Lilian Freeman Clarke, November 27, 1875, in Perry-Clarke Collection: James Freeman Clarke papers. Ms. N-2155.1. Lilian Freeman Clarke correspondence. Ms. N-109, Massachusetts Historical Society.

28. Luggers are small sailing ships, often employed for fishing and widely used in France, England, and Scotland. Cornish pilot gigs are 28- to 32-foot long, narrow, six-oared rowing boats made of Cornish elm; though intended for use in taking pilots out to vessels and as general workboats, they have been utilized since the late 17th century as agile, shore-based rescue lifeboats for vessels in distress. These gigs are popular for sporting races today, especially in Cornwall and the Isles of Scilly.

29. Hugh Town still has most of the same rough-hewn stone buildings as it did in 1875. The two inns where survivors were housed in 1875 exist today as the Atlantic and Treygarthen, while one of the pier-side warehouses used as makeshift morgues may have been the current Mermaid Tavern.

30. Amanda Martin (curator), interview with author, Isles of Scilly Museum, St. Mary's, Isles of Scilly, June 17, 2018.

31. *New York Times*, May 9, 1875.

32. *Boston Evening Transcript*, May 10, 1875.

33. Salvor's warrant by the Receiver of Wrecks, Public Record Office, in Austin, *The Victorian Titanic,* 150; "Received of Mr. George Hoggan," letter from London dated May 15, 1875, Susan Dimock file, Brown Library Archives, Washington, North Carolina; and Richard Larn OBE, *The Wrecks of Scilly, Fifth Revised* Edition (Shipwreck & Marine, Isles of Scilly, 2015), 35.

34. Married in 1874, Frances Morgan and George Hoggan established the first husband-and-wife medical practice in Britain.

35. Lilian Freeman Clarke, "The Story of an Invisible Institution," *Outlook*, December 15, 1906, 934.

36. George Hoggan to Mrs. Dimock, May 15, 1875, in Cheney, *Memoir*, 63–64, 96–97.

37. Cheney, *Memoir*, 96.

38. S.S. *Schiller* exhibit at the Isles of Scilly Museum; and Austin, *The Victorian Titanic*, 159–164.

39. Austin, *The Victorian Titanic*, 151–155.

40. Mary M. Dimock to Lilian Freeman Clarke, November 7, 1875, in, Perry-Clarke Collection: James Freeman Clarke papers, Ms. N-2155.1, Lilian Freeman Clarke correspondence, Ms. N-109, 2–3, Massachusetts Historical Society.

41. Signed, handwritten statement from John Dunn, Penzance, August 9,

1875, Crane Family Papers, 1819–1944, Correspondence, 1875, New York Public Library, Manuscripts and Archives Division.

42. *Ibid.* Ambassador George Perkins Marsh was devastated by the death and loss at sea of his beloved niece Carrie Crane; he died just three years after the Schiller shipwreck. "Next to the loss of you, there can be in store for me no greater affliction than the death of Carrie," he often told his wife, Caroline Crane Marsh. David Lowenthal, *George Perkins Marsh: Prophet of Conservation* (Seattle, University of Washington Press, 2000), 377.

43. Todd Stevens (diver), interview with author, St. Mary's, Isles of Scilly, June 16, 2018; Richard Larn (diver/shipwreck expert), interview with author, St. Mary's, Isles of Scilly, June 18, 2018. The barrels of gold coins were addressed to "E.S. Baillin & Co., Paris." Eugene S. Baillin was on the Finance Committee of the New York Gold Exchange and had offices at 24 Exchange Place in New York City and 28 Boulevard Haussmann in Paris.

44. Mary M. Dimock to Lilian Freeman Clarke, November 7, 1875.

45. Health Department, Bureau of Vital Statistics, 301 Mott Street, New York City, Permit No. 30920, June 2, 1875; Forest Hills Cemetery, order of interment for lot No. 3056, June 3, 1875; courtesy Forest Hills Cemetery, Jamaica Plain, Massachusetts; George Hoggan M.D. to Mrs. Dimock, May 15, 1875, in Cheney, *Memoir*, 65.

46. Clarke, "The Story of an Invisible Institution," 934.

47. Wm. B. (William Batchelder) Greene to "My Dear Mrs. Dimock," May 21 and May 23, 1875, Brown Library Archives, Washington, North Carolina.

48. Cheney, *Memoir*, 102; "Funeral of the late Dr. Susan Dimock," *Boston Globe*, June 5, 1875, 5; "Funeral of a Victim of the Schiller Disaster," *New York Times*, June 7, 1875, 2.

49. Cheney, *Memoir*, 102.

50. "Funeral of a Victim of the Schiller Disaster," 2.

51. Cheney, *Memoir*, 94–95.

52. *Ibid.*, 98.

53. *New York Times*, June 7, 1875, 2; *Boston Globe*, June 5, 1875, 5; Cheney,

Memoir, 100. Mary Roth Walsh, *Doctors Wanted: No Women Need Apply* (New Haven and London: Yale University Press, 1977), 157.

54. Cheney, *Memoir*, 100–101.

55. Article from *The Washington Echo*, N.C., in Cheney, *Memoir*, 91. Ednah Dow Cheney, "An Irreparable Loss," in Cheney, *Memoir*, 75. Letter from Anne Whitney, May 19, 1875, "Anne Whitney," unpublished manuscript by Elizabeth Rogers Payne, Anne Whitney papers, Wellesley College Library (archives 2128), 1009.

56. Mary Putnam Jacobi, MD, "An Obituary of the Author [Susan Dimock, M.D.]." *The Medical Record: A Weekly Journal of Medicine and Surgery* 10 (January 2–December 25, 1875): 358.

57. Margaret Fuller (1810–50) was a powerful, highly respected, and sometimes feared intellectual, journalist, and transcendentalist who intersected with Boston's literary elite and defied feminine stereotypes. She died in a shipwreck off Fire Island, New York, while returning from Italy with her husband and infant child.

58. John Greenleaf Whittier, *The Letters of John Greenleaf Whittier*, Vol. 1 (Cambridge: Belknap Press of Harvard University Press, 1975), 334.

59. Sarah Orne Jewett to Annie Adams Fields, May 20, 1875 [mislabeled 1874], in the Sarah Orne Jewett Text Project, http://contrun.libertarian-labyrinth. org/2005/11/ Accessed April 5, 2017.

60. E.D.C., "The Index," in Cheney, *Memoir*, 77. The phrase "even in their death they were not divided" was borrowed from the tale of David and Jonathan as told in the book of Samuel, Chapter 2, Verse 24.

61. "November Publications," *The Literary World; a Monthly Review of Current Literature*, Dec. 1, 1875, 6–7.

62. "Literature of the Day," *Lippincott's Magazine of Popular Literature and Science* 35 (February 1885): 214.

63. Cheney, *Memoir*, 48.

64. *Ibid.*, 49.

65. In 1995, author Susan Wilson was given a copy of the Boston ambrotype by Kay Hicks of Lynchburg, Virginia, a distant cousin of Dr. Dimock's. Since then, with Hicks' permission, the author has shared digital copies of that image

with various historical outlets around the world.

66. Cheney, *Memoir*, 67; Anna H. Clarke to Mrs. Dimock, January 22, 1876; in the private collection of Kay Hicks, Lynchburg, Virginia.

67. *The Boston Evening Transcript*, January 10, 1881, 4.

68. Cheney, *Memoir*, 67.

69. Anna H. Clarke to Mrs. Dimock, Feb. 20, 1876, in the private collection of Kay Hicks, Lynchburg, Virginia; accessed 1995.

70. Carol Driscoll (stone carver), email message to author, June 3, 2016. In 2005, Driscoll was hired in to recreate Susan Dimock's badly decaying headstone with a more durable granite replica.

71. Cheney, *Memoir*, 59.

72. "City and Suburbs: Notes of the Day About Town," *Boston Daily Globe*, July 29, 1875, 8.

73. Cheney, *Memoir*, 59.

74. *Annual Report of the New-England Hospital for Women and Children for the Year Ending September 30, 1875* (Boston: Press of W.L. Deland, 1876), 9–11.

75. "EDITORIAL: WOMEN IN MEDICINE," *Philadelphia Medical Times (1871–1889)*, July 3, 1875; 5, 40; American Periodicals, 632.

76. Marie Zakrzewska, "In Memoriam," in Cheney, *Memoir*, 83; Jacobi, MD, "An Obituary of the Author," 358.

77. *History of the New England Hospital for Women and Children, 1859–1899: Fair at the Hotel Vendome, Dec. 4–9, 1899* (Boston, 1899), 52.

78. Susan Dimock to Dr. Samuel Cabot, October 25, 1868, in New England Hospital for Women and Children Records, MS 339, Sophia Smith Collections, Smith College, Northampton, Massachusetts.

79. Walter Lincoln Burrage, *A History of the Massachusetts Medical Society: With Brief Biographies of the Founders and Chief Officers, 1781–1922* (Norwood, Massachusetts: Plimpton Press, 1923), 143–149.

80. In the decades after Susan Dimock's death, the New England Hospital for Women and Children produced or employed an unusual number of exceptional female doctors: The first five women surgeons admitted to the newly created American College of Surgeons in 1913 were all affiliated with the New England Hospital. Carol E.H. Scott-Conner, MD, PhD, FACS and Ingrid M. Lizarraga, MBBS, FACS, "The first women elected to College Fellowship," *Bulletin of the American College of Surgeons*, September 1, 2019. https://bulletin.facs.org/2019/09/the-first-women-elected-to-college-fellowship.

81. *The New England Hospital, 1862–1962: One Hundred Years* (Boston, 1962), 18.

82. M.M.D. (Mary Malvina Dimock) to Susan Dimock, May 2, 1875, in the private collection of Kay Hicks, Lynchburg, Virginia; accessed 1995.

83. Mary M. Dimock to Lilian Freeman Clarke, November 7, 1875, in Perry-Clarke Collection: James Freeman Clarke papers. Ms. N-2155.1. Lilian Freeman Clarke correspondence. Ms. N-109, 3–4, Massachusetts Historical Society.

New research by Stephen Farrell of the Brown Library shows that Mrs. Dimock had an active and productive business life in Washington, North Carolina, for more than two decades after her daughter's tragic death. Her varied ventures included school teaching, real estate, and tending her orchards.

Stephen Farrell, interviews with author, March 7–14, 2023. See also Clark Curtis, "The Real History Behind 328 W. Main Street Revealed," The Washington Daily News, March 11–12, 2021, 1B.

84. North Carolina, Wills and Probate Records, 1665–1998 for Mary M. Dimock, 1061; 1910 United States Federal Census for Mary M. Dimmock [sic], North Carolina, Guilford, Greensboro Ward 3, District 0105; Kay and Mary Hicks (Dimock distant cousins), email message to author, December 6, 2020.

85. *The Fiftieth Anniversary of the New England Hospital for Women and Children, Dimock Street, Boston, Mass., October twenty-nine, Nineteen Hundred Twelve* (Boston: Press of Geo. H. Ellis Co., 1913).

86. Pauline Marion Worthy, "Susan Dimock, Pioneer in Medicine," *Raleigh News & Observer*, April 25, 1937. The longest single piece created in Dimock's memory was compiled by Ednah Dow Cheney and published six months after Dimock's death: *Memoir of Susan Dimock* (Boston: Press of J. Wilson, 1875). In 1878,

a six-page chapter on Dimock was included in James Freeman Clarke's *Memorial and Biographical Sketches* (Boston: Houghton, Osgood and Company, 1878). In 1906, the Reverend Clarke's daughter, Lilian Freeman Clarke, included substantial personal biographical material on Dimock in "The Story of an Invisible Institution," *Outlook*, December 15, 1906, 932–936.

87. Claude Hodges, "Tombstone Comes Home to Rest," *Washington Daily News*, October 23, 1996, 6A; "Presentation Exercises, North Carolina Historical Commission of Markers to Historic Beaufort County and the Town of Washington, January 19, 1940," typed program from Susan Dimock file, Brown Library Archives, Washington, North Carolina.

88. *The Fiftieth Anniversary of the New England Hospital*, 51.

89. In the wake of the Mass Medical Society's opening up to women, Marie Zakrzewska was told she could take an examination to once again apply. Having been turned down three times in the past, she declined, arguing that after 27 years of practice and the creation of a successful women's hospital, asking her to take an examination was a "condescending proposal." "[T]his venerable Society ... must give me an honorary membership if it wants me at all," Zak insisted, adding that she was "happy that the younger women can have the benefit of an association which is very desirable for all beginners, and most desirable in assisting women to gain the position for which they strive." Agnes C. Vietor, M.D., F.A.C.S., *A Woman's Quest: The Life of Marie E. Zakrzewska, M.D.* (New York: D. Appleton and Company, 1924), 395.

90. These five inaugural fellows of the ACS were Alice G. Bryant, Emma V.P.B. Culbertson, Florence West Duckering, Jane D. Kelly Sabine, and Mary Almira Smith. Scott-Connor and Lizarraga, "The first women elected to College Fellowship."

91. Herbert Black, "Roxbury Health Center to Be Formed from N.E. Hospital," *The Boston Globe*, March 19, 1969, 21.

92. "New England Hospital Proud of Its Long Medical History," *A Feature Publication of The Tribune Publishing Company* (Hyde Park, Massachusetts, May 31, 1954), 1.

93. The definitive study of the hospital, including the success and ultimate failure of its policy of separatism, is Virginia G. Drachman's *Hospital with a Heart: Women Doctors and the Paradox of Separatism at the New England Hospital, 1862–1969* (Ithaca NY: Cornell University Press, 1984).

94. Undated promotional brochure, circa 1970s, from the archives of the Dimock Center, Roxbury, MA.

95. Radical journalist and editor Karl Heinzen (1809–80) and printer, lithographer, and publisher Louis Prang (1824–1909) were both part of the tight-knit community of progressive German immigrants who regularly socialized with German-born Marie Zakrzewska. Heinzen, his wife, and children, also lived at Dr. Zak's Roxbury home for many years. A cenotaph is a cemetery memorial that does not include the actual body of the person commemorated.

96. Forest Hills Cemetery Service Order to Mrs. Beatrice M. Bonnevie, Administrator of the New England Hospital for Women and Children, June 8, 1964; lot plan for Lot No. 3085, Sweetbrier Path, Original Proprietor, Marie E. Zakrzewska; courtesy Forest Hills Cemetery, Jamaica Plain MA.

97. Susan Wilson, "History Notebook: A selfless pioneer in Boston medicine," *The Boston Sunday Globe*, Night & Day section (Boston: Sunday, May 8, 1994), 264–265.

98. "Susan Wilson Heads Dimock Heritage Fund," *The ProclaimHer* (Boston Women's Heritage Trail, April 1995), 1–3. The Dimock Heritage Fund initially included Jackie Jenkins-Scott, Carneice Goode Pierce, Ediss Gandelman, and Victoria Jones of the Dimock Community Health Center; project leader Susan Wilson; conservators Carol Driscoll and Scott Wall; president Erling A. "Bud" Hanson of Forest Hills Cemetery; landscape architect Richard Heath of the Boston Greenspace Alliance; Michael Reiskind of the Jamaica Plain Historical Society; Boston College nurse historian Mary Ellen Doona; Cecilia Joseph of the New England Regional Black Nurses Association; Mary Smoyer of the Boston Women's Heritage Trail; Kathy Kottaridis and Stanley Smith of the Bostonian Society; Beth Shepard of the

Historic Burying Grounds Initiative; Ann Wadsworth of the Boston Athenaeum; Alice Krapf of Krapf Associates; Tufts University history professor Virginia Drachman, author of *Hospital with a Heart*; and Kay Hicks of Lynchburg, Virginia, a distant cousin of Susan Dimock.

99. Carol Driscoll to the author, July 31, 2016.

100. In addition to being used to create positives for small-scale casting, sodium alginate is utilized as an impression-making material in dentistry, prosthetics, and life-casting.

101. Carol Driscoll to the author.

102. Boston-based pianist Amy Cheney Beach (Mrs. H.H.A. Beach, 1867–1944) was America's first successful female composer. She composed works in a variety of genres including a Mass, a symphony, a piano concerto, and works for chamber ensembles, piano, mixed chorus, and solo voice. In the year 2000, she became the first woman composer to have her name added to the engraved names of 86 male composers on Boston's Hatch Shell on the Charles River Esplanade.

103. Drachman, *Hospital with a Heart: Women Doctors and the Paradox of Separatism at the New England Hospital, 1862–1969* (Ithaca NY: Cornell University Press, 1984).

104. Erling A. Hanson, Jr. (president of Forest Hills Cemetery) to Carolyn Stroud (Public Affairs Director, City of Washington), March 28, 1996; courtesy Forest Hills Cemetery, Boston, Massachusetts.

105. Johanna Huber, email message to author, February 9, 2017.

106. *Ibid.*; signed document for release of the Dimock monument, October 15, 1996; courtesy Forest Hills Cemetery, Boston MA; Hodges, "Tombstone Comes Home to Rest."

Bibliography

Archival Collections

Archival Center. Newburyport Public Library. Newburyport, Massachusetts.

Baugeschichtliches Archiv (BAZ). Zurich, Switzerland.

Beaufort County Register of Deeds. Beaufort County Courthouse. Washington, North Carolina. Book 29.

Biermer, Anton; Escher von der Linth, Arnold; Gusserow, Adolf, Heer, Oswald; Dimock, Susan diploma, faculty of medicine. Universität Zürich, University Archives. Zurich, Switzerland.

Birney Mann File. Sterling Historical Society. Sterling, Massachusetts.

The Boston Evening Transcript; *The North State Whig*. American Antiquarian Society. Worcester, Massachusetts.

Boston Street ledger, 1863, 1874, Ward 9. City of Boston Archives. West Roxbury, Massachusetts.

Crane Family Papers, 1819–1944. Manuscripts and Archives Division. New York Public Library. New York, New York.

Dr. Marie E. Zakrzewska Medical Building, 55 Dimock Street, Roxbury. Building Information Form #11168. Boston Landmarks Commission. Boston, Massachusetts.

Du Bois, W.E.B. (William Edward Burghardt), 1868–1963. The war to preserve slavery, February 1960. W.E.B. Du Bois Papers (MS 312). Special Collections and University Archives. University of Massachusetts Amherst Libraries.

Forest Hills Cemetery. Jamaica Plain, Massachusetts.

Form B-Building, Community: Hopkinton; No: G-407; Property name: 112 Main Street, recorded by A. Forbes for the Hopkinton Historical Commission, 6/89. Massachusetts Historical Commission. Boston, Massachusetts.

Harvard Medical School. Office of the Dean. Records, 1828–1904 (inclusive), 1869–1874 (bulk). Harvard Medical School Papers re: admission of women, 1847, 1850, 1866–1868, 1878. RG M-DE01 Series 00266 Box 4, Folder 5. Countway Library of Medicine. Boston, Massachusetts.

Hicks, Kay. Private family collection of letters, photos, and official papers. Lynchburg, Virginia.

Hoboken Public Library. Hoboken, New Jersey.

Illustrated London News. Morrab Library. Penzance, Cornwall, U.K.

Isles of Scilly Museum. Hughtown, St. Mary's, Isles of Scilly, Cornwall, U.K.

Library of Congress Prints and Photographs Division. Washington, D.C.

Local History Room, Treasure Room Collection. Hopkinton Public Library. Hopkinton, Massachusetts.

Massachusetts Department of Corrections. Charlestown State Prison records, 1805–1930 [Massachusetts] (Salt Lake City, UT: Filmed by the Genealogical Society of Utah, 1994). https://www.familysearch.org/ark:/61903/3:1:3Q9M-CSFH-4SDX-S?i=580&cat=730034.

New England Hospital for Women and Children. Records of Medical Wards and Surgical

Wards. Boston Medical Library in the Francis A. Countway Library of Medicine. Harvard University. Boston, Massachusetts.

New England Hospital for Women and Children Records, 1792–1994. Sophia Smith Collection of Women's History. Smith College. Northampton, Massachusetts.

New England Hospital Record of Interments; Anna B.S. Greene Family Record of Interments.

North Carolina Collection. University of North Carolina at Chapel Hill.

Perry-Clarke Collection: James Freeman Clarke papers; Lilian Freeman Clarke correspondence; William Lloyd Garrison Papers; Caroline Wells Healey Dall Papers. Massachusetts Historical Society. Boston, Massachusetts.

Privatarchiv Auguste Forel. Archiv für Medizingeschichte Universität Zürich. Zurich, Switzerland.

Promotion File, Susan Dimock. Staatsarchiv des Kantons Zürich. Zurich, Switzerland.

Susan Dimock Papers; Wiswall Papers; Satchwell genealogy; Washington, N.C. Census Records; Schools—Private & Public; Dave Fowle's General Store Ledger, Henry Dimock rolling account, 1856–59. George H. & Laura E. Brown Library Archives. Washington, North Carolina.

Tagblatt, 1868–1871, Theater AG. Stadtarchiv Zürich. Zurich, Switzerland.

Waltham City Directories. Waltham Public Library. Waltham, Massachusetts.

W.B. Nickerson Cape Cod History Archives. *Account Book of Francis Jackson, Treasurer, The Vigilance Committee of Boston, The Boston Vigilance Committee, Appointed at the Public Meeting in Faneuil Hall, October 21st 1850 to Assist Fugitive Slaves.* Dr. Irving H. Bartlett collection, 1830–1880. Cape Cod Community College. West Barnstable, Massachusetts.

19th Century Newspapers, Journals and Magazines

The Boston Daily Advertiser
The Boston Daily Globe
The Boston Post
The Boston Sunday Globe
The Boston Transcript
Frank Leslie's Illustrated Newspaper
Harper's New Monthly Magazine
Harper's Weekly
The Illustrated London News
The Jersey Journal (New Jersey)
Lippincott's Magazine of Popular Literature and Science (Philadelphia)
The New York Times
The Newburyport Daily Herald (Massachusetts)
The North State Whig (North Carolina)
The Saturday Review
The Springfield Republican (Massachusetts)
Tagblatt (Zürich)
The Woman's Journal

Unpublished Theses, Papers, and Dissertations

Catalano, Megan. "Oh, I could not go to a man: The Experiences of Health, Medicine and Surgery at the New England Hospital for Women and Children from 1862–1875." Senior Thesis, Faculty of the School of Arts and Sciences, Brandeis University, May 2021.

Dimock, Susan J. "Ueber die verschiedenen Formen des Puerperalfiebers. Nach Beobachtungen in der Züricher Gebaranstalt." Inaugural-Dissertation, Zürich, Druck von Zürcher und Furrer, 1871.

Goldstein, Linda Lehmann. "Roses Bloomed in Winter: Women Medical Graduates of

Western Reserve College, 1852–56." Submitted in partial fulfillment of the requirements for the Degree of Doctor of Philosophy, Case Western Reserve University, May 14, 1989.

Jex-Blake, Sophia. "Puerperal Fever: An Enquiry into Its Nature and Treatment, with an historical retrospect of some of the chief epidemics recorded under that name, and of the principal theories successively entertained respecting it. With notes of personal observations." Graduation Thesis, Medical Faculty of the University of Bern, 1877.

King, William Randall. "Ghost Dance: The Legacy of Susan Dimock, Nineteenth Century Surgeon." Thesis submitted to the Yale University School of Medicine, 1997.

Meyer, Paulette Ann. "Women Doctors Refashion a Men's Profession: Medical Careers of Nineteenth-Century Zurich University Graduates in Germany." University of Minnesota Graduate School, 1997.

Salzman, Franklyn. "Gay or Nay, Modern Readings of the David and Jonathan Narrative." Winner 2015 Henry A. Bern Memorial Essay Competition. Indiana University, Bloomington, Indiana.

Books

Absolon, Karel B. *The Surgeon's Surgeon: Theodor Billroth 1829–1894*. 2 vols. Lawrence, KS: Coronado Press, 1981.

Alonso, Harriet Hyman. *Growing Up Abolitionist: The Story of the Garrison Children*. Amherst and Boston: University of Massachusetts Press, 2002.

Annual Report of the School Committee of the City of Boston. Boston: Geo. C. Rand & Avery, 1874.

Annual Reports of the New-England Hospital for Women and Children, 1866–84. Boston: Press of W.L. Deland and Press of Geo. H. Ellis Company

Austin, Keith. *The Victorian Titanic: The Loss of the S.S Schiller in 1875*. Tiverton, Devon, Great Britain: Halsgrove House, 2001.

Barker-Benfield, G.J. *The Horrors of the Half-Known Life: Male Attitudes Toward Women and Sexuality in Nineteenth-Century America*. New York: Harper and Row, 1976.

Barrett, John G. *The Civil War in North Carolina*. Chapel Hill: University of North Carolina Press, 1963.

Bonner, Thomas Neville. *To the Ends of the Earth: Women's Search for Education in Medicine*. Cambridge: Harvard University Press, 1992.

Burrage, Walter Lincoln. *A History of the Massachusetts Medical Society: With Brief Biographies of the Founders and Chief Officers, 1781–1922*. Norwood, MA: Plimpton Press, 1923.

Cecelski, David S. *The Waterman's Song: Slavery and Freedom in Maritime North Carolina*. Chapel Hill: University of North Carolina Press, 2001.

Channing, William Ellery. *The Wanderer: A Colloquial Poem*. Boston: James R. Osgood and Company, 1871.

Cheney, Ednah Dow (anon.). *Memoir of Susan Dimock*. Boston: Press of J. Wilson, 1875.

______. *Reminiscences of Ednah Dow Cheney*. Boston: Lee & Shepard, 1902.

Clarke, Edward H., M.D. *Sex in Education; or, A Fair Chance for the Girls* second edition. Boston: James R. Osgood and Company, 1873.

Clarke, James Freeman. *Autobiography, Diary and Correspondence*, edited by Edward Everett Hale. Boston: Houghton, Mifflin and Company, 1891.

______. *Memorial and Biographical Sketches*. Boston: Houghton, Osgood and Company, 1878.

Clarke, Louise Brownell. *The Greenes of Rhode Island, With Historical Records of English Ancestry, 1534–1902. Compiled from the Mss. of the Late Major-General George Sears Greene, U.S.V.* New York: The Knickerbocker Press, 1903.

Cochran, Betty, and C.A. Mann. *On This Rock: A History of St. Peter's Church*. Washington, North Carolina, 1997.

Coltrane, Jenn Winslow. *Lineage Book—National Society of the Daughters of the American Revolution*. Washington, D.C.: Judd & Detweiler, 1922.

Coon, Charles L. *Facts About Southern Education Progress*. Durham, NC: The Campaign Committee of the Southern Education Board, 1905.

Craig, Gordon A. *The Triumph of Liberalism: Zurich in the Golden Age, 1830–1869*. New York: Charles Scribner's Sons, 1988.

Creese, Mary R.S. *Ladies in the Laboratory? American and British Women in Science, 1800–1900*. Lanham, MD: Scarecrow Press, 2000.

Crosby, Alice B. (Mrs. William O.). *The Story of the New England Hospital for Women and Children through Seventy-Five Years, 1862–1937*. Boston: New England Hospital for Women and Children, 1937.

Cyclopedia of Eminent and Representative Men of the Carolinas of the Nineteenth Century. Madison, WI: Brant & Fuller, 1892.

Dally, Ann. *Women Under the Knife: A History of Surgery*. New York: Routledge, 1992.

Daniels, Josephus. *Tar Heel Editor*. Chapel Hill: University of North Carolina Press, 2012. Reprint of 1939 original.

Dobson, Mary. *Disease: The Extraordinary Stories Behind History's Deadliest Killers*. London, England: Quercus Books, 2008.

Drachman, Virginia G. *Hospital with a Heart: Women Doctors and the Paradox of Separatism at the New England Hospital, 1862–1969*. Ithaca NY: Cornell University Press, 1984.

Edmonson, James M., Ph.D. *Nineteenth Century Surgical Instruments: A Catalogue of the Gustav Weber Collection at the Howard Dittrick Museum of Historical Medicine*. Cleveland, OH: Historical Division, The Cleveland Health Sciences Library, 1986.

The Fiftieth Anniversary of the New England Hospital for Women and Children, Dimock Street, Boston, Mass., October Twenty-Nine, Nineteen Hundred Twelve. Boston: Press of Geo. H. Ellis Company, 1913.

Forel, August. *Briefe Correspondence 1864–1927*, edited by Hans H. Walser. Bern: Verlag Hans Huber, 1968.

______. *Out of My Life and Work*, translated by Bernard Miall. New York: W.W. Norton, 1937.

Genealogy of the Caverly Family, from the Year 1116 to the Year 1880, Made Profitable and Exemplified by Many a Lesson of Life. Lowell, MA: George M. Elliott, Publisher, 1880.

Grodzins, Dean. *American Heretic: Theodore Parker and Transcendentalism*. Chapel Hill: University of North Carolina Press, 2002.

Haycock, David Boyd, and Sally Archer, eds. *Health & Medicine at Sea, 1700–1900*. Woodbridge, Suffolk UK: Boydell Press and National Maritime Museum, 2009.

History and Description of the New England Hospital for Women and Children, Codman Avenue, Boston Highlands, Prepared by a Committee of the Board of Directors for the Massachusetts Exhibit in the Department of Education and Science and for the Women's Department of Massachusetts, at the International Exhibition in Philadelphia, 1876. Boston: Press of W.L. Deland, 1876.

History of the New England Hospital for Women and Children, 1859–1899; and *Fair at the Hotel Vendome for the Benefit of the New England Hospital for Women and Children, December 4th to 9th, 1899*. Boston, 1899.

History Project. *Improper Bostonians: Lesbian and Gay History from the Puritans to Playland*. Boston: Beacon Press, 1998.

Holmes, Richard. *This Long Pursuit: Reflections of a Romantic Biographer*. New York: Vintage Books, 2016.

Jabour, Anya. *Topsy-Turvy: How the Civil War Turned the World Upside Down for Southern Children*. Lanham, MD: Rowman & Littlefield, 2010.

James, Edward T., ed. *Notable American Women, 1607–1950: A Biographical Dictionary*. Cambridge, MA: Belknap Press of Harvard University Press, 1971.

Jones-Rogers, Stephanie E. *They Were Her Property: White Women as Slave Owners in the American South*. New Haven: Yale University Press, 2019.

Larn, Richard OBE. *The Wrecks of Scilly*, 5th ed. Isles of Scilly: Shipwreck & Marine, 2015.

Larson, Kate Clifford. *Bound for the Promised Land: Harriet Tubman, Portrait of an American Hero*. New York: One World/Ballantine Books, 2004.

Lesky, Erna. *The Vienna Medical School of the 19th Century*. Baltimore: Johns Hopkins University Press, 1976.

Lowenthal, David. *George Perkins Marsh: Prophet of Conservation*. Seattle: University of Washington Press, 2000.

Loy, Ursula, and Pauline Worthy. *Washington and the PamliCompany* Washington, NC: Washington-Beaufort County Bicentennial Commission, 1976.

Maygrier, Jacques-Pierre. *Nouvelles démonstrations d'accouchements*, Forestier, graveur; A. Chazal, dess. Paris, 1822.

McCullough, David. *The Greater Journey: Americans in Paris*. New York: Simon & Shuster, 2011.

Merrill, Walter M., ed. *The Letters of William Lloyd Garrison, Volume 5, 1861–1867*. Cambridge, MA: Belknap Press of Harvard University Press, 1979.

Moore, Wendy. *No Man's Land: The Trailblazing Women Who Ran Britain's Most Extraordinary Military Hospital During World War I*. New York: Basic Books, 2020.

Müller, Verena E. *Marie Heim-Vögtlin—die erste Schweizer Ärztin (1845–1916): Ein Leben zwischen Tradition und Aufbruch* (Baden 2007, vierte Auflage 2016). Kindle. Select translations by Inez Hedges and Aina Lagor.

The New England Hospital, One Hundred Years, 1862–1962. Boston: 1962.

New England Hospital for Women and Children: Fair at Tremont Temple, December 1–6, 1896. Souvenir booklet. Boston: 1897.

Nimura, Janice P. *The Doctors Blackwell: How Two Pioneering Sisters Brought Medicine to Women—And Women to Medicine*. New York: W.W. Norton and Company, 2021.

Nineteenth Annual Catalogue and Report of the New England Female Medical College. Boston: Published by the Trustees, Wright & Potter Printers, 1867.

Pierce, Edward L., ed. *Memoir and Letters of Charles Sumner*. Boston: Roberts Brothers, 1893.

Rennell, James, Esq. F.R.S. *Observations on a Current That Often Prevails to the Westward of Scilly; Endangering the Safety of Ships That Approach the British Channel*. London: Philosophical Transactions of the Royal Society of London, 1793. Vol. 83, 182–200.

Richards, Linda. *Reminiscences of Linda Richards, America's First Trained Nurse*. Boston: Whitcomb & Barrows, 1911.

Rodgers, Bradley A. et al. *Research Report No. 14: The Castle Island Ships' Graveyard: The History and Archeology of Eleven Wrecked and Abandoned Watercraft*. Greenville, NC: East Carolina University Program in Maritime Studies, 2006.

Roe, Alfred S. *The Twenty-Fourth Regiment Massachusetts Volunteers, 1861–1866, "New England Guard Regiment."* Worcester, MA: Twenty-Fourth Veteran Association, 1907.

Safford, Mrs. Frances A. *A Brief History of Hopkinton, Prepared for the Town's Bicentennial Celebration in 1915*. Hopkinton, MA: Hopkinton Public Library, 1915.

Showalter, Elaine. *The Civil Wars of Julia Ward Howe*. New York: Simon & Schuster, 2016.

Sparrow, Joy W., ed. *Sparrows' Nest of Letters*. Wake Forest, N.C.: The Scuppernong Press, 2011.

Stanbrook, Elisabeth. *Bishop Rock Lighthouse*. Truro, Cornwall: Twelveheads Press, 2016.

Stanton, Elizabeth Cady, Susan Brownell Anthony and Matilda Joslyn Gage, eds. *History of Woman Suffrage*, Volume III. 1876–1885. Rochester, NY: Charles Mann Printing Company, 1886.

Sterling, Massachusetts: A Pictorial History. The Sterling Historical Society, 1981.

Strother, David Hunter ["Crayon, Porte"]. *The Old South Illustrated*. Chapel Hill: University of North Carolina Press, 1959.

Taylor, Robert L. *Early Families of Limington, Maine*. Bowie, MD: Heritage Books, 1991.

Ticknor, Carolyn, ed. *Dr. Holmes's Boston*. Boston: Houghton Mifflin Company, 1915.

Todd, Margaret, M.D. *The Life of Sophia Jex-Blake*. London: Macmillan and Company, 1918.

Transactions of the Nineteenth Annual Meeting of the Medical Society of the State of North Carolina, Held at Newbern, N.C., May, 1872. Raleigh: Edwards & Broughton, Book and Job Printers, 1872.

Tuchman, Arleen Marcia. *Science Has No Sex: The Life of Marie Zakrzewska, M.D.* Chapel Hill: University of North Carolina Press, 2006.

Turnbull, Laurence, M.D., PhG. *The Advantages and Accidents of Artificial Anaesthesia. A Manual of Anaesthetic Agents and Their Employment in the Treatment of Disease.* Philadelphia: P. Blakiston, Son & Company, 1885.

Van Camp, Louis. *Images of America: Washington, North Carolina.* Charleston, SC: Arcadia Publishing, 2000.

Vietor, Agnes C., M.D., F.A.C.S. *A Woman's Quest: The Life of Marie E. Zakrzewska, M.D.* New York: D. Appleton and Company, 1924.

Walker, Francis. A., ed. *United States Centennial Commission. International Exhibition, 1876. Reports and Awards, Vol. VII, Groups XXI–XXVII.* Washington, D.C.: Government Printing Office, 1880.

Walsh, Mary Roth. *Doctors Wanted: No Women Need Apply.* New Haven and London: Yale University Press, 1977.

The Waltham and Watertown Directory, 1888–89, Of the Inhabitants, Institutions, Manufacturing Establishments, Societies, Business, Business Firms, State Census, Map, Etc., Etc. Boston: W.A. Greenough & Company, 1888.

The Waltham and Watertown Directory, 1893, Of the Inhabitants, Institutions, Manufacturing Establishments, Societies, Business, Business Firms, State Census, Map, Etc., Etc. Boston: W.A. Greenough & Company, 1893.

The Waltham City Directory, 1890, Of the Inhabitants, Institutions, Manufacturing Establishments, Societies, Business, Business Firms, State Census, Map, Etc., Etc. Boston: Littlefield Directory Publishing Company, 1893.

Waltham Directory, 1908–9, Of the Inhabitants, Business Firms, Institutions, Societies, Streets, Map, State Census, Etc., No. XVIII. Boston: W.A. Greenough & Company, 1908.

Ward, James F. *The Common Uncommon: Stories of the Past, Hopkinton, Massachusetts.* Framingham, MA: Damianos Publishing, 2014.

Whittier, John Greenleaf. *The Letters of John Greenleaf Whittier,* Vol. 1. Cambridge: Belknap Press of Harvard University Press, 1975.

Winsor, Justin, ed. *The Memorial History of Boston: Including Suffolk County, Massachusetts, 1630–1880.* 4 vols. Boston: Ticknor and Company, 1881.

Worcester, Alfred, A.M., M.D. *Nurses for Our Neighbors.* Boston: Houghton Mifflin Company, 1914.

Articles

"American Nursing: An Introduction to the Past." University of Pennsylvania School of Nursing. https://www.nursing.upenn.edu/nhhc/american-nursing-an-introduction-to-the-past/ Accessed November 20, 2020.

"Another Lady-Doctor." *The British Medical Journal* 2, no. 568 (November 18, 1871): 588.

Bonner, Thomas Neville. "Medical Women Abroad: A New Dimension of Women's Push for Opportunity in Medicine, 1850–1914." *Bulletin of the History of Medicine* 62, no. 1 (Johns Hopkins University Press, Spring 1988): 58–73.

__________. "Pioneering in Women's Medical Education in the Swiss Universities 1864–1914." *Gesnerus 45: Swiss Journal of the history of medicine and sciences* (1988): 461–474.

__________. "Rendezvous in Zurich: Seven Who Made a Revolution in Women's Medical Education, 1864–1874." *Journal of the History of Medicine and Allied Sciences* 44, no. 1 (Oxford University Press, 1989): 7–27.

Bourne, Jenny. "Slavery in the United States." *EH.Net Encyclopedia,* edited by Robert Whaples. (March 26, 2008). http://eh.net/encyclopedia/slavery-in-the-united-states/

Brouwer, Marilyn. "The Paris Morgue: A Gruesome Tourist Attraction in the 19th Century." *Bonjour Paris: The Insider's Guide* (Oct. 7, 2019). https://bonjourparis.com/history/the-paris-morgue-a-gruesome-tourist-attraction-in-19th-century/?utm_source=Bonjour+Paris&utm_campaign=0ba6be207a-EMAIL_CAMPAIGN_2019_03_07_02_50_COPY_01&utm_medium=email&utm_term=0_306bdf7563-0ba6be207a-294026465&mc_cid=0ba6be207a&mc_eid=b555450a09.

Bushee, Frederick A. "The Growth of the Population of Boston." *Publications of the American Statistical Association* 6, no. 46 (1899): 239–74.

Call, Emma L., M.D. "Evolution of Modern Maternity Technique. Illustrated by Records of the New England Hospital for Women and Children, Boston, from 1862 to 1907." *The American Journal of Obstetrics and Diseases of Women and Children*, 58, no. 1, edited by Brooks H. Wells, M.D. (New York: William Wood and Company July–December 1908): 392–404.

Campbell, Olivia. "The Queer Victorian Doctors Who Paved the Way for Women in Medicine." *History Stories*, June 1, 2021. The History Channel, A+E Networks. https://www.history.com/news/queer-victorian-doctors-women-medicine.

Carter, K. Codell, PhD. "Leechcraft in Nineteenth Century British Medicine." *Journal of the Royal Society of Medicine* 94 (January 2001): 38–42.

Cheney, Ednah Dow Littlehale. "Moses." *The Freedmen's Record* 1, no. 3 (Boston: March 1865): 34–38.

[Clarke, James Freeman] J.F.C. and *Boston Advertiser*, "Susan Dimock." *Woman's Journal*, May 22, 1875. Nineteenth Century Collections Online. https://link.gale.com/apps/doc/GKKHFF010031398/NCCO?u=mlin_m_brandeis&sid= NCCO&xid=e58128e2. Accessed May 29, 2020.

Clarke, Lilian Freeman. "The Story of an Invisible Institution." *The Outlook* 84 (December 15, 1906): 932–936. https://www.libertarian-labyrinth.org/the-sex-question/lilian-freeman-clarke-the-story-of-an-invisible-institution-1906/

Columbus, Cristie. "In a World with No Antibiotics, How Did Doctors Treat Infections?" *The Conversation*, Texas A&M University (January 29, 2016). https://theconversation.com/in-a-world-with-no-antibiotics-how-did-doctors-treat-infections-53376.

deLue, Willard, "Footloose in Eastern Carolina: First Woman Physician." *The State*, September 10, 1955.

______. "Roaming South with Willard deLue—XI: A Courageous Woman and Dimock St., Roxbury." *Boston Globe*, January 5, 1955.

______. "Roaming South with Willard de Lue—XII: When Bay State Troops Burned Carolina Town." *Boston Globe*, January 7, 1955.

Devine, Shauna. "Health Care and the American Medical Profession, 1830–1880." *The Journal of the Civil War Era* (July 6, 2017). https://www.journalofthecivilwarera.org/2017/07/health-care-american-medical-profession-1830-1880/.

Diggs, Marylynne. "Romantic Friends or a 'Different Race of Creatures'? The Representation of Lesbian Pathology in Nineteenth-Century America" 21, no. 2 (Feminist Studies, Summer 1995): 317–340.

Dimock, Susan, M.D. "A Case of Congenital Anal Occlusion of an Unusual Kind." *The Medical Record* 10, edited by George F. Shrady (January 2, 1875–December 25, 1875): 357–358.

______. "A Case of Successful Operation for Recto-Vaginal Fistula." *The Medical Record* 9, edited by George F. Shrady (January 1, 1874–December 15, 1874): 458.

______, Student of Medicine. "Messrs. Editors," *Boston Medical and Surgical Journal* 7, no. 3 (January 19, 1871): 50.

______. "Two Cases of Rudimentary Uterus." *The Medical Record* 9, edited by George F. Shrady (January 1, 1874–December 15, 1874): 423–424.

"Dr. Susan Dimock." *The New England Journal of Medicine* 92, no. 23 (June 10, 1875): 695–696.

Du Bois, W.E.B., ed. *The Brownies' Book* 1, no. 11 (November, 1920): 339. https://www.loc.gov/resource/rbc0001.2004ser01351/?sp=361.

Ehrhardt, J. D., Jr., J. P O'Leary, and D. K Nakayama. "Yes, I Shot the President, but His Physicians Killed Him." The Assassination of President James A. Garfield. *The American surgeon*, 84, no. 11 (2018): 1711–1716.

Elinder, Mikael, and Oscar Erixson. "Gender, Social Norms, and Survival in Maritime Disasters." *Proceedings of the National Academy of Sciences* 9, no.33 (August 14, 2012): 13220–13224.

Frangos, Steve. "Captain Costentenus: The Tattooed Greek of New York City." *The National*

Herald, Feature 7, June 3, 2006. http://hellenicgenealogygeek.blogspot.com/2017/09/captain-costentenus-tattooed-greek-of.html.

Gritz, Jennie Rothenberg. "But Were They Gay? The Mystery of Same-Sex Love in the 19th Century." *The Atlantic,* September 7, 2012. https://www.theatlantic.com/national/archive/2012/09/but-were-they-gay-the-mystery-of-same-sex-love-in-the-19th-century/262117/.

Hawthorne, Nathaniel. "Chiefly About War Matters." *Atlantic Monthly* 10 (July 1862): 43–61. https://www.theatlantic.com/magazine/archive/1862/07/chiefly-about-war-matters/306159/.

Hendersen-Smathers, Irma, M.D., ed. "History of Women in Medicine—Medical Women of North Carolina: Dr. Susan Dimock." *Medical Woman's Journal* (November 1949): 38–40.

Hodges, Claude. "Tombstone Comes Home to Rest." *Washington Daily News,* October 23, 1996.

Kreitner, Richard. "When the North Almost Seceded." *Boston Globe,* October 28, 2016.

Lane, Hilary J., MLS, Nava Blum, PhD, and Elizabeth Fee, PhD. "Oliver Wendell Holmes (1809–1894) and Ignaz Philipp Semmelweis (1818–1865): Preventing the Transmission of Puerperal Fever." *American Journal of Public Health* 100, no. 6 (June 2010): 1008–9.

Lowell, Josephine. Untitled Letter, *Century Illustrated Magazine* 41, no. 4 (February 1891): 634.

Ludmerer, Kenneth M. "Reform at Harvard Medical School, 1869–1909." *Bulletin of the History of Medicine* 55, no. 3 (Johns Hopkins University Press, 1981): 343–70.

Luola. "Jennie's Tooth-ache." *North Carolina Presbyterian,* August 10, 1858.

Midgett, Ray. "Pamlico's Past: The Burning of Washington." *The Washington Daily News,* April 29, 2014.

"New England Hospital Proud of Its Long Medical History." *A Feature Publication of The Tribune Publishing Company,* May 31, 1954.

Norton, Scott A. "Whither medical botany?" *CMAJ: Canadian Medical Association Journal* 174, June 20, 2006. https://www.ncbi.nlm.nih.gov/pmc/articles/PMC1475913/.

"The Ocean Steamer." *Harper's New Monthly Magazine* 41, no. 242 (August 1870): 185–198.

Osanec, Jiri. "All About LV Holzmaister, Widower of Louise," translated by Miroslav Koudelka. *The Scillonian,* no. 264 (Winter 2006/7): 141–145.

Petro, Jane, MD, FACS, Susan Wilson, and Megan Catalano. "Susan Dimock, Pioneering American Physician." *Bulletin of the American College of Surgeons* 106, no. 3 (March 2021): 27–34. https://www.facsbulletin.com/acsbulletin/march2021/MobilePagedReplica.action?pm=2&folio=26#pg28.

Petro, Jane, MD, FACS, Susan Wilson BA, MA History, and Megan Catalano BS, MS Health Policy. "Susan Dimock, Pioneering 19th Century American Surgeon/Physician." *Annals of Surgery Open* 3, no. 4 (December 2022): e208. https://journals.lww.com/aosopen/Fulltext/2022/12000/Susan_Dimock,_Pioneering_19th_Century_American.5.aspx?context=LatestArticles.

Pula, James S. "A Passion for Humanity: Founding the New England Hospital for Women and Children." *The Polish Review* 57, no. 3 (2012): 67–82.

Putnam-Jacobi, Mary, MD. "An Obituary of the Author [Susan Dimock, M.D.]." *The Medical Record: A Weekly Journal of Medicine and Surgery* 10 (January 2-December 25, 1875).

Rabinovitch, Eyal. "Gender and the Public Sphere: Alternative Forms of Integration in Nineteenth-Century America." *Sociological Theory* 19, no. 3 (November 2001): 344–370.

Richards, Linda. "Early Days in the First American Training School for Nurses." *The American Journal of Nursing* 16, no. 3 (December 1915): 174–179.

Rosenberg, Charles E. "And Heal the Sick: The Hospital and the Patient in the 19th Century America." *Journal of Social History* 10, no. 4 (Summer 1977): 428–447.

The Saturday Review of Politics, Literature, Science, and Art 40 (1875). https://archive.org/details/sim_saturday-review_1875-08-07_40_1032.

Scott-Conner, Carol E.H., MD, PhD, FACS, and Ingrid M. Lizarraga, MBBS, FACS. "The First Women Elected to College Fellowship." *Bulletin of the American College of Surgeons* (September 1, 2019). https://bulletin.facs.org/2019/09/the-first-women-elected-to-college-fellowship/.

Slawson, Robert G., MD, FACR. "Medical Training in the United States Prior to the Civil War." *Journal of Evidence-Based Complementary & Alternative Medicine* 17, no. 1 (September 28, 2011): 11–27. https://journals.sagepub.com/doi/full/10.1177/21565 87211427404.

Smith, Philip W., MD, Kristin Watkins, MBA, and Angela Hewlett, MD. "Infection Control Through the Ages." *American Journal of Infection Control* 40 (2012): 35–42.

Speaker, Susan. "The Question of Rest for Women." *Circulating Now: From the Historical Collections of the National Library of Medicine,* July 29, 2014.

"Susan Wilson Heads Dimock Heritage Fund." *The ProclaimHer,* Boston Women's Heritage Trail, April 1995.

Wall, L. Lewis, M.D., PhD. "The medical ethics of Dr J Marion Sims: a fresh look at the historical record." *Journal of Medical Ethics* 32, no. 6 (June 2006): 346–50. https://www.ncbi.nlm.nih.gov/pmc/articles/PMC2563360/.

"Washington, North Carolina." *Frank Leslie's Illustrated Newspaper,* May 16, 1863.

Wilson, Susan. "History Notebook: A Selfless Pioneer in Boston Medicine." *The Boston Sunday Globe,* May 8, 1994.

Worthy, Pauline Marion. "Susan Dimock, Pioneer in Medicine." Raleigh *News & Observer,* April 25, 1937.

Online Resources

Craven County Marriage Bonds. North Carolina, U.S. Marriage Records, 1741–2011. https://www.ancestry.com/discoveryui-content/view/64671:60548?_phsrc=uCX130&_phstart=successSource&gsfn=Henry&gsln=Dimock&ml_rpos=1&queryId=b726f11895 ee767de4b2c91ee0dc3831.

Digital Library on American Slavery, Gateway, UNC Greensboro Libraries https://gateway.uncg.edu/dlas Accessed November 4, 2022.

Dunn, Adrienne, "Contraband Camps," The North Carolina History Project, Encyclopedia. John Locke Foundation. Raleigh, North Carolina, 2016. https://northcarolinahistory.org/encyclopedia/contraband-camps/ Accessed November 3, 2022.

Fitzharris, Dr. Lindsey. "An appointment at the house of death: the horror of the early Victorian hospital." *History Extra: The official website for BBC History Magazine, BBC History Revealed and BBC World Histories.* https://www.historyextra.com/period/victorian/an-appointment-at-the-house-of-death-the-horrors-of-the-early-victorian-hospital/ Accessed November 3, 2022.

Heath, Richard. "The Architectural History of Egleston Square," August 14, 2017; editorial assistance provided by Kathy Griffin. https://www.jphs.org/locales/2005/9/30/egleston-square-by-richard-heath.html Accessed November 3, 2022.

Lewis, J.D. *A History of Washington, North Carolina.* Little River, South Carolina, 2007. https://www.carolana.com/NC/Towns/Washington_NC.html.

Linder, Professor Douglas O. "Famous Trials: The Three Trials of Oscar Wilde (1895)." University of Missouri–Kansas City School of Law. https://famous-trials.com/wilde Accessed November 3, 2022.

Martin, Jonathan. "Susan Dimock (1847–1875)." North Carolina History Project. Raleigh, NC: John Locke Foundation, 2016. https://northcarolinahistory.org/encyclopedia/susan-dimock-1847-1875/ Accessed November 4, 2022.

Massachusetts, U.S. State Census, 1865. Middlesex, Hopkinton. https://www.ancestry.com/imageviewer/collections/9203/images/41265_316179-00163?ssrc=&backlabel=Return.

Morgan, Keith N. "Dimock Community Health Center (New England Hospital for Women and Children)." [Boston, Massachusetts], *SAH (Society of Architectural Historians) Archipedia,* edited by Gabrielle Esperdy and Karen Kingsley, Charlottesville: UVaP, 2012_____, https://sah-archipedia.org/buildings/MA-01-RX26 Accessed November 3, 2022.

"North Carolina Highway Historical Marker Program." North Carolina Office of Archives & History—Department of Cultural Resources, 2008. http://www.ncmarkers.com/Markers.aspx?MarkerId=B-14. Accessed November 4, 2022.

"Sheriffs Throughout History." Sheriff. Beaufort County. Beaufort County Sheriff's Office. Washington, North Carolina, 2022 https://www.beaufortcountysheriff.org/2015/10/14/sheriff/. Accessed November 4, 2022.

"Ship Incident & Shipwreck List for Scilly." Scillypedia: Encyclopedia of the Isles of Scilly, Shipwreck Listings http://scillypedia.Companyuk/ShipwreckListing.htm#S. Accessed November 4, 2022.

Smith, Tara. "The 1872 Equine Influenza Epidemic That Sickened Most U.S. Horses." July 1, 2015. https://www.mentalfloss.com/article/65528/1872-equine-influenza-epidemic-sickened-most-us-horses. Accessed February 1, 2020.

Snyder, Charles. "Massachusetts Eye and Ear Infirmary: Studies on Its history." Boston: Massachusetts Eye and Ear Infirmary, 1984. https://archive.org/details/massachusettseye00snyd. Accessed November 3, 2022.

U.S. Census Bureau. 1850 U.S. Federal Census—Slave Schedules for Henry Dimock. Washington, Beaufort, North Carolina. https://www.ancestry.com/imageviewer/collections/8055/images/NCM432_650-0147?ssrc=&backlabel=Return&pId=91441313 Accessed November 4, 2022.

U.S. Census Bureau. 1860 U.S. Federal Census—Slave Schedules for F L Owens. Washington, Beaufort, North Carolina. https://www.ancestry.com/imageviewer/collections/7668/images/ncm653_920-0215?ssrc=&backlabel=Return&pId=2050479 Accessed November 4, 2022.

"Washington Historic District." Washington City, Beaufort County, NC. LivingPlaces.com, 1997–2022. http://www.livingplaces.com/NC/Beaufort_County/Washington_City/Washington_Historic_District.html. Accessed November, 4, 2022.

Winer, Samantha. "A Brief History of Slavery in North Carolina," Walter Clinton Jackson Library, The University of North Carolina at Greensboro (UNCG) https://dlas.uncg.edu/notices/history/ Accessed November 4, 2022.

"Women Gaining Access to Medical Education." *Johns Hopkins Medicine, History* https://www.hopkinsmedicine.org/about/history/women-med-ed.html Accessed November 4, 2022.

Index

Numbers in **_bold italics_** indicate pages with illustrations